Management of Bleeding Disorders in Surgical Practice

The only weapon with which the unconscious patient can immediately retaliate upon the incompetent surgeon is haemorrhage

William Stewart Halsted (1852–1922)
Bulletin of the Johns Hopkins Hospital (1912) **23**, 191

Management of Bleeding Disorders in Surgical Practice

C.D. FORBES
MD DSc FRCP (Glas. Edin. Lond.) FRS (Edin.)
Ninewells Hospital
Dundee

A. CUSCHIERI
MD ChM FRCS (Edin. Glas. Eng.)
Ninewells Hospital
Dundee

OXFORD
BLACKWELL SCIENTIFIC PUBLICATIONS
LONDON EDINBURGH BOSTON
MELBOURNE PARIS BERLIN VIENNA

Editorial Offices:
Osney Mead, Oxford OX2 0EL
25 John Street, London WC1N 2BL
23 Ainslie Place, Edinburgh EH3 6AJ
238 Main Street, Cambridge
Massachusetts 02142, USA
54 University Street, Carlton
Victoria 3053, Australia

Other Editorial Offices:
Librairie Arnette SA
2, rue Casimir-Delavigne
75006 Paris
France

Blackwell Wissenschafts-Verlag
Meinekestrasse 4
D-1000 Berlin 15
Germany

Blackwell MZV
Feldgasse 13
A-1238 Wien
Austria

First published 1993

Set by Setrite Typesetters, Hong Kong
Printed and bound in Great Britain
at the University Press, Cambridge

DISTRIBUTORS

Marston Book Services Ltd
PO Box 87
Oxford OX2 0DT
(*Orders*: Tel: 0865 791155
Fax: 0865 791927
Telex: 837515)

USA
Blackwell Scientific Publications, Inc.
238 Main Street
Cambridge, MA 02142
(*Orders*: Tel: 800 759–6102
617 876–7000)

Canada
Times Mirror Professional Publishing, Ltd
5240 Finch Avenue East
Scarborough, Ontario M1S 5A2
(*Orders*: Tel: 800 268–4178
416 298–1588)

Australia
Blackwell Scientific Publications
(Australia) Pty Ltd
54 University Street
Carlton, Victoria 3053
(*Orders*: Tel: 03 347–0300)

A catalogue record for this book is available from the British Library.

ISBN 0–632–03368–1

Contents

Contributors

BRUCE BENNETT MD FRCP FRCPath, *Reader in Medicine, Department of Medicine and Therapeutics, Medical School, Aberdeen University, Aberdeen AB9 2ZD, Scotland*

DANIEL BLOCKMANS PhD MD, *Resident Division of Bleeding and Vascular Disorders, Center for Thrombosis and Vascular Research, University of Leuven, Herestraat 49, B-3000 Leuven, Belgium*

JOHN D. CASH BSc MB ChB PhD FRCP FRCPath, *Professor, National Medical and Scientific Director, Scottish National Blood Transfusion Service, Headquarters Unit, Ellen's Glen Road, Edinburgh EH17 7QT, Scotland*

JAMES M. COURTNEY PhD, *Professor, University of Strathclyde, Bioengineering Unit, Wolfson Centre, 106 Rottenrow, Glasgow G4 0NW, Scotland*

ALFRED CUSCHIERI MD ChM FRCS (Edin., Glas., Eng.), *Professor and Head, Department of Surgery, Ninewells Hospital and Medical School, Dundee DD1 9SY, Scotland*

J. ANDREW DAVIES MD FRCP, *Senior Lecturer in Medicine, The University of Leeds, and Consultant Physician, The General Infirmary, Leeds LS1 3EX, England*

MARK DEAKIN MB ChM FRCSE FRCS, *Senior Registrar in Surgery, Hepatobiliary and Liver Transplantation Unit, The Queen Elizabeth Medical Centre, Edgbaston, Birmingham B15 2TH, England*

DAVID W. EASTER MD FACS, *Associate Professor of Surgery, University of California, San Diego Medical Centre, San Diego, California 92093, USA*

PATRICK FITCH BSc, *Research Assistant, Department of Medicine, Aberdeen Royal Infirmary, Foresterhill, Aberdeen AB9 2ZD, Scotland*

CHARLES D. FORBES DSc MD MB ChB FRCP (Edin., Glas., Lond.) FRSE, *Professor of Medicine, Ninewells Hospital, Dundee DD1 9SY, Scotland*

BRENDA GIBSON MB ChB FRCP MRCPath DFM, *Consultant in Charge of Haematology, Royal Hospital for Sick Children, Yorkhill, Glasgow G3 8SJ, Scotland*

IAN S. GRANT MB ChB FRCP FFARCS, *Medical Director, Intensive Therapy Unit, Western General Hospital, Crewe Road, Edinburgh EH4 2XU, Scotland*

PETER J. GRANT MD MRCP, *Senior Lecturer in Medicine, University of Leeds, and Consultant Physician, The General Infirmary, Leeds LS1 3EX, England*

IAN A. GREER MD MRCP (UK) MRCOG, *Clinical Consultant, MRC Reproductive Biology Unit, University of Edinburgh, 37 Chalmers Street, Edinburgh EH3 9EW, Scotland*

JENNIFER L. HANSLIP MB ChB MRCP, *Lecturer, Section of Ageing and Health, Department of Medicine, Ninewells Hospital and Medical School, Dundee DD1 9SY, Scotland*

SUSAN K. HAWLEY MB ChB FFARCS, *Lecturer, The University of Liverpool, The University Department of Anaesthesia, Liverpool Hospital, Prescot Street, PO Box 147, Liverpool L69 3BX, England*

MARK N. LEVINE MD MSc FRCP(C), *Chief Executive Officer, The Ontario Cancer Treatment and Research Foundation, Hamilton Regional Cancer Centre, Henderson Clinic, 699 Concession Street, Hamilton, Ontario L8V 5C2, Canada*

GORDON D.O. LOWE MD FRCP (Edin., Glas., Lond.), *Reader and Consultant Physician, University Department of Medicine, Royal Infirmary, 10 Alexandra Parade, Glasgow G31 2ER, Scotland*

MICHAEL J. MACKIE MD FRCP FRCPath, *Head, Department of Clinical and Laboratory Haematology, Western General Hospital, Crewe Road, Edinburgh EH4 2XU, Scotland*

PAUL McMASTER MB ChM FRCS FICS, *Consultant Surgeon, Hepatobiliary and Liver Transplantation Unit, The Queen Elizabeth Medical Centre, Edgbaston, Birmingham B15 2TH, England*

CHARLES P.J. MORTON MB BS FRCAnaes., *Registrar, Intensive Therapy Unit, Western General Hospital, Crewe Road, Edinburgh EH4 2XU, Scotland*

WILLIAM G. MURPHY MB ChB MD MRCP, *Senior Lecturer, Department of Medicine, University of Edinburgh and South East Scotland Blood Transfusion Service, Royal Infirmary, Lauriston Place, Edinburgh EH3 9HB, Scotland*

VILMA E. QUIJADA MD, *Fellow in Renal Disease, Georgetown University Medical Center, Department of Medicine, Division of Nephrology, 3800 Reservoir Road NW, Washington DC 20007, USA*

MIN HONG SAW MB ChB MRCP (UK), *Department of Clinical and Laboratory Haematology, Western General Hospital, Crewe Road, Edinburgh EH4 2XU, Scotland*

R. ALEXANDER SHARP MB ChB MRCP MRCPath, *Department of Haematology, University of Dundee, Ninewells Hospital and Medical School, Dundee DD1 9SY, Scotland*

RICHARD SOUTAR MB ChB, *Royal Hospital for Sick Children, Yorkhill, Glasgow G3 8SJ, Scotland*

SUMUK SUNDARAM MB BS MSc, *Bioengineering Unit, University of Strathclyde, Wolfson Centre, 106 Rottenrow, Glasgow G4 0NW, Scotland*

JOHN E. UTTING MA MB BChir FFARCS, *Professor of Anaesthesia, University of Liverpool, The University Department of Anaesthesia, Royal Liverpool Hospital, Prescot Street, PO Box 147, Liverpool L69 3BX, England*

JOS VERMYLEN MD, *Professor of Medicine, Division of Bleeding and Vascular Disorders, Center for Thrombosis and Vascular Research, University of Leuven, Herestraat 49, B-3000 Leuven, Belgium*

JAMES F. WINCHESTER MD FRCP (Glas.), *Professor of Medicine, Georgetown University Medical Center, Department of Medicine, Division of Nephrology, 3800 Reservoir Road NW, Washington DC 20007, USA*

Preface

The ability to control blood loss is one of the most basic protective mechanisms of the body's defences. This has evolved in humans into an extremely complex interaction of vessel wall, plasma coagulation factors, platelets and fibrinolysis. The molecular mechanisms are now relatively well understood and the reasons that individual patients bleed can be investigated easily by specialist laboratories.

Excess bleeding remains a threat to the success of surgery both directly by reducing circulating blood volume and indirectly by interfering with wound healing.

This volume has been written for surgeons in a range of specialties to explain the mechanisms of bleeding in general, and also in particular diseases of different organs. Sections on diagnosis and treatment offer valuable specialist advice in the management of bleeding disorders.

C.D. Forbes
A. Cuschieri

Part 1
Pathophysiology of Bleeding

Chapter 1
Normal haemostasis

BRUCE BENNETT AND PATRICK FITCH

Maintenance of a normal blood volume circulating within the vascular compartment is critical for normal tissue function. Any significant breach of the integrity of this compartment may result in death when perfusion of vital organs becomes significantly impaired. Haemostatic mechanisms have evolved to ensure (a) that any injuries are efficiently sealed to maintain the circulating blood volume, and (b) that thereafter patency of damaged blood vessels is restored. The first aim is achieved by three basic mechanisms:

1 Vasoconstriction.

2 Platelet plug formation.

3 Fibrin formation and coagulation.

The second aim is achieved by one principal mechanism, namely:

4 Fibrinolysis.

These four mechanisms are intimately linked one with another and have evolved into a highly efficient system for ensuring the maintenance of our circulating blood volume and the patency of the vascular system. A considerable amount of knowledge has accrued as to how the systems operate and interrelate though complete understanding of their interactions has not yet been achieved. Failure of any component to maintain a balance may result in haemorrhage or thrombosis. The defects which lead to haemorrhage are fairly well understood. In contrast, the abnormalities responsible for thrombosis are less well defined.

This chapter outlines the four principal components of the haemostatic system and the checks and balances to which they are subject.

Vasoconstriction

Damage to a blood vessel results in a vasoconstrictive response. This is mediated through the muscle layers of the walls of arteries and veins. Capillary walls do not contain significant contractile muscle elements but blood flow in capillaries may be modified by contraction of precapillary sphincters. Such constriction of vascular muscle layers can be mediated via two pathways:

1 Neurogenic constriction of blood-vessel muscle occurs via intact reflexes and is normally very transient.

2 Muscle spasm, mediated by direct stimulation of vascular muscle layers during injury is more sustained and lasts up to an hour.

Neither of these pathways, being relatively transient, plays a major role in the severe bleeding encountered in medical practice and as a result they have not been subject to the detailed examination devoted to the other three mechanisms listed above. Agents produced by the other three processes, for example thromboxane, bradykinin and fibrinopeptide, all act as vasoconstrictors and may contribute to haemostasis in this way. Adequate support or pressure on injured vessels by surrounding connective tissue is also necessary for haemostasis; defects in this, for example Ehlers–Danlos syndrome, in which connective tissue is abnormally elastic, may result in abnormal bleeding.

Platelet plug formation

Circulating platelets produce clumps or aggregates when subjected to a wide variety of stimuli. In normal circumstances they are inhibited from doing so by a number of factors including the flow properties of the blood and the antiaggregating effect of prostacyclin which is synthesized by vascular endothelial cells from arachidonic acid by the cyclo-oxygenase pathway.

When the vascular endothelium is disrupted by injury, however, flowing blood contacts subendothelial tissues from which it is normally separated. This initiates a series of reactions leading to platelet plug formation. The first such reaction is *adhesion* of platelets to the subendothelium. Individual platelets adhere to exposed collagen and elastic fibres in a process that depends upon their own intrinsic properties, the properties of the tissue exposed and a number of additional plasma factors. The platelet membrane agent identified as participating in adhesion reactions in glycoprotein 1b though other platelet constituents may participate. The plasma component identified as of major importance in adhesion is von Willebrand Factor (vWF) which is produced by the endothelium itself and circulates in a number of macromolecular forms in plasma. Absence of vWF is responsible for the long bleeding time in von Willebrand's disease in which platelet adhesion, the initiating event in platelet plug formation, cannot occur normally. Glycoprotein 1b acts as the platelet receptor for vWF and defects in this receptor, such as those which occur in Bernard–Soulier syndrome, account for defective adhesion and the long bleeding time in that disorder.

Physical factors influence platelet adhesion. Blood-flow velocity and blood viscosity, critically influenced by the haematocrit and the consequent shear forces at the blood–tissue interface, all influence adhesion.

Subsequent to adhesion of platelets to exposed subendothelial tissues on injury, the second component of platelet plug formation, namely *platelet aggregation*, occurs (Fig. 1.1a,b). This is the accumulation of platelets one to another. Platelets adherent to subendothelial tissues alter their shape from a spherical to a discoid conformation and a number of chemical factors then promote aggregation of further platelets from the circulation to form a platelet mass. Principal among the recruiting mechanisms is the one which depends on arachidonic acid metabolism products generated by adherent platelets. Arachidonic acid is generated from platelet membrane phospholipid by phospholipase and under the influence of platelet cyclo-oxygenase, generates the unstable prostaglandins PGG_2 and PGH_2, which are then converted by platelet thromboxane synthetase to thromboxane A_2. This acts as a potent aggregating agent recruiting circulating platelets to enlarge the growing platelet plug at the site of injury. The *platelet release reaction* occurs in which platelets discharge the content of their endogenous granules, notably adenosine diphosphate and serotonin which further promote the aggregation reaction. Additional agents which enhance platelet aggregation at the site of injury are fibrinogen, adenosine diphosphate from damaged red cells, traces of thrombin generated by the coagulation mechanism (see below), platelet aggregating factor (PAF), released from platelets themselves on thrombin stimulation, serotonin and, under some circumstances, catecholamines.

The consequence of the two sequential processes, adhesion and aggregation, is the production of a platelet plug which is sufficient to stop bleeding from injuries to small blood vessels but insufficient to secure permanent sealing of these or larger wounds. Such permanent sealing requires reinforcement of the platelet plug by the formation of fibrin described below (Fig. 1.2).

The integrity of the sequence of reactions leading to platelet plug formation is detected by the simple clinical test known as the bleeding time. This is normally carried out by making a small cut on the skin of the forearm, finger or ear and recording the time taken for bleeding to stop. If this time is normal platelet plug formation is intact. If it is

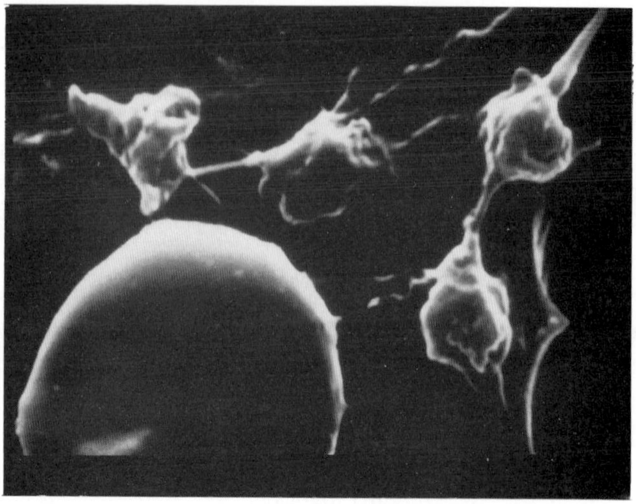

(a)

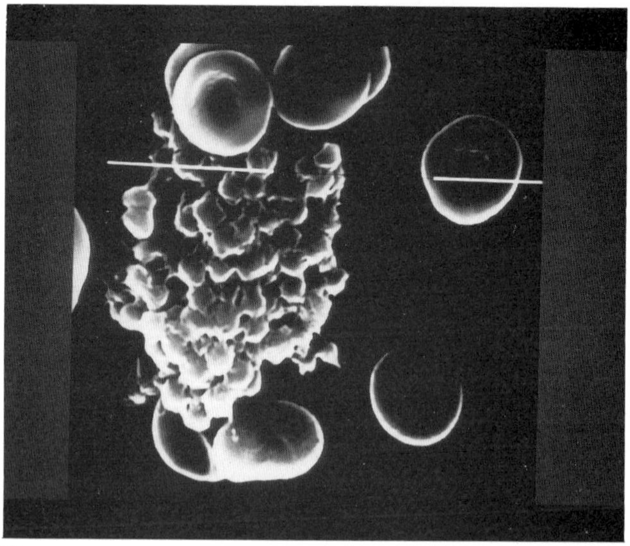

(b)

Fig. 1.1 (a) SEM of platelets which have adhered, changed shape, thrown out pseudopodia and initiated the reaction that leads to aggregation (b) of platelets into a clump. This rapid process is primary haemostasis.

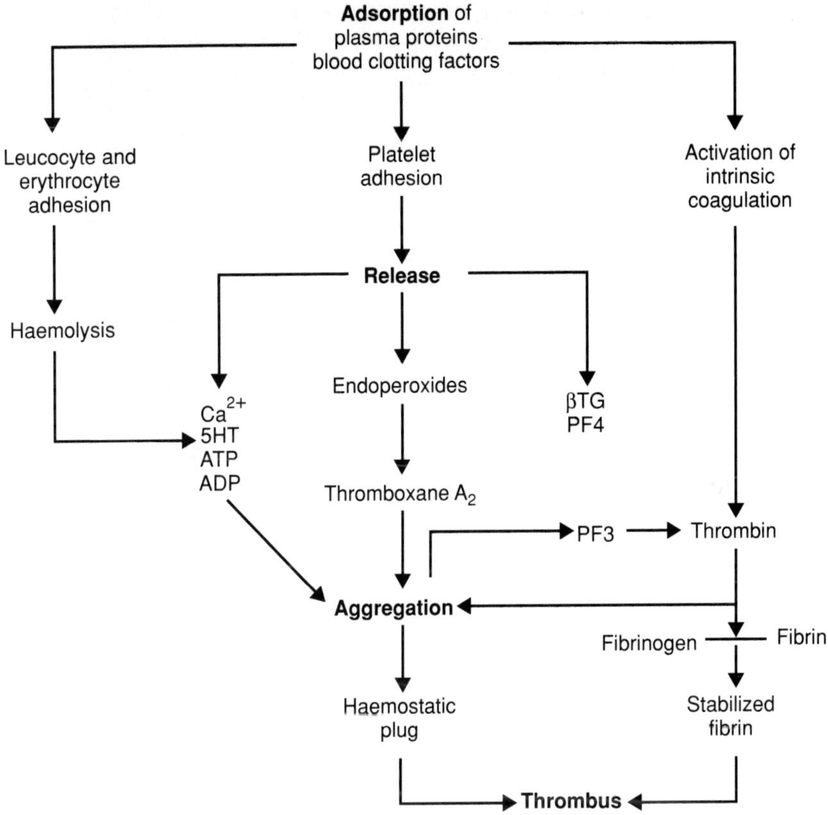

Fig. 1.2 Schema for the interaction of platelets and coagulation in the production of a platelet–fibrin plug which stops further bleeding.

prolonged, a component of the adhesion and aggregation sequence is abnormal and more complex tests are required to define the precise site and nature of the deficit.

Fibrin formation and coagulation

Platelet plug formation is sufficient to secure temporary cessation of bleeding from small blood vessels. Such wounds will thus cease to bleed temporarily even if major disorders of coagulation such as haemophilia exist. However, unless fibrin formation occurs concurrently or very shortly after platelet plug formation, bleeding tends to *recur* within an hour or so. In the presence of more major injury, if fibrin formation is defective for any reason, bleeding becomes a major problem from the outset. This section discusses the physiological mechanisms leading to fibrin formation.

Fibrin forms as a dense network of insoluble strands, reinforcing any platelet plug that has already formed and producing an efficient seal to wounds to ensure maintenance of the vascular tree's integrity and prevent further loss of circulating blood volume. Circulating fibrinogen is a soluble dimeric molecule, each component of the dimer having three polypeptide subunits known as the α-, β- and γ-chains. Under the action of thrombin a peptide fragment, fibrinopeptide A, is split from the α-chain followed by a further fragment, fibrinopeptide B which is removed from the β-chain. These apparently minor losses from the molecule produce firstly fibrin monomer which remains soluble, but rapidly polymerizes to form fibrin strands which seal wounds *in vivo* by incorporating the platelet plug, further platelets, red and white cells and anchoring these to the edges of the injured area. Fibrin polymer thus formed efficiently seals wounds but will break down unless a further chemical event takes place. This is the crosslinking of adjacent fibrin molecules via amide linkages between γ- and later α-chains of the adjacent molecules. These bonds, particularly those between α-chains, stabilize the insoluble fibrin and render it much less susceptible to attack by plasmin generated via the fibrinolytic system. Factor XIII (fibrin stabilizing factor), one of the inert circulating clotting factors, is converted by thrombin to an active enzyme capable of forging the crosslinks. This end stage of the production of a stable fibrin wound seal is summarized in Fig. 1.3.

The thrombin time is the simple test that establishes whether fibrinogen levels and fibrin formation occur normally. In this test plasma is clotted by addition of a small amount of purified thrombin and the time for this is recorded in seconds. The normal range is 10–12 s. In normal circumstances thrombin is not generated in the body as this would rapidly produce widespread intravascular coagulation.

Haemostatic mechanisms have evolved to generate thrombin and hence fibrin formation *locally* at the site of injury and prevent its action throughout the circulation. Two pathways have evolved, each leading to production of active thrombin. In each an initial stimulus, usually local injury, triggers a series of cascade reactions which amplify locally the effect of the initial stimulus, thus leading to the explosive generation of thrombin. How this phenomenon is kept local will be dealt with later. The two pathways referred to were defined in the 1960s and are known as the *extrinsic* and *intrinsic pathways*. These have several unique initial stages but thereafter share a final common pathway (Fig. 1.4).

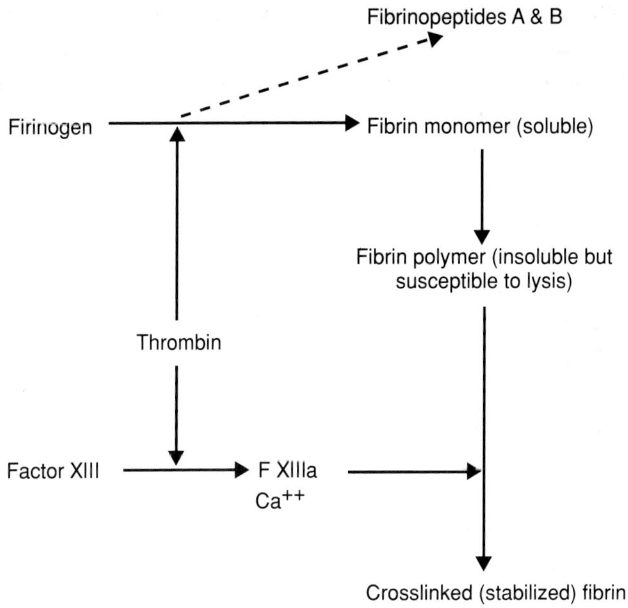

Fig. 1.3 Fibrin formation and stabilization by thrombin and Factor XIII.

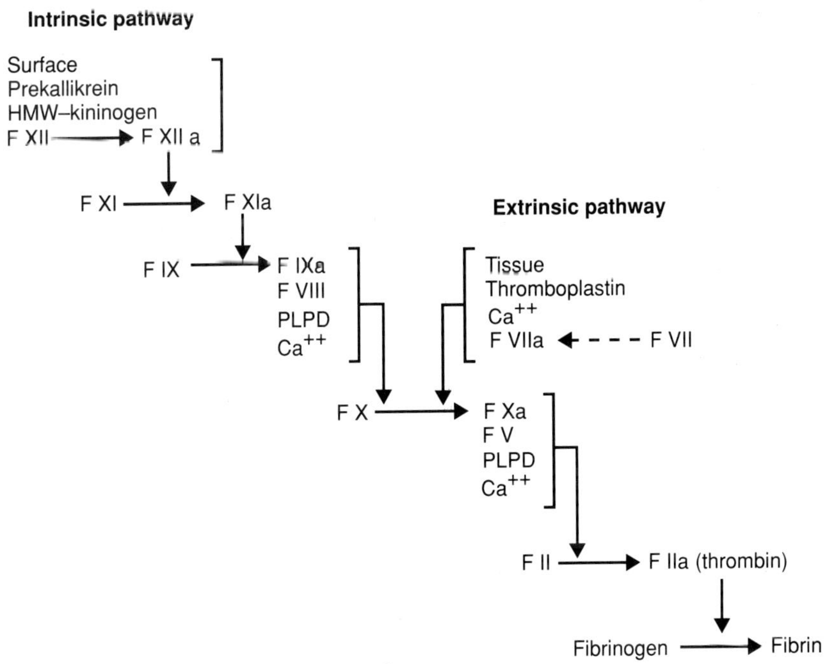

Fig. 1.4 The intrinsic and extrinsic pathways.

The reactions illustrated all share the common principle that the clotting factor circulates in an inactive or proenzyme form which is converted by the product of the preceding reaction in the cascade to an active enzyme and this in turn attacks the inert circulating agent in the next reaction, converting it to its active form, and so on. Each conversion of proenzyme to enzyme involves the modification of the molecule which results in the release of a fragment of the molecule or the conversion of the molecule from a single to a two-chain form. This modification of configuration with the exposure of the critical active enzyme site allows it to catalyse the next reaction in the series. It is not proposed to define the molecular nature of each of these reactions in detail but all follow the same basic pattern.

Extrinsic pathway

Activity in this pathway is initiated when thromboplastins, which are derived from damaged extravascular tissue, come into contact with the blood (Fig. 1.4). Blood exposed to these agents clots within a few seconds. Tissue thromboplastin occurs in all tissues and has a lipid and a protein component both of which are necessary for expression of its function. In the absence of lipid the protein has little activity. Phosphatidylethanolamine is the most effective agent in conferring activity on the purified protein, a negative surface charge on the phospholipid being critical for such activity and it probably functions by enhancing interaction of the protein component with its substrate, Factor VII. This plasma protein, with a molecular weight of 48 kDa, forms a complex with tissue factor and calcium and in the process is converted from a single-chain relatively inert factor to a two-chain active enzyme. This complex, now powerfully catalytically active, converts Factor X, the next proenzyme in the cascade, to its active form. In this process Factor X, a two-chain 60 kDa protein, is converted to its active form by cleavage of a peptide bond in the heavy chain which exposes the active enzyme site. Factor Xa alone is able to activate prothrombin but at a slow rate. Prothrombin activation by Factor Xa is markedly accelerated if Factor V, phospholipid and calcium are present. The presence of these allow prothrombin and Factor Xa to bind to the phospholipid and Factor V also associates with this complex. The juxtaposition of these proteins on the surface of phospholipid greatly increases the rate of their interaction and also shelters them from the inhibitory effect of antithrombin III. The role of Factor V, a large 250 kDa protein, is incompletely understood but when activated by traces of thrombin it is able to bind to the prothrombin part of the complex and this enhances prothrombin activation considerably. Prothrombin, a single-chain 70 kDa protein, when incorporated in the above complex is cleaved with the release of active thrombin which generates fibrin from fibrinogen as described above.

Integrity of this extrinsic pathway is tested by the prothrombin time which measures the clotting time of plasma after tissue factor from a brain source is added. The time of a normal test is about 14–16 s. The test plasma is always compared to a control done at the same time. This simple test, if prolonged, indicates that there is deficiency of fibrinogen, Factor II, V, X or VII.

Intrinsic pathway

Activity of this pathway is triggered by the contact of blood with a foreign surface, that is, a surface other than the normal vascular endothelium (Fig. 1.4). In wounds this is normally collagen, elastic fibres, muscle, fat or skin. Such contact brings together Factor XII (Hageman factor), prekallikrein, high-molecular-weight kininogen and Factor XI. The consequence of the adhesion of the four factors to negatively-charged surfaces is the conversion by Factor XIIa of Factor XI, a two-chain plasma protein of 160 kDa to its active enzymic form Factor XIa.

Factor IX (Christmas factor), a 55 kDa single-chain polypeptide, is then converted to its active form by Factor XIa which cleaves the molecule releasing small molecular fragments and generates the two-chain active form of the enzyme.

Thereafter Factor IXa converts Factor X to its active form. This conversion is markedly enhanced by the presence of phospholipid, Factor VIII (antihaemophilic factor) and calcium ions. These form with Factor IXa and Factor X a multimolecular complex approximating the participants and enhancing their interaction. Factor VIII, the agent deficient in classic haemophilia, normally circulates in a large molecular complex with vWF. It catalyses activation of Factor X by Factor IX in a manner similar to that of Factor V in the generation of thrombin from prothrombin by Factor Xa. Like Factor V, Factor VIII activity is markedly enhanced by traces of thrombin.

The activated partial thromboplastin time is the screening test that examines integrity of the intrinsic pathway, its prolongation indicating deficiency in fibrinogen, Factor II, V, X, VIII, IX, XI or XII. In this test, plasma clotting times are measured after plasma is activated (usually with kaolin) and an additional source of lipid is added. The time for normals is approximately 45–55 s. The test samples from patients are always compared to normal controls.

Although it is convenient to distinguish the extrinsic and intrinsic pathways for conceptual and investigation purposes it is known that considerable interaction between the pathways occurs. It should also be noted that a number of feedback loops exist in the system influencing its function. Most notable of these is the fact that, when traces of thrombin have been generated this markedly enhances (many thousand-fold) the activity of Factors V and VIII thus encouraging generation of further thrombin. Once large concentrations of thrombin are present, activity of Factors V and VIII is destroyed. It seems likely that these and other feedback loops play a role in local fine-tuning of fibrin formation.

The role of the liver

Virtually all the coagulation factors are synthesized in the liver with the exception of the vWF which is synthesized by vascular endothelial cells. Coagulation factor synthesis is part of the overall protein synthetic role of the liver. When this function of the liver is reduced in hepatic failure, synthesis of all coagulation factors is reduced and if sufficiently severe a global reduction in clotting factors ensues. This results in non-specific prolongation of all the screening coagulation tests: the prothrombin time, the thrombin time and the partial thromboplastin time are thus all prolonged. Acute hepatic damage, for instance, by viruses as in hepatitis or in acute paracetamol overdosage, results in an acute bleeding disorder.

In addition, under the influence of vitamin K, the liver attaches specific γ-carboxyglutamic acid side-chains to four coagulation factors—Factors II (prothrombin), VII, IX and X. These side-chains bind calcium and are necessary for the procoagulant actions of the factors. In vitamin K deficiency from whatever cause, be it intestinal malabsorption or be it due to warfarin therapy, these side-chains are not attached to the protein skeletons and the functional activity of these four clotting factors is significantly reduced and results in a bleeding tendency. Because the half-life of Factor VII is the shortest of the four clotting factors, Factor VII activity levels are reduced first in vitamin K deficiency, the disorder being characterized initially by prolongation of the prothrombin time. If vitamin K deficiency persists longer or is severe, prolongation of the partial thromboplastin time will also occur.

If the protein synthetic role of the liver is intact and the disorder is simply vitamin K deficiency, it is rapidly reversed by injection of vitamin K; however, if liver cell damage is extensive, injection of vitamin K has little effect.

Control of coagulation in the circulation

Unrestricted activation of clotting factors does not occur in the body normally. As indicated above, the coagulation cascade is triggered locally by injury. Disseminated activation of coagulation throughout the circulation is prevented by a number of inhibitors of activated clotting factors. Principal among these is antithrombin III (ATIII) which complexes with, and inhibits, the activity of a number of activated clotting factors, principally thrombin and Factor Xa. Thus, traces of these activated factors, should they gain access to the general circulation, are rapidly neutralized. Other major inhibitors are proteins C and S. These two proteins are produced by the liver under the influence of vitamin K but, unlike the other vitamin K-dependent agents, act as inhibitors of coagulation. Normally they are inert but if activated by traces of thrombin will, in combination, neutralize the activity of Factors V and VIII. An additional inhibitor has recently been identified which neutralizes the activity of the tissue factor-dependent (extrinsic) pathway. Its role in the control of haemostasis is as yet not fully defined. Other inhibitory proteins exist in the circulation which may inhibit activated coagulation factors. Examples of these are C1 inhibitor, α_2-macroglobulin and α_1-antitrypsin. These agents inhibit activated clotting factors *in vitro* and act as subsidiary inhibitors when the principal inhibitors have been exhausted in disseminated intravascular coagulation.

The action of all these inhibitors therefore is to ensure that a stimulus promoting fibrin formation remains local at the site of injury and that the body is thus protected from widespread intravascular coagulation.

Role of the endothelium in coagulation

Blood-vessel endothelium functions primarily as a barrier between the circulating blood and the extravascular tissues. Endothelium also produces glycosaminoglycans, heparin-like agents with anticoagulant function which protect the body from unwanted fibrin formation in the circulation and thrombomodulin which enhances thrombin-induced conversion of protein C to its anticoagulant form. Finally, endothelium produces prostacyclin (via the arachidonic acid pathway) which is a potent inhibitor of platelet aggregation and a powerful vasodilator.

Role of platelets in coagulation

Blood platelets are not essential for fibrin formation but their presence considerably enhances the rate at which fibrin formation occurs by contributing phospholipid from the platelet membrane which acts at several stages in the coagulation cascade. Thrombocytopenic bleeding is primarily due to the failure to produce a normal platelet plug rather than due to a failure of fibrin formation.

The fibrinolytic system

The fibrinolytic system is responsible for removal of fibrin when its wound-sealing function is over and for restoring patency to injured blood vessels occluded by haemostatic clot.

The system (Fig. 1.5) operates ultimately by the action of the proteolytic enzyme, plasmin, on the formed fibrin thrombus. Free plasmin is rarely present in the circulation but is generated and exerts its action locally on the surface of fibrin deposits. The first component of this system is plasminogen, which is an inert single-chain proenzyme with a molecular weight of approximately 80 kDa. Several internal disulphide bonds create looped or 'kringle' structures in the chain which confer its unique properties. Rupture of a single bond (Arg-560–Val-561) converts it to the two-chain molecule plasmin, a protease with serine at its active centre, now exposed on the light or β-chain. The heavy chain contains the kringles responsible for the interaction between the molecule and substrate fibrin and its major inhibitor, α_2-antiplasmin.

Two principal physiological activators have been identified which convert plasminogen to plasmin. The first recognized, urokinase or uPA, was identified initially in urine but is now known to circulate in small quantities in the blood. It exists in two forms, a proenzyme (pro-uPA) with fibrin affinity but little enzymic activity, and as the active enzyme which may exist in 50 or 30 kDa forms. Conversion of the proenzyme to the active enzyme is promoted by traces of plasmin itself. uPA converts plasminogen to plasmin, is non-antigenic in man,

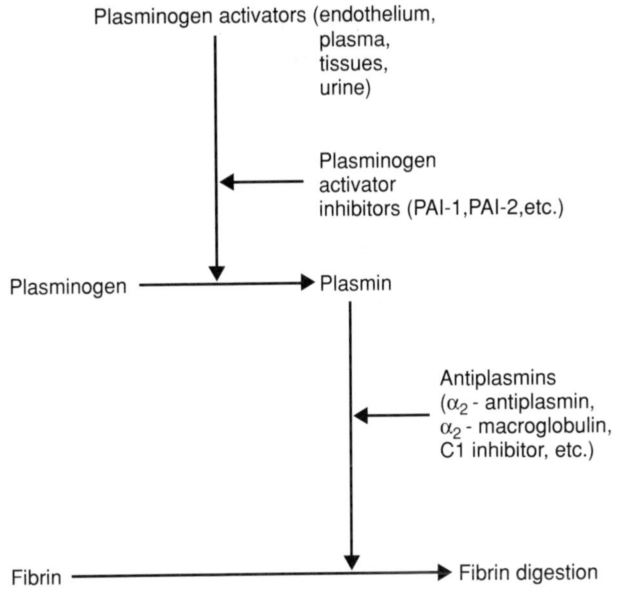

Fig. 1.5 The fibrinolytic system in plasma. Note that the function of formed fibrin in specifically adsorbing plasminogen activators and plasminogen itself is not illustrated but is described in the text.

being a human protein, and has been used therapeutically. The active form, unlike the proenzyme, has little specific fibrin affinity which represents a disadvantage to its therapeutic use.

Many solid tissues contain a plasminogen activator that is similar to the one produced by vascular endothelium. This is now known as tissue plasminogen activator or tPA. It has a molecular size of approximately 70 kDa, and is the principal circulating plasminogen activator. Normally levels are low in the blood, but they show a diurnal rhythm and tPA is released into the circulation by stimuli such as exercise and acute venous occlusion. The principal property of tPA is its marked affinity for fibrin onto which it is absorbed rapidly by virtue of its possessing a kringle structure similar to those present on plasminogen. This fibrin affinity confers considerable theoretical advantage on its use as a thrombolytic agent.

Control of the fibrinolytic system in the circulation

The active enzymes of the fibrinolytic pathway are held in check in the circulating blood by the influence of inhibitory proteins. The principal antiplasmin is known as α_2-antiplasmin. This protein, of molecular weight 70 kDa, forms a 1 : 1 molecular complex with plasmin. This reaction takes place very rapidly so that any plasmin generated in the circulation is immediately neutralized thus protecting circulating coagulation proteins such as fibrinogen and other clotting factors from digestion by plasmin. Interaction between α_2-antiplasmin and plasmin takes place at specific 'lysine binding sites' on the plasmin molecule located on the kringle structures. Plasmin–α_2-antiplasmin complexes once formed are rapidly cleared from the circulation. Inhibitors of plasminogen activator have recently been identified and are two in number. The principal one is known as plasminogen activator inhibitor-1, or PAI-1, and is present in circulating blood where it rapidly complexes with any circulating tPA. Normally, the bulk of circulating tPA is present in complexes with this inhibitor and is not available to convert plasminogen to plasmin. In addition to its presence in plasma, PAI-1 is present in large quantities in circulating platelets, though platelet PAI-1 seems a much less active molecule than that free in plasma. The large quantity present in platelets means that haemostatic plugs are rich in inhibitors of plasminogen activator and are relatively resistant to lysis. A second inhibitor of plasminogen activator, PAI-2, is generated in the placenta and is present in large quantities in the blood of pregnant women. Traces of this inhibitor are present in lymphoid cells of non-pregnant individuals but its function there is unknown.

A unique property of the proteins of the fibrinolytic system is their affinity for fibrin. Plasminogen and tissue plasminogen activator are absorbed onto the surface of formed fibrin via the lysine binding sites. When bound to fibrin they are not susceptible to binding by their respective inhibitors at the lysine binding sites are occupied by the fibrin link. Thus, on the surface of fibrin, plasminogen and plasminogen activator are placed in close proximity and generate plasmin locally which digests the fibrin deposit. This allows the powerful activity of the system to be localized to the surface of fibrin deposits. Plasminogen activators and any plasmin formed in the circulation are rapidly complexed with their inhibitors at the lysine binding sites. Thus, any unwanted proteolytic activity of plasmin is neutralized in the circulating blood. Occasionally, if large quantities of plasminogen activator are introduced into the circulation, usually as a result of major tissue injury, the controlling inhibitors are overwhelmed and some free plasmin is generated. This results in a proteolytic state with digestion of fibrinogen and other clotting factors, notably Factors V and VIII, with production of a haemorrhagic stage. This situation is rare, but may occur in association with disseminated intravascular coagulation, worsening the haemorrhagic state generated by that process. Occasionally a pure fibrinolytic state may result from release of activators from cancers and this produces systemic proteolysis with a resultant bleeding disorder. When the principal inhibitors of fibrinolysis, α_2-antiplasmin and PAI-1 are overwhelmed in this way, certain other inhibitors are called into play, neutralizing the action of plasminogen activators and plasmin; examples of these are α_2-macroglobulin and C1-esterase inhibitor.

Role of the liver in fibrinolysis

As in the coagulation system the liver plays a crucial role in the control of the fibrinolytic mechanism. Plasminogen, α_2-antiplasmin, PAI-1 are synthesized in the liver. Defects in the protein synthetic capability of the liver therefore result in reduced levels of all these agents and may result in abnormal fibrinolysis, the type of abnormality depending on the relative reduction in the various components. Additionally, the liver is responsible for clearance of plasminogen activator and probably plasmin from the circulation. It does this by mechanisms as yet incompletely defined. Plasminogen activator and plasmin are cleared by the liver principally after they are complexed to their respective inhibitors but clearance of free tPA also occurs. Reduced hepatocellular function such as occurs in hepatic failure results in defective clearance of activators from the circulation and this may be partially responsible for the enhanced fibrinolytic state seen in cirrhosis.

Role of the endothelium in fibrinolysis

Blood-vessel endothelium plays a unique role in the fibrinolytic mechanism. Tissue plasminogen activator is synthesized by blood-vessel endothelium and probably represents the principal source in the circulation. It is normally released into the circulation only in trace amounts in normal individuals. In certain circumstances however, enhanced release of tissue plasminogen activator may occur especially after strenuous physical activity and acute venous obstruction. The former may result in strikingly enhanced fibrinolytic activity being present in circulating blood. The latter is only a very transient event. The role of endothelial tissue plasminogen activator is primarily a local one, tPA being released from damaged endothelium at the site of injury, where it will have maximum access to fibrin formed as a result of the injury.

Role of platelets in fibrinolysis

It is physiologically desirable that rapid lysis of fibrin formed in wounds should not occur but that lysis should be delayed till the haemostatic function is no longer necessary. Platelets are an integral part of all fibrin formation and their high content of PAI-1 ensures considerable resistance to immediate lysis by tPA. Other than this crucial role platelets do not appear to influence fibrinolysis greatly.

Conclusion

The expertly applied ligature remains the mainstay of surgical haemostasis. In cases of postoperative bleeding, defects in the haemostatic mechanisms may be identified by simple screening tests and the defect readily corrected.

Further reading

Bennett, B. and Ogston, D. Fibrinolytic bleeding syndromes. In: *Disorders of Hemostasis* (Eds Ratnoff, O.D. & Forbes, C.D.), pp. 321–350. Grune & Stratton, London (1991).

Biggs, R. and Rizza, C.R. (Eds) *Human Blood Coagulation, Haemostasis and Thrombosis*. Blackwell Scientific Publications, Oxford (1984).

Bloom, A.L. and Thomas, D.P. (Eds) *Haemostasis and Thrombosis*. Churchill-Livingstone, Edinburgh (1987).

Ratnoff, O.D. The evolution of knowledge about hemostasis. In: *Disorders of Hemostasis* (Eds Ratnoff, O.D. & Forbes, C.D.) pp. 1–22. Grune & Stratton, London (1991).

Saito, H. Normal hemostatic mechanisms. In: *Disorders of Hemostasis* (Eds Ratnoff, O.D. & Forbes, C.D.), pp. 23–42. Grune & Stratton, London (1991).

Chapter 2
Inherited bleeding disorders

R. ALEXANDER SHARP AND CHARLES D. FORBES

Genetically determined defects of haemostasis have been identified in relation to all four components of the haemostatic process (vascular, platelet, coagulation and fibrinolytic systems). However, the clinical incidence of significant disorders is in fact very low. The three conditions most frequently encountered are haemophilia A, Christmas disease (also referred to as haemophilia B) and von Willebrand's disease. Haemophilia A has a reported incidence in the UK of approximately 5 per 100 000, Christmas disease 1 per 100 000 and von Willebrand's disease 2.5 per 100 000. These figures are derived from patients registered with designated haemophilia centres and therefore reflect those patients with clinically significant bleeding disorders. It is probable many more individuals exist with more minor expressions of the disorders. The relevance of these genetic defects is greater than their rarity might suggest in view of the major expenditure on provision of the plasma-derived therapeutic materials required to treat and prevent bleeding complications. A major component of the function of the National Blood Transfusion Service is the collection of plasma from the donor population and its subsequent fractionation into Factor VIII and Factor IX concentrates as well as other products. The current problems related to HIV and hepatitis have led to this process becoming even more complex and expensive in recent years in order to ensure a supply of products with as high a safety profile as possible.

In the UK, most of the day-to-day clinical care of bleeding patients is organized through designated haemophilia centres, the directors of which are usually haematologists or physicians with appropriate expertise. These centres exist in most large general hospitals. In addition, there are several supraregional Haemophilia Reference Centres which can provide more sophisticated diagnostic and clinical services when required and it is usually to such centres that patients requiring elective major surgical procedures such as joint replacement are referred. It is important, however, for practising surgeons to be aware of the nature and some aspects of the management of inherited bleeding disorders for the following reasons:

1 They may well be required to give surgical opinions and perhaps perform various surgical procedures in this group with advice and assistance from their local haemophilia expert.

2 Surgical bleeding, of course, may also be one way in which some of these patients may present.

3 Finally, acute surgical bleeding can occur unpredictably in any subject at any location. If it does so incidentally in a haemophiliac, urgency may dictate that the surgeons on hand would have to operate.

In this chapter, the pathophysiology and main clinical features of the commoner inherited haemostatic disorders will be described with particular reference to clinical management required in a surgical setting.

Inherited coagulation disorders

The inherited disorders of the coagulation system most frequently encountered are haemophilia A, Christmas disease (haemophilia B) and von Willebrand's disease, which are discussed below. Those encountered less frequently are listed in Table 2.1 along with brief relevant details.

Haemophilia

Jewish writings in the 2nd century refer to the genetic and surgical aspects of a bleeding disorder likely to be haemophilia with references to fatal bleeding following circumcision in brothers and serious bleeding following minor surgery in male cousins [1]. The X-linked recessive fashion of inheritance of both haemophilia A and Christmas disease as well as their similar clinical features is of course now well recognized.

Haemophilia A is due to deficiency of the procoagulant portion of the coagulation Factor VIII complex (referred to as FVIII Act) which plays a key role in the intrinsic system of blood coagulation. Christmas disease is due to deficiency of Factor IX, also a key factor in the intrinsic system. The genes for both these factors are located on the X-chromosome and hence the classic pattern of inheritance with affected males and female carriers. Clinical problems are largely confined to the affected males; however, in certain circumstances, if the surgical challenge is a major one, female carriers may have bleeding problems. The diagnosis is usually suspected initially on clinical or genetic grounds. Investigations reveal a prolongation of the activated partial thromboplastin time

Table 2.1 Less frequent hereditary coagulation disorders

Disorder	Bleeding tendency	Replacement therapy and comments
Afibrinogenaemia	Mild to moderate	FFP, cryoprecipitate
Dysfibrinogenaemia	Rare	May have thrombotic tendency
Factor II (prothrombin) deficiency	Mild to moderate	FFP, prothrombin concentrate
Factor V deficiency	Variable	FFP
Factor VII deficiency	Variable, some asymptomatic	FFP, prothrombin complex
Factor X deficiency	Variable, some asymptomatic	FFP, prothrombin concentrate
Factor XI deficiency	Mild	FFP
Factor XII deficiency	Usually asymptomatic	
Factor XIII (fibrin-stabilizing factor) deficiency	Severe in homozygote, often bleed from umbilical cord	FFP, 7-day half-life of Factor XIII makes once-weekly therapy adequate. Poor wound healing a feature

FFP, fresh frozen plasma.

(APTT) and a normal prothrombin time (PT) and the diagnosis is established by specific assay of Factor VIII and IX levels. It is usual to classify patients as suffering severe, moderate or mild disease states. Those severely affected usually have factor levels of <1% of normal, moderately affected, 1–5%, and mildly affected, 5–20%. However, occasionally moderately affected individuals run a severe course or vice versa. Those with factor levels of ≥20% rarely have any problems. Sufferers within any one family tend to be affected to a similar degree.

Clinical features

The classic clinical picture of the severely affected individual is of recurrent incapacitating and painful bleeds (Fig. 2.1) into muscles and joints with consequent sequelae of contractures and arthropathy. It is often stated that bleeding episodes are rare until haemophiliac children have the usual falls whilst first starting to walk, although a recent review indicates that up to 20% have bleeding episodes in the neonatal

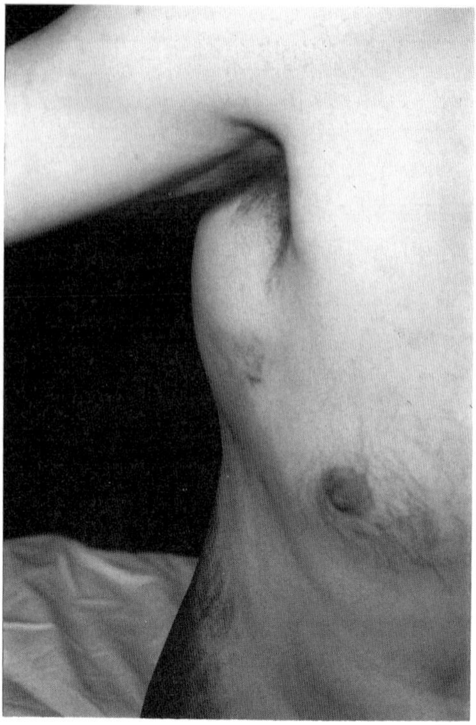

Fig. 2.1 Large haematoma in right axilla resulting from use of a crutch. Note the tracking of blood down into the subcutaneous tissues.

period and the mean age at diagnosis for severe cases was 9 months [2] (Fig. 2.2).

As platelet function is unaffected, it is reasonable to say that mucosal bleeding is infrequent; however, serious bleeding can occur in any site, muscles, joints, renal and gastrointestinal tract, and the mouth following dental extraction being the areas most frequently affected. Those with milder disease may only develop problems following trauma or surgical challenge and in fact may present in this way. Bleeding in haemophiliacs in these circumstances does tend to occur after initial vasoconstriction has passed, therefore recurrence and persistence of bleeding 1 or 2 h later is a recognized feature.

It is more convenient to consider the clinical features of bleeding in various sites and situations along with its treatment under specific headings. This follows on after some more general discussion on management.

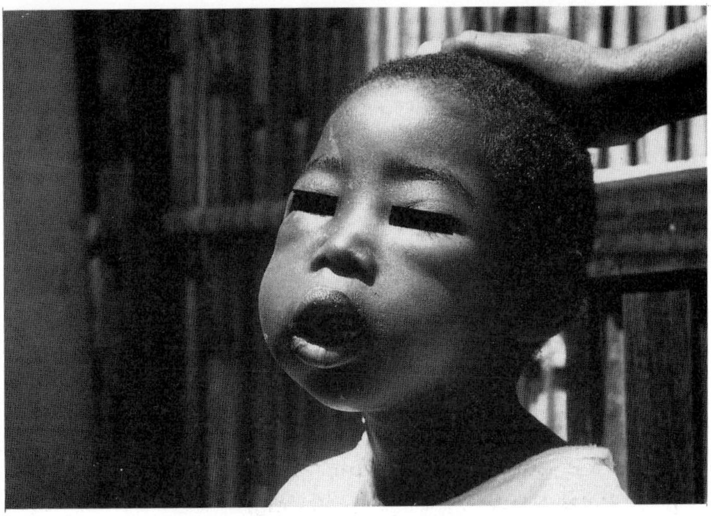

Fig. 2.2 This child presented with massive swelling of the face following a trivial injury. The haematoma tracked into the soft tissues of the neck. Before adequate treatment, this type of injury could result in asphyxia due to tracheal compression.

Treatment of haemophilia and Christmas disease

Replacement therapy and dosage

Haemostatic levels of the deficient coagulation factor are achieved usually by the intravenous infusion of human plasma-derived Factor VIII or IX concentrates. The doses of concentrate required, the frequency and duration of administration and other adjunctive measures to aid haemostasis will depend on:

1 The severity of the defect.
2 The nature and site of injury (or proposed surgery).
3 The presence of any acquired coagulation inhibitors.

For minor bleeds involving non-weight-bearing muscles or joints or whenever the early warning signs of an incipient bleed are experienced, the achievement of level of 15–20% of the relevant factor is probably adequate and many haemophiliacs treat themselves at home in these circumstances. Moderate to severe haemarthroses, mucosal bleeding (e.g. haematuria) or moderate surgical challenge such as dental extraction require levels in the region of 20–70% and in the case of more major surgery or trauma 50–100% is recommended initially. The biological half-life of Factor VIII in the plasma is from 8 to 12 h, therefore twice-

Table 2.2 Formula for calculating dose of concentrate required (calculation of dosage of Factor VIII or IX)

$$\text{Dose in units} = \frac{\%\ \text{rise desired} \times \text{weight (kg)}}{K}$$

Where K = 1.5 for Factor VIII concentrates
1.5 for cryoprecipitate
0.7 for Factor IX concentrates
2.0 for FFP (ml)

Problem	*Factor level (%)*	*Dose (iu/kg)*
1 Minor bleed	10–20	10–15
2 Dental extraction Haemarthrosis Haematuria	20–70	15–50
3 Major surgery or trauma	70–100	50–70

daily administration is usually required to maintain therapeutic levels in severe bleeds or for surgical prophylaxis. Factor IX has a plasma half-life of 18–24 h, therefore administration more frequently than once a day is only rarely necessary.

Calculation of required dosage should take into account the patient's baseline factor level, the desired peak and trough levels required in the relevant situation, their plasma volume and the 'recovery' of activity from the therapeutic material used. There is also a patient-to-patient variation in the levels achieved following a standard dose of concentrate infused and previous response to treatment forms an important part of the dosage calculation with some individuals. Dosage calculation formulae, of which there are many, are useful on a day-to-day basis. The one we use locally is illustrated in Table 2.2.

Following major surgery, it is necessary to maintain haemostatic factor levels until wound healing is complete by continuing replacement therapy for 10 to 14 days, although if antifibrinolytic agents (see later) are employed dental extractions can be carried out safely following a single adequate dose of factor concentrate.

Therapeutic materials

1 *Whole-blood and red-cell concentrates.* Historically, whole blood was once the sole means of improving haemostasis in haemophiliacs.

This has long since been abandoned on account of the fact that volume requirements are excessive and also it is a wasteful use of resources. In fact very little 'fresh whole blood' is held by transfusion centres and hospital blood banks nowadays. Red-cell concentrates which have a haematocrit of approximately 65%, and in particular red-cell concentrates supplemented with an optimal additive system, should be considered as having little or no useful content of coagulation factors.

2 *Fresh frozen plasma (FFP).* This is issued as a pack containing approximately 200 ml of plasma separated within 6 h of collection from a donor unit of whole blood, or alternatively larger volumes are collected from individual donors using plasmapheresis machines. At least 70% of the plasma Factor VIII (0.7 iu/ml) and normal levels of the more stable clotting factors (including Factor IX and fibrinogen) are present. Although there may be some circumstances in mild haemophilia or von Willebrand's disease where FFP might be used, as a rule, for reasons of volume overload and economic use of resources, it is reserved for replacement of multiple clotting-factor deficiencies and some other special indications.

3 *Cryoprecipitate.* This is prepared in transfusion centres by resuspending the precipitate formed during controlled thawing in a small volume of plasma. It is usually supplied as a pool from six or eight donor units and supplied in a pack in a volume of approximately 100 ml. It is rich in Factor VIII (approximately 100 iu per pack), fibrinogen and fibronectin. It contains no Factor IX. It is used particularly in the management of von Willebrand's disease and as an alternative to Factor VIII concentrates in haemophilia in some areas. Unlike the latter it can be produced relatively simply in transfusion centres and does not require a complex fractionation process. In addition, the total donor pool to which recipients are exposed is very much less than those given concentrates, which has led to its use in milder haemophiliacs in an attempt to minimize the risk of exposure to hepatitis and HIV.

4 *Factor VIII concentrates.* Intermediate and high-purity concentrates are prepared by fractionation from large donor pools of cryoprecipitate. In the UK, this is carried out by the National Blood Transfusion Service. The two products are considered as having 'intermediate purity' and come under the code numbers 8Y and Z8. The products are all heat treated to inactivate HIV-1 and are provided as vials of lyophilized powder containing in the region of 250 iu of Factor VIII which is reconstituted with 10 ml of water for injection. A variety of other commercially produced concentrates are also available.

5 *Factor IX concentrates.* Partially purified Factor IX concentrates are used for replacement therapy in Christmas disease. These also contain large amounts of prothrombin and Factor X, some may also contain Factor VII. Again they are now all treated to inactivate HIV-1 and are available in vials of about 300 iu. Activation of some of the clotting factors within these preparations has led to anxieties regarding thrombotic risks with their use.

Reactions and complications of replacement therapy

All of the above are plasma-derived products and therefore can lead to allergic reactions ranging from urticaria, which is relatively common, to anaphylaxis which is extremely rare. Volume overload if FFP is required must be guarded against and non-cardiogenic pulmonary oedema due to donor plasma antileucocyte antibodies leading to the pulmonary trapping of leucocyte aggregates has been reported, albeit extremely rarely. The thrombotic potential of Factor IX concentrates has already been mentioned.

The transmission of viral infections, particularly hepatitis B, hepatitis C and HIV-1, from plasma products is a well-recognized problem despite the routine testing of all blood and plasma donations for hepatitis B surface antigen (HBsAg) and HIV antibodies. No screening test for hepatitis C is in routine use although these are currently being assessed within the National Blood Transfusion Service. Up to 90% of haemophiliacs have antibodies to HBsAg and are therefore immune; however, a few patients (1–5%) have persisting HBsAg. There is now evidence implicating hepatitis C as the main agent responsible for the majority of blood product-associated hepatitis (previously referred to under the blanket term of 'non-A, non-B hepatitis'). Almost all treated haemophiliacs have some evidence of disturbed liver function and of particular anxiety is the high risk of progression to chronic active hepatitis and cirrhosis [3–5]. Assessment of liver function preoperatively and identification of any incidental hepatic coagulation defect is therefore important.

Contamination of Factor VIII and IX concentrates with HIV-1 virus occurred initially probably in 1980–81 and led subsequently to widespread HIV infection in haemophiliacs, those treated with Factor VIII showing a very much higher level of seroconversion than those requiring Factor IX. There is wide regional variation in the prevalence depending on the quantities and variety of therapeutic materials used. The overall incidence of HIV positivity amongst UK haemophiliacs is approximately 40% but this ranges from <15% in Scotland to 60% in Newcastle and London. These figures are now falling as increasing numbers of those infected are dying from AIDS [6].

In addition to screening all donor plasma for HBsAg and HIV-1 antibodies, all concentrates are heat treated to inactivate HIV. Methods of modifying the process to reduce the chances of hepatitis transmission are also being explored. All newly diagnosed haemophiliacs can, and should, now of course be immunized against hepatitis B.

Antibodies to Factor VIII develop in 6–12% of haemophiliacs, which can lead to resistance to conventional treatment. Management of these patients is difficult and is discussed briefly later in the chapter.

Haemarthroses, muscle bleeds and haematomas

Acute haemarthroses are common and a major problem affecting all severe haemophiliacs (Fig. 2.3a,b). Knees, elbows, ankles and wrists are most frequently affected although bleeding can occur into any joint. Bleeding is often spontaneous with no preceding history of trauma. Premonitory symptoms of a sensation of warmth and tingling in the affected joint are often experienced and early therapy with modest doses of concentrate (usually self-administered at home) is thought to prevent many of these episodes developing into full-blown haemarthroses, which are extremely painful. Examination reveals a hot, swollen, tense and extremely tender joint usually held in a relatively immobile, flexed position. Signs may be modified in patients who have experienced many previous episodes which have resulted in synovial hypertrophy, muscle wasting, capsular fibrosis and chronic arthropathy. Radiographic examination is rarely indicated unless a history of trauma raises the suspicion of fracture. Joint aspiration is usually unnecessary. Muscle bleeding, either following trauma or spontaneous, is also common. Superficial bruising may be apparent. Clinical features as one might expect are those of pain, tenderness, swelling and inability to use the affected muscle group. Adjacent joints are often held in a neutral position to minimize discomfort. Some muscle necrosis inevitably occurs during such episodes with subsequent muscle wasting, fibrosis and contraction. Large muscle haematomas can lead to peripheral nerve or vascular compression. Iliopsoas haematoma may present with acute lower abdominal or inguinal pain. Right-sided episodes may mimic acute appendicitis. On examination the hip and knee are held partially flexed and passive movement is

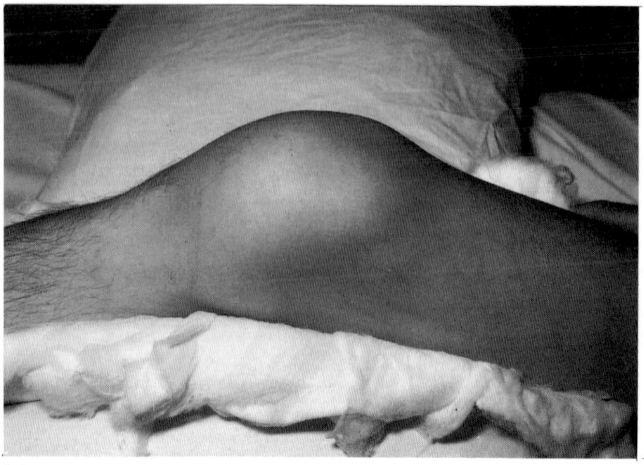

(a)

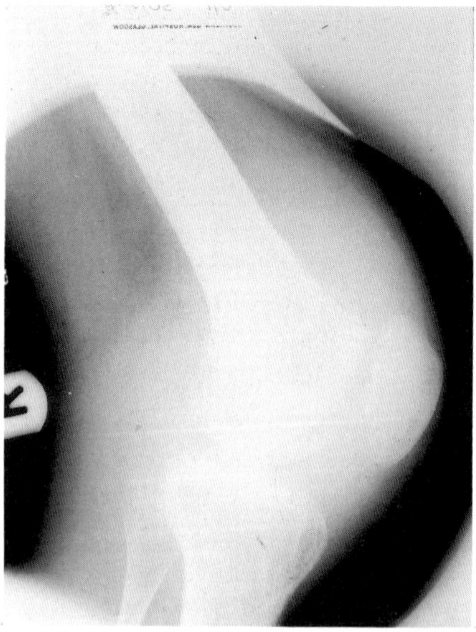

(b)

Fig. 2.3 (a) A spontaneous haemarthrosis in a severely affected patient. This joint had been the site of several previous bleeds and there was evidence of residual synovium hypertrophy and hyperaemia long after the acute episode settled down. (b) X-ray of acute bleed into the knee showing the soft-tissue swelling. There is a denser shadow resulting from the presence of haemosiderin in the joint capsule due to previous bleeds.

Table 2.3 Preparation of the haemophiliac for surgery—general history and examination

Routine investigations	Haemoglobin, full blood count, platelets Urea, electrolytes Liver function tests and prothrombin time Blood group plus check for irregular antibodies Crossmatch as required
Specific investigations	Baseline coagulation factor assays (to confirm diagnosis) Inhibitor screening test HBsAg, HIV-1 antibody
Preoperative therapy	Tranexamic acid (if indicated) intravenously, 1 h preoperatively Replacement therapy (see text), first dose approximately 1 h preoperatively followed by blood sample for factor assay 15–30 min later to ensure level adequate for surgery to proceed
Postoperative management	Factor assay immediately postoperatively and subsequent replacement therapy and laboratory monitoring as required Tranexamic acid (oral or intravenous) continued for 7–10 days

resisted. Lower abdominal tenderness and guarding may be noted. Femoral nerve compression leads to reduced sensation over the anterior aspect of the thigh to the knee and a reduced knee jerk. Retroperitoneal haematomas also present with acute abdominal signs. Ultrasound, computed tomography (CT) [7] and measurement of the muscle enzymes [8] creatine phosphokinase and aldolase can be of some diagnostic help. This clinical situation may be a trap for the unwary surgeon.

Coagulation factor replacement therapy (see Table 2.3), partial immobilization with the use of splints or slings where appropriate, analgesia (see below), ice packs and physiotherapy following resolution of the initial acute signs are the key features of treatment. Joint aspiration is of marginal benefit only in the relief of symptoms and aspiration of haematomas in the absence of life-threatening compression complications should be avoided. Peripheral nerve compression should also be treated conservatively. Lingual and sublingual haematomas occasionally occur but usually respond promptly to replacement therapy, although in the past they have led to asphyxia.

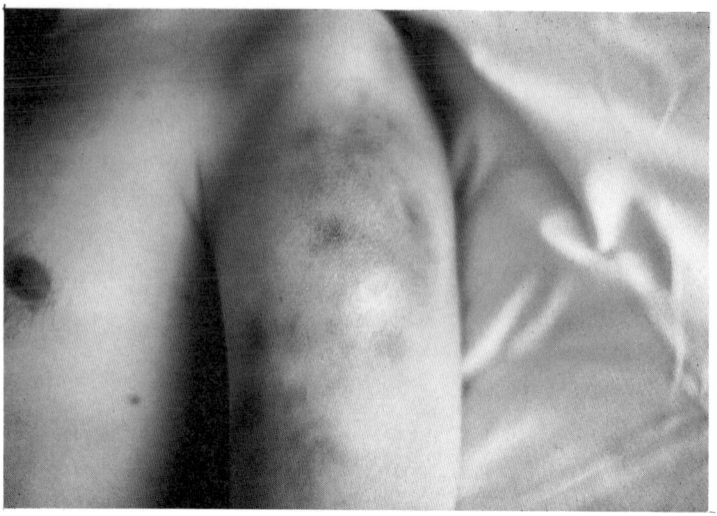

Fig. 2.4 Haematoma in the left deltoid muscle resulting from an intramuscular injection of pethidine. Intramuscular injections should be avoided in patients with a bleeding tendency.

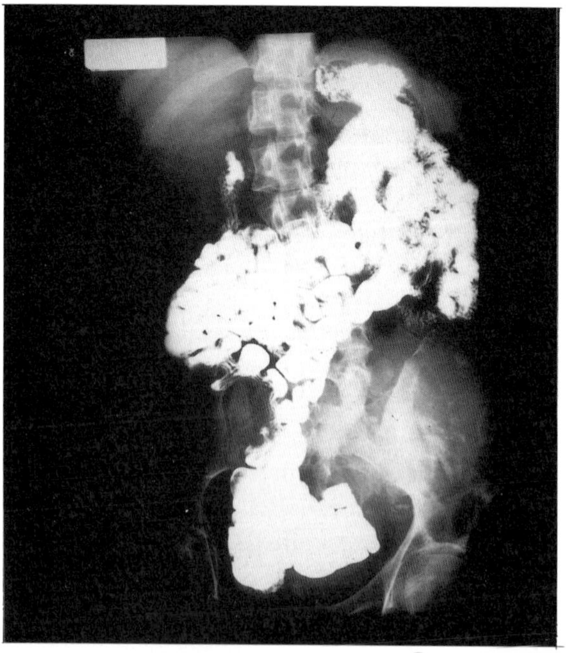

Fig. 2.5 Barium meal and follow through in a patient with obstruction as a result of massive bilateral pseudotumours of the pelvis. Erosion of the left ilium can be seen.

Recurrent intramuscular bleeding may lead to the formation of blood cysts or pseudotumours [9] (Fig. 2.4). With the early use of replacement therapy these are now extremely rare. Recurrent bleeding within the cyst leads to its gradual expansion with pressure on surrounding structures (Fig. 2.5). Erosion of bone and pathological fractures can occur. Heroic surgical resection and even amputations have been required in the past, often with disastrous results. Fortunately this complication is seldom seen nowadays.

Haematuria

Haematuria is fairly common in severe haemophiliacs, occurring in >90% on at least one occasion. It does not necessarily imply other underlying pathology. It may be painless or associated with symptoms of ureteric colic (Fig. 2.6). Management is conservative with high fluid

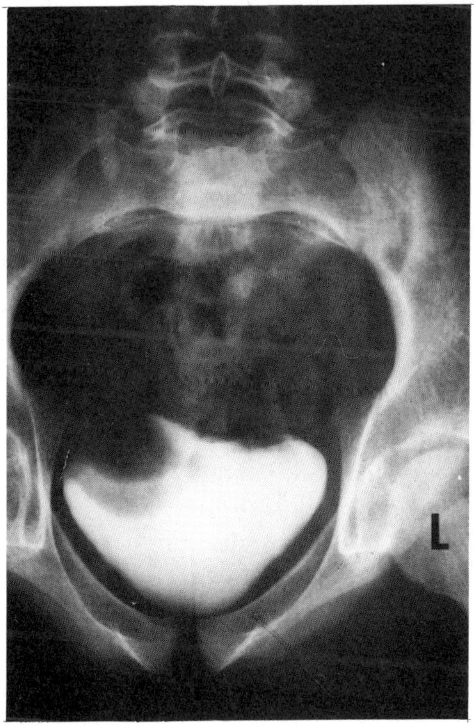

Fig. 2.6 An IVU showing a large haematoma around the orifice of the right ureter in a haemophiliac with recurrent haematuria. The kidney on this side showed obstructive features. L, left side.

intake accompanied by clotting-factor replacement therapy until the urine is clear. Recurrent or protracted episodes and episodes in milder haemophiliacs should be investigated along standard lines with the advice of a urologist. Replacement therapy cover will be required if intravenous urography with abdominal compression or cystoscopy are to be performed but not for ultrasound, isotopic renography and CT scanning.

Dental procedures

Haemophiliacs, as others, are likely to require dental extractions and other procedures. In fact bleeding following dental extraction is a well-recognized mode of presentation, particularly in less severely affected patients who may have remained relatively free from spontaneous bleeding episodes previously. Characteristically, the bleeding occurs some hours after the extraction. Examination may reveal superficial loose clot with blood oozing from the underlying socket. Fibrinolysis mediated by plasminogen activator present in saliva may further encourage bleeding in this site. Routine fillings can be safely carried out under local anaesthetic following a single dose of concentrate sufficient to give a Factor VIII (or IX) level of 50% (0.5 iu/ml). More recently, local anaesthetic injection via the periodontal ligament has been used in the absence of replacement therapy cover for minor dental procedures without any bleeding complications [10]. The extraction of one or two teeth can also be safely done on an outpatient basis. If antifibrinolytic therapy with tranexamic acid is used, a single dose of concentrate preoperatively to raise the factor level to 50–70% is usually all that is required. For adults, tranexamic acid (1 g) preoperatively followed by 1 g three times a day for the subsequent 7 days is given (appropriate dosage reduction is required for children). When this strategy of management is used, post-extraction bleeding complications are rare [11,12]. More elaborate dental work should be carried out in hospital and the patient managed along the guidelines given for major surgical procedures. The importance of good surgical technique to ensure local haemostasis cannot be over-emphasized, with the use of suturing, surgical packs, splints and protective plates as appropriate. Topical styptics such as thrombin and silver nitrate are recommended by some but of little or no proven benefit. Topical tranexamic acid has also been used. Desmopressin (DDAVP) will raise Factor VIII levels in selected patients with mild or moderate haemophilia A and its use is discussed later in the section on von Willebrand's disease.

Gastrointestinal bleeding

Acute upper gastrointestinal bleeding in haemophiliacs is usually associated with an underlying lesion such as peptic ulceration, oesophagitis, gastritis, etc. An increased incidence of peptic ulcer disease in haemophiliacs has been noted [13]. Aspirin or other non-steroidal anti-inflammatory drugs are likely to lead to major gastrointestinal bleeding and all haemophiliacs are warned at diagnosis to avoid these completely. Paracetamol or dihydrocodeine are of value for pain relief. Investigation and management is along conventional lines with the use of replacement therapy as necessary and to cover invasive investigative procedures. Variceal bleeding of course can occur in the setting of transfusion-related liver disease and its management may be desperately difficult, with the incidental problems of deficiency of other liver-derived clotting factors and thrombocytopenia.

Acute abdominal pain mimicking appendicitis, cholecystitis, pancreatitis, etc. can be a difficult diagnostic problem and is more likely due to bleeding into the bowel wall, mesentery or retroperitoneal space. Ultrasound and CT scanning may be helpful in diagnosis. Initially a conservative approach assessing the response to replacement therapy is advised.

Rectal bleeding is fairly common and should be investigated in the usual manner with replacement therapy required for endoscopy or barium enema examination [14].

Head injury and intracranial bleeding

Cerebral haemorrhage remains a common cause of death in haemophiliacs and up to 5% may suffer intracranial bleeding as neonates [2]. This may occur in cerebral, subarachnoid or subdural sites. Subdural haematomas (Fig. 2.7) occur fairly frequently and may arise in the setting of minor trauma. The clinical progression is usually fairly rapid with onset of headache followed by other signs of increased intracranial pressure and falling level of consciousness. The classic fluctuating neurogical signs associated with subdural haematoma are rarely seen. It is essential to give replacement therapy immediately in such circumstances, with doses of concentrate sufficient to achieve levels approaching 100% (1 iu/ml) before proceeding with CT and other diagnostic investigations (Fig. 2.8). Craniotomy with evacuation of haematoma when indicated should be done following appropriate patient preparation (Fig. 2.9). Factor levels should be maintained at no less than 50% (0.5 iu/ml) postoperatively

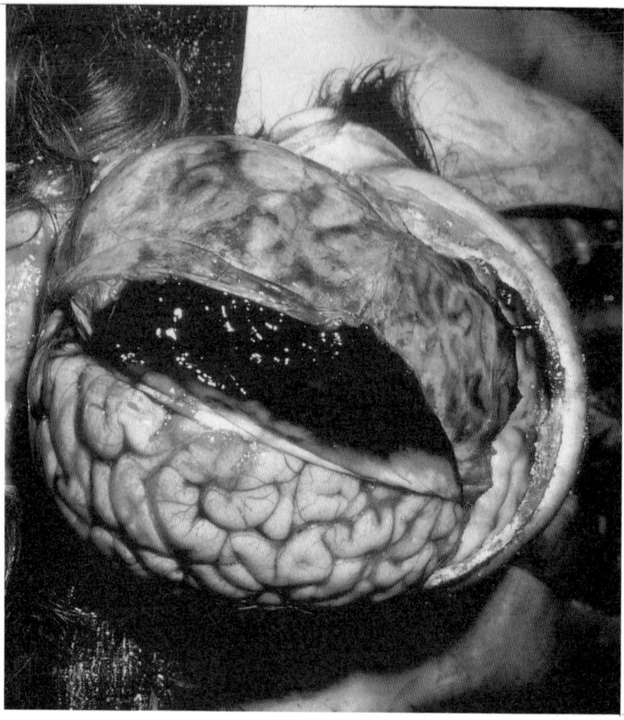

Fig. 2.7 Subdural haematoma in a severely affected haemophiliac who died suddenly in hospital after admission for a minor haemarthrosis of the knee resulting from a fall. There was no history of head injury.

for at least 10 days and tranexamic acid is also given. Anticonvulsant prophylaxis is also recommended as there is a high risk of intracranial bleeding during convulsions. In addition, 2 or 3 weeks of prophylaxis with replacement therapy to maintain factor levels of 10–15% is recommended.

Head injury in the absence of neurological signs must also be treated with prophylactic replacement therapy even in the absence of loss of consciousness. Each case has to be considered on its own merits of course. However, several days of hospital supervision and replacement therapy are recommended.

Bleeding into the spinal canal is rare but when it occurs the effects are usually catastrophic, with rapidly developing paraplegia or tetraplegia. Replacement therapy and decompression has been successful in a few cases.

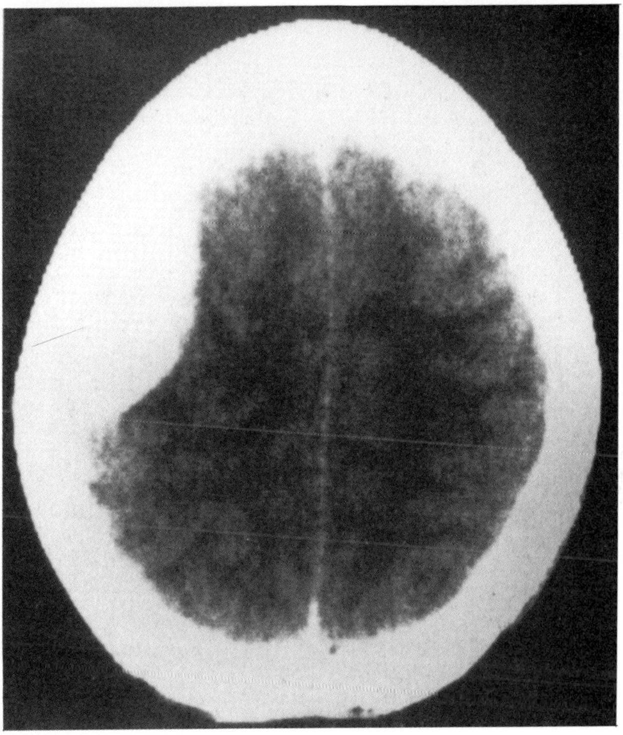

Fig. 2.8 CT head scan showing a massive subdural haematoma with midline shift in a 23-year-old patient with moderately severe Christmas disease.

Other bleeding sites

Epistaxes occur but are more frequently seen in von Willebrand's disease. Treatment again is along conventional lines with replacement therapy. We have seen spontaneous haemothorax occurring in a young man with severe Christmas disease. This was treated by insertion of a wide-bore chest drain and aggressive factor replacement therapy.

Chronic arthropathy

Recurrent intra-articular bleeding leads to chronic arthropathy, usually seen at its most advanced stages in larger weight-bearing joints (Fig. 2.10). Pathological features include synovial thickening, thinning of

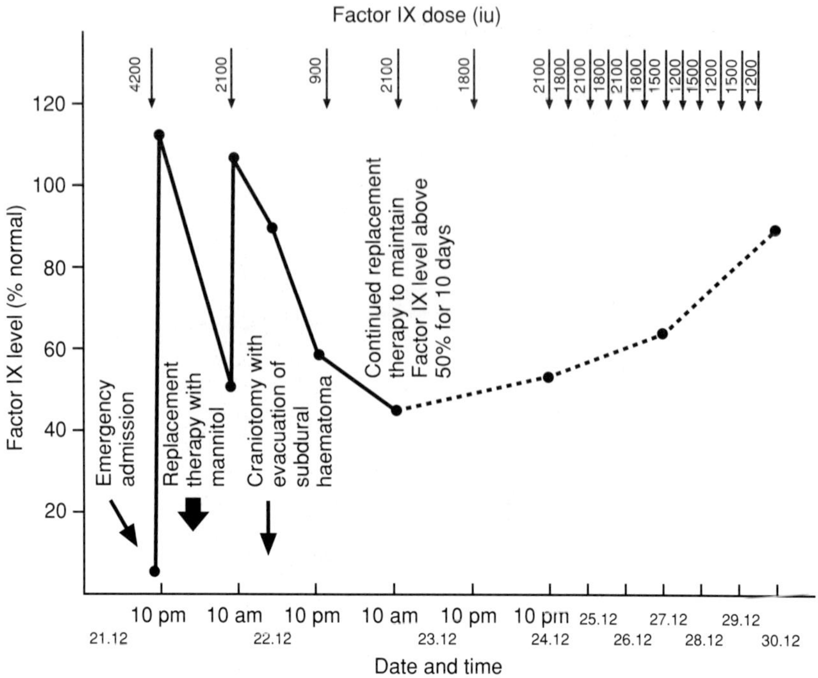

Fig. 2.9 Management of the patient whose CT scan is illustrated in Fig. 2.8. He presented comatosed with a non-reacting left pupil and a decerebrate posture with hemiplegia on the left. Prompt replacement therapy to achieve a Factor IX level of 100% was given along with mannitol to reduce cerebral oedema. Craniotomy and evacuation of the haematoma was carried out early the following morning. The patient made a full recovery.

cartilage, subchondral cysts and osteoporosis. There is extensive peri-articular fibrosis. The thickened synovium is often very vascular and a site of recurring haemorrhage. This results in severe deformity with limited range of movement and muscle wasting. Analgesia, prompt replacement therapy for acute episodes, physiotherapy and the use of lightweight orthotic devices as indicated are the mainstays of therapy. Serial splinting to gradually correct flexion deformities is sometimes helpful. Synovectomy, arthrodesis and arthroplasty may be indicated. Results can be excellent [15,16] and such procedures are best undertaken by orthopaedic specialists experienced in the management of haemophiliacs in conjunction with a haemophilia centre.

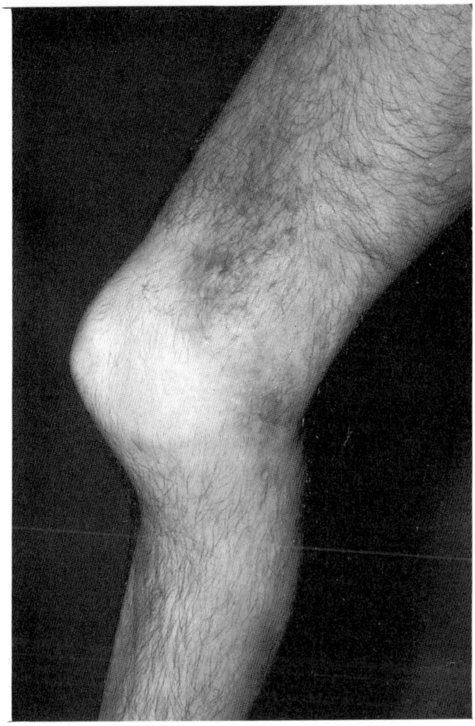

Fig. 2.10 Chronic degenerate haemophilic arthritis with severe deformity of knee joint.

Preparation and management of the haemophiliac undergoing major surgery

This requires close collaboration between the surgical and haemophilia centre teams. In the case of elective surgery all parties concerned should be given several weeks' notice, during which time many of the pre-operative checks listed in Table 2.3 can be carried out and the availability of adequate coagulation factor concentrate assured. The large amount of replacement therapy required to cover surgery may have considerable resource management implications and it therefore may be advantageous to attempt to schedule surgery during a period in time when the stocks are relatively high. A coagulation-inhibitor screening test is particularly important as their presence makes correction of factor levels extremely difficult and surgery particularly hazardous (see later section on inhibitors).

Replacement therapy

A dose of concentrate sufficient to achieve a preoperative factor level of approximately 100% is required. This must be checked by laboratory assay before surgery can commence. It is reasonable to plan to give this dose 1 h before the time scheduled for surgery to allow sufficient time for the analysis of a blood sample taken 30 min following this initial dose. Surgery should be scheduled reasonably early in the day and last-minute rearrangements of the surgical list should be discouraged. A postoperative factor assay should be done and further replacement therapy given as required to maintain a level >40% for the next 10 days or so. Factor assays should be repeated periodically pre- and post-dose over the first 3 or 4 days postoperatively (Fig. 2.9). Depending on the nature of the surgery, further replacement therapy may be required to cover the removal of sutures, drains, etc. or physiotherapy.

It is important to remind those medical and nursing staff involved, who deal infrequently with haemophiliacs, of the fact that intramuscular injections should not be given and aspirin and other non-steroidal anti-inflammatory drugs are contraindicated.

Analgesia in the haemophiliac

Aspirin and other non-steroidal anti-inflammatory drugs are dangerous in the haemophiliac and all patients are warned to avoid taking them. For mild-to-moderate pain, paracetamol, if necessary in combination with codeine or dextropropoxyphene may be adequate. For severe pain, the rational use of stronger opiate derivatives is often necessary in the short term. There are major concerns about drug dependence in this patient group.

Coagulation inhibitors in haemophiliacs

Inhibitors to Factor VIII are found in 6–12% of patients with haemophilia A. These are thought to be iso-antibodies which have developed as a result of exposure to 'foreign' transfused Factor VIII. Similar inhibitors can also rarely develop in 'normal' individuals, leading to an acquired haemophilia-like state. In haemophiliacs their presence may be suspected by an increase in frequency and severity of bleeds with apparent failure to respond to conventional doses of concentrates. Post-dose assays demonstrate poor 'recovery' of Factor VIII levels. Diagnostic tests reveal the presence of an inhibitor by the failure of the addition of normal plasma to correct the deficiency. Management is difficult even in expert centres. Factor VIII replacement may be withheld for all but the most serious of bleeding episodes in the hope that antibody titres would decline and the subsequent use of high doses of concentrate would achieve an albeit temporary haemostatic level before excess antibody levels developed. Therapeutic options for the most difficult cases include the use of porcine Factor VIII [17] or activated prothrombin concentrates.

Attempts to reduce the level of inhibitors over the longer term by immunosuppressive therapy, plasmapheresis and the induction of immunological tolerance have had some success [18]. Similar inhibitors to Factor IX have also been reported, albeit less frequently.

von Willebrand's disease

In 1926, von Willebrand identified a familial bleeding disorder in inhabitants of the Åland Islands. Unlike haemophilia, both sexes were equally affected. The skin bleeding time was prolonged but the platelet count and clot retraction were normal. Deficiency of a plasma factor (now called von Willebrand factor) required for platelet adhesion to the subendothelium was subsequently noted.

von Willebrand factor and Factor VIII

von Willebrand factor (vWF) has two main functions:

1 It is required for the adhesion of platelets to the subendothelium exposed after blood-vessel injury with consequent platelet aggregation and formation of the haemostatic plug.

2 It is also serves as a carrier molecule for Factor VIII and as such has a protective and stabilizing role. Table 2.4 lists the current terms used for the component parts of the Factor VIII complex as measured in the laboratory by various methods.

vWF is produced in the endothelial cell and the megakaryocyte and is present in both plasma and platelets as high-molecular-weight multimeric molecules of varying sizes, the largest of which are most effective in promoting platelet adhesion.

Clinical features

Inheritance is typically autosomal dominant although recessively inherited variants have been described. If severe the disease may present in early childhood. Mucocutaneous bleeding is common; haemarthroses

Table 2.4 Factor VIII and von Willebrand factor (vWF) terminology

Factor VIII/vWF	The Factor VIII procoagulant and vWF complex
FVIII Act	The procoagulant activity of Factor VIII (antihaemophilic factor, formerly referred to as Factor VIIIc) as measured by standard coagulation assays
Factor VIII Ag	Factor VIII antigen measured by immunological methods using homologous or monoclonal antibodies. This measurement normally correlates closely with FVIII Act and used to be called Factor VIIIcAg
vWFRCo	vWF measured using its requirement as a cofactor for the platelet aggregation induced by the antibiotic ristocetin
vWF Ag	vWF antigen measured by immunological methods using heterologous antibodies to Factor VIII/vWF. This measurement correlates to vWFRCo and was formerly termed Factor VIII RAg or 'related antigen'

are rare. More commonly, the disease may present as bleeding following surgical procedures, particularly dental extractions or ear, nose and throat surgery. In women menorrhagia is fairly common. There is wide variation in the severity of the disorder even within any one family.

Diagnosis

Typically, there is prolongation of the skin bleeding time, prolongation of the APTT with a normal PT and reduction of the FVIII Act, vWF Ag and vWFRCo (see Table 2.4). In contrast, in haemophilia there is a normal bleeding time, reduced FVIII Act and normal or even increased levels of vWFRCo and vWF Ag. However, many variants of von Willebrand's disease are now recognized. In the classic type IA, there is a uniform decrease in the quantity of vWF multimers but other types show more selective reduction of the larger multimers, qualitative disorders in structure and discordance in plasma and platelet patterns of distribution [19].

Management

FFP, cryoprecipitate and some intermediate-purity Factor VIII concentrates will correct both the bleeding time and coagulation defects found in von Willebrand's disease. Transfusion of these products not only produces an immediate rise in FVIII Act but also produces a secondary rise at

18–24 h due to increased release of endogenously produced Factor VIII in response to the vWF infused. Some intermediate-purity and the higher-purity concentrates have insufficient vWF and may be relatively ineffective in correcting the bleeding time. Preparation of the patient for surgery and estimation of the doses of replacement therapy required are along the same lines as those for haemophilia. DDAVP in therapeutic doses will lead to an increse in FVIII Act and vWF levels in selected patients with type I von Willebrand's disease (and mild haemophiliacs) and can be used as an alternative to replacement therapy [20,21]. As it also stimulates release of plasminogen activator, it is used in conjunction with an inhibitor of fibrinolysis such as tranexamic acid. DDAVP (0.3 μg/kg is diluted in 100 ml of saline and given by intravenous infusion over 30 min). Maximal correction of the bleeding time is usually achieved in 30 min but may be delayed for up to 2 h. Laboratory measurement of FVIII Act preoperatively is essential. The response may be suboptimal with repeated doses. Adverse effects are uncommon but in view of the drug's antidiuretic effect, excessive fluid intake should be avoided and the blood pressure monitored. A single dose used in this fashion is suitable for covering dental extraction and some minor surgical procedures. However, for more major procedures, close laboratory monitoring, repeated doses and possibly supplementary replacement therapy will be necessary.

Again, it is imperative that good local haemostasis be effected surgically. In view of the nature of the defect, cautery or cryosurgical techniques seem attractive.

Inherited vascular and connective-tissue disorders

The hereditary conditions in which bleeding on account of a primarily vascular defect can occur are listed in Table 2.5. Hereditary haemorrhagic

Table 2.5 Inherited vascular and connective-tissue disorders associated with bleeding

Hereditary haemorrhagic telangiectasia (Osler–Weber–Rendu syndrome)
Ehlers–Danlos syndrome
Marfan's syndrome
Osteogenesis imperfecta
Pseudoxanthoma elasticum

telangiectasia is the commonest of these. This disorder is characterized by the presence of numerous thin-walled telangiectases in skin and mucous membranes which bleed easily, and is inherited in an autosomal dominant fashion. The lesions become more apparent, enlarge and bleed more readily as the patient becomes older and bleeding problems tend to become more troublesome from early adult life onwards. Epistaxes, gastrointestinal bleeding and iron-deficiency anaemia are common. Lesions can also be present in other organs such as lungs, brain, uterus, liver, etc. Larger arteriovenous malformations may arise and if present in the lung may cause a significant degree of right-to-left shunting. The typical mucocutaneous lesions (which characteristically blanch on pressure) are illustrated in Fig. 2.11.

Management of specific bleeding episodes can be difficult. Epistaxes are managed along conventional lines with packing and cautery as appropriate. Oestrogen therapy, which promotes squamous metaplasia, and septal dermatoplasty can be helpful in those with very frequent toublesome epistaxes, although results may be disappointing. Gastrointestinal bleeding is managed conservatively in the first instance with transfusion and H_2-receptor blockers. There is usually extensive involvement of the gastrointestinal tract with multiple lesions although

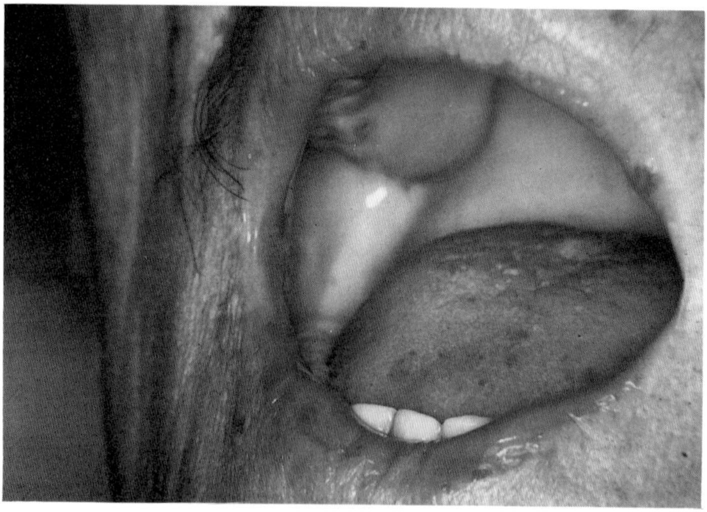

Fig. 2.11 Hereditary haemorrhagic telangiectasia of lips, tongue and face. These lesions may be found in any organ. The common presentations are recurrent epistaxis or chronic iron-deficient anaemia.

occasionally cautery, cryotherapy or even surgical resection can be helpful if an isolated bleeding site is identified. Great caution is necessary if endoscopy is to be performed in view of the ease with which lesions may bleed on contact.

Defective collagen structure in Ehlers–Danlos syndrome, Marfan's syndrome and osteogenesis imperfecta may lead to bleeding as a consequence of increased vascular fragility. Poor wound healing may also be a problem. Defective platelet function has been noted in some cases and should be excluded prior to surgery.

Inherited disorders of platelet function

A variety of inherited functional disorders of platelets have been described, the best known of which are listed in Table 2.6. Both disorders of the platelet membrane and its receptors and disorders of the secretory granules (storage pool disorders) are recognized. The possibility of such a disorder should be considered if a patient with a suggestive history has a prolonged bleeding time but normal coagulation screening tests (PT, APTT and fibrinogen). Glanzmann's disease [22] is probably the commonest of these rare disorders. In this condition platelets lack the glycoprotein IIb and glycoprotein IIIA membrane glycoproteins and show defective aggregation in response to the aggregating agents adenosine diphosphate (ADP), adrenaline and thrombin. The clinical pattern is variable although mucocutaneous bleeding, particularly from the nose and gastrointestinal tract, is common. Menorrhagia can be a problem

Table 2.6 Hereditary disorders of platelet function

Disorder	Comment
Membrane defects	
Glanzmann's syndrome (thrombasthenia)	See text
Bernard–Soulier syndrome	See text
Defects in secretory granules	
Grey platelet syndrome Chediak–Higashi	α-granule deficiency
Hermansky–Pudlak TAR (thrombocytopenia absent radii) Wiscott–Aldrich	δ-granule deficiencies all associated with a variety of other congenital disorders

but can be managed with hormonal therapy. Inexplicably, the patients seem to have fewer bleeding episodes as they grow older. Bernard–Soulier syndrome [23] is due to absence of the glycoprotein Ib membrane glycoprotein, the vWF receptor. This leads to defective platelet adhesion to exposed subendothelial collagen. Bleeding problems are similar to those seen in Glanzmann's disease. Although platelet transfusions will initially correct the bleeding defect in these patients, alloimmunization usually occurs fairly rapidly and patients subsequently become resistant to transfused platelets. Platelet transfusions should therefore be reserved for life-threatening bleeding episodes and ideally they should be as HLA (human leucocyte antigen) compatible as possible to limit HLA immunization.

References

1 Ingram, G.I.C. (1976) The history of haemophilia. *J. Clin. Pathol.*, **29**, 469–479.

2 Ljung, R., Petrini, P. and Nilsson, I.M. (1990) Diagnostic symptoms of severe and moderate haemophilia A and B. A survey of 140 cases. *Acta Paediatr. Scand.*, **79**(2), 196–200.

3 Preston, F.E., Triger, D.R., Underwood, J.C.E. *et al.* (1978) Percutaneous liver biopsy and chronic liver disease in haemophilia. *Lancet*, **ii**, 592–594.

4 Hay, C.R.M., Preston, F.E., Triger, D.R. *et al.* (1985) Progressive liver disease in haemophilia: an understated problem? *Lancet*, **i**, 1495–1498.

5 Underwood, J.C.E. (1990) Hepatitis C virus and transfusion transmitted liver disease: review. *J. Clin. Pathol.*, **43**, 445–447.

6 Madhok, R. and Forbes, C.D. (1990) HIV-1 infection in haemophilia. *Baillière's Clin. Haematol.*, **3**(1), 79–101.

7 Shirkoda, A., Mauro, M.A., Staab, E.V. *et al.* (1982) Soft tissue haemorrhage in hemophilic patients: computed tomography and ultrasound study. *Radiology*, **147**, 811–814.

8 Forbes, C.D., King, I., Prentice, C.R.M. *et al.* (1972) Serum enzyme changes after intramuscular bleeding in patients with haemophilia and Christmas disease. *J. Clin. Pathol.*, **25**, 1034–1037.

9 Gilbert, M.S. (1990) The hemophilic pseudotumour. *Prog. Clin. Biol. Res.*, **324**, 257–262.

10 Spuller, R.L. (1988) Use of the periodontal ligament injection in dental care of the patient with haemophilia—a clinical evaluation. *Spec. Care Dentist*, **8**(1), 28–29.

11 Walsh, P.N., Rizza, C.R., Matthews, J.M. *et al.* (1971) Epsilon-aminocaproic acid therapy for dental extraction in haemophilia and Christmas disease: a double blind controlled study. *Br. J. Haematol.*, **20**, 463–475.

12 Forbes, C.D., Barr, R.D., Reid, G. *et al.* (1972) Tranexamic acid in control of haemorrhage after dental extraction in haemophilia and Christmas disease. *Br. Med. J.*, **2**, 311–313.

13 Forbes, C.D., Barr, R.D., Prentice, C.R.M. *et al.* (1973) Gastrointestinal bleeding in haemophilia. *Quart. J. Med.*, **42**, 503–511.

14 Orangio, G.R. and Lucas, G.W. (1989) Management of hemophilia in colon and rectal surgery. *Dis. Colon Rectum*, **32**(10), 878–883.

15 Wiedel, J.D. (1990) Arthroscopy of the knee in haemophilia.. *Prog. Clin. Biol. Res.*, **324**, 231–239.

22 Caen, J.P. (1989) Glanzmann's thrombasthenia. *Baillière's Clin. Haematol.*, **2**(3), 609–625.

23 Berndt, M.C., Fournier, D.J. and Castaldi, P.A. (1989) Bernard–Soulier syndrome. *Baillière's Clin. Haematol.*, **2**(3), 585–607.

Chapter 3
Acquired bleeding disorders

J. ANDREW DAVIES AND PETER J. GRANT

The circumstances under which acquired abnormal bleeding occurs tend to be unexpected and often severe. Management can often be difficult because the patient is ill, with diminished capacity to maintain circulatory homeostasis and the bleeding disorder is poorly characterized. Appropriate laboratory techniques may not be available to monitor response to treatment, and measures to reverse the haemostatic defect may be unavailable or ineffective. This chapter aims to provide an overview of mechanisms of bleeding in the acquired haemostatic disorders, since lack of understanding compounds the other management problems. Here pathophysiology of bleeding disorders is related to the basic mechanisms of haemostasis (Table 3.1), linking it with the physiology covered in Chapter 1.

Table 3.1 Classification of the acquired bleeding disorders according to haemostatic function

Function affected	Condition leading to bleeding
Platelet adhesion	Uraemia, drugs
Platelet aggregation	Uraemia, liver disease, leukaemias, myelodysplastic syndromes, extracorporeal circulation, drugs
Platelet number	Malignancies, liver disease, idiopathic thrombocytopenic purpura, drugs, transfusion, disseminated intravascular coagulation
Blood coagulation	Liver disease, coumarin anticoagulants, malignancies, disseminated intravascular coagulation, massive transfusion
Coagulation inhibitors	Autoimmune diseases, lymphomas, heparin
Fibrinolysis	Drugs, disseminated intravascular coagulation

Platelet adhesion

Platelets contribute to haemostasis broadly in three ways. They stop bleeding in the injured microcirculation by adhering to non-endothelial surfaces, and then through cell–cell aggregation, a platelet-rich microthrombus is built up. With more severe injury coagulation is initiated, and platelets provide a crucial lipoprotein template on which coagulation proteins assemble, as well as interacting at a number of points in the coagulation cascade to accelerate thrombin generation. Platelets also affect fibrinolysis in poorly understood ways, for example by releasing an inhibitor of plasminogen activator, and possibly modulating the susceptibility of fibrin to lysis by variation in the extent of clot contraction. The majority of acquired bleeding disorders involve an element of impaired platelet function, though mechanisms may be poorly characterized.

Platelets adhere to any surface exposed to blood which is not covered by endothelium. At high shear rate, under conditions of arterial flow, this involves binding of plasma von Willebrand factor (vWF) to collagen and other matrix proteins of the vessel wall, which serves as a ligand by binding to the surface membrane glycoprotein 1b, on the platelet and joining it to the surface by a molecular bridge. In addition platelets can interact directly with collagen and other extracellular matrix proteins, which fulfil a similar function to that of vWF, and these mechanisms are probably more important at low shear rates.

The bleeding disorder of von Willebrand's disease (Chapter 2) illustrates the adverse effects on haemostasis when this process breaks down. Acquired forms of von Willebrand's disease have been described in association with collagen vascular diseases and with the lymphoproliferative disorders. These cases are characterized by a low plasma concentration of vWF and prolongation of the bleeding time. Unless (rarely) due to an inhibitor to vWF, they respond to treatment with cryoprecipitate, which restores the missing ligand.

Bleeding in renal disease is largely due to impaired platelet function, the favoured concept involving one or more dialysable plasma factors present in uraemic plasma which inhibit several steps in platelet activation. There is accumulating experimental evidence that platelet adhesion is specifically affected. Plasma concentration of vWF, and its multimeric structure, are both normal. However, transient improvement in bleeding and shortening of the bleeding time can be obtained by raising plasma vWF concentrations either by administration of cryoprecipitate, which contains vWF, or by infusion of deamino-D-arginine vasopressin (DDAVP) which raises the level of vWF by release from endothelial cells. Early studies showed rather inconsistent abnormalities in platelet adhesion to glass beads and in platelet agglutination to ristocetin (an *in vitro* test of the ability of platelets to interact with vWF). Recently it has been shown that platelet adhesion to subendothelium is impaired in uraemic plasma because of a functional defect in the interaction between vWF and the platelet surface receptor. It seems likely that this defect can be overcome by increasing the plasma concentration of vWF. An unexplained facet of the bleeding tendency of uraemia is its relation to haematocrit. The bleeding time correlates inversely with the haematocrit and a prolonged bleeding time can be shortened by transfusion of washed red cells. It is likely that this effect is mediated by the mechanical action of red cells on platelet adhesiveness, platelets depending on collision with red cells to bring them in contact with the vessel wall.

Defects in primary platelet adhesion probably do not play a significant part in other acquired bleeding disorders. However, adhesion is also inhibited by a number of drugs. At high plasma concentrations in the pharmacological range, adhesion is impaired by dipyridamole and PGI_2 (epoprostenol), though neither drug is associated with significant bleeding in clinical practice in patients with otherwise normal haemostasis. Antibiotics with a β-lactam ring can also interfere with platelet adhesion at the concentrations achieved in plasma in the treatment of fulminating infection, and may contribute to bleeding in some cancer patients and in syndromes of disseminated intravascular coagulation (DIC) associated with severe infection under treatment.

Platelet aggregation

Aggregation physiologically is initiated by adhesion but it also occurs following exposure to several soluble agonists, for example adenosine diphosphate (ADP). Following activation of one or more receptors on the platelet surface, the processes of the release reaction, and exposure of the glycoprotein complex IIb/IIIa on the platelet surface, prime the cell to bond to neighbouring platelets through fibrinogen bridges. The biochemistry of platelet aggregation involves at least three independent second messenger systems, which converge on a final pathway involving internal calcium mobilization, cytoskeletal contraction, and formation of the glycoprotein IIb/IIIa complex. It is not surprising that in such a complicated process defects can develop and impairment of platelet aggregation contributes to many acquired bleeding disorders.

In bleeding associated with renal failure, there are probably multiple defects in platelet function [1–3]. Studies of platelet aggregation *in vitro*, although not invariably consistent, have usually shown impaired aggregation in response to several agonists. Platelets from uraemic patients have reduced levels of serotonin and ADP in storage organelles, which further impairs function. Platelets in uraemic plasma have a reduced capacity to synthesize thromboxanes following platelet activation, and this inhibits platelet microthrombus formation. The defects in uraemia are almost fully reversed by dialysis, indicating that plasma factor(s) are responsible, but how these affect biochemical pathways in platelets is not understood.

Bleeding in liver disease is multifactorial, involving all aspects of the haemostatic mechanism [4,5]. Thrombocytopenia is often a prominent feature of advanced liver disease and a large part of the platelet component of the haemostatic defect is simply due to lack of platelets. However, plasma bilirubin levels, as well as the platelet count, correlate with prolonged bleeding times in patients with cirrhosis, indicating that other factors are affecting platelet function. Because of the heterogeneity of liver disease, and the frequency of associated renal impairment, it is impossible to establish a consistent pattern of abnormality, with some studies indicating impaired aggregation responses while in others, aggregation *in vitro* has been normal. Amongst factors proposed to account for diminished platelet function are the presence of fibrin(ogen) degradation products which inhibit platelet–platelet interactions, structurally abnormal fibrinogen which weakens the molecular bonds between aggregating platelets and, in some cirrhotics, the direct effects of alcohol [6] The mechanisms leading to thrombocytopenia are similarly poorly understood, but include adhesion on necrotic hepatocytes, involvement in consumption coagulopathy, and premature senescence due to the presence of increased surface-bound immunoglobulins [7].

Bleeding in cancer similarly involves multiple abnormalities in the haemostatic mechanism. The most striking abnormalities have been described in patients with haematological malignancy and particularly in the myeloproliferative disorders, amongst whom 15–20% have prolonged bleeding time. In these patients, platelet aggregation is usually abnormal to a range of agonists, a variety of abnormalities in surface membrane receptors has been described, and decreased numbers of dense granules, resulting in reduced platelet content of serotonin and ADP, are almost invariable. Platelets from patients with myelodysplasia also are liable to show impaired ability to synthesize thromboxanes. An apparent paradox in the myeloproliferative syndromes is the bleeding associated with very high platelet counts in patients with thrombocythaemia. The bleeding is thought to be due to functional defects, similar to those just described, resulting from abnormal platelet maturation, but for reasons which are not understood the bleeding tendency can often be diminished by lowering the platelet count, for example by plasmapheresis.

In some cancers, particularly lymphomas, production of abnormal immunoglobulins which bind to platelet surface receptors can induce a syndrome of immune thrombocytopenic purpura, in which the antibody-coated cells are removed by the monocyte–macrophage system at an accelerated rate. Thrombocytopenia can similarly occur in myeloma and macroglobulinaemia, in which, in addition, there can be non-specific inhibition of platelet function due to interference with agonist–receptor binding by the abnormal plasma proteins. Bleeding problems are more marked in myeloma patients with an excess of κ-light chains, though this has not been related to any functional abnormality. Platelet aggregation abnormalities are rarely found in association with solid tumours, though abnormalities due to actions of cytotoxic, or other drugs, are not uncommon. Bleeding related to thrombocytopenia tends to indicate advanced disease, usually, though not invariably, related to tumour invasion of the bone marrow.

Many drugs inhibit platelet function and some can cause thrombocytopenia. Drugs used therapeutically to inhibit platelet function do not produce a significant bleeding tendency in otherwise normal individuals. Aspirin, which inhibits platelet prostaglandin synthesis and thereby impairs aggregation, only slightly prolongs the bleeding time. Increased bleeding from the stomach is probably due to loss of mucosal resistance factors, rather than an action on platelets. There is a small excess risk of haemorrhagic stroke in individuals taking aspirin, the precise mechanism of which is unknown. Other non-steroidal anti-inflammatory drugs have similar actions to aspirin, and the newer inhibitors of thromboxanes are also likely to have a similar profile of bleeding complications. Ticlopidine results in a risk of bleeding equivalent to that with aspirin at therapeutic levels. Its mechanism of action is not fully understood but it probably interferes with receptor function. Unlike aspirin, as the dose is increased, bleeding time is progressively prolonged and a profound inhibition of platelet activation can be induced. Dipyridamole does not

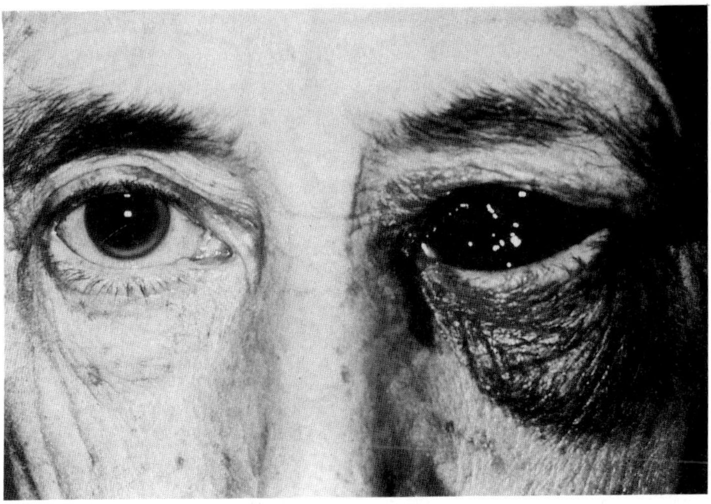

Fig. 3.1 Periorbital bleeding at presentation in a 65-year-old woman with acquired platelet storage pool disease.

create a bleeding tendency. β-Lactam antibiotics can inhibit aggregation as well as platelet adhesion, and may contribute to bleeding if used in very high doses.

Platelet storage pool disease (SPD) is a rare disorder due to absence of the dense storage granules in platelets. These contain adenine nucleotides, serotonin and other agonists, which are released by activated platelets and cause aggregation of surrounding platelets in the immediate environment. Bleeding in SPD is usually relatively mild but often patients have prominent purpura and surface bruising (Fig. 3.1). Most cases are congenital, but acquired SPD occurs in a range of conditions, for example, myelodysplastic syndromes, leukaemias and DIC amongst others. Occasionally SPD occurs without any other apparent disorder.

Platelet number

Idiopathic thrombocytopenic purpura (ITP) occurs in two forms, acute and chronic. Acute ITP is a disease of young children, usually self-limiting over 4–6 weeks. Platelet count falls suddenly following an infective illness, probably due to platelet damage caused by binding to the platelet surface of immune complexes formed in response to the infective agent. A minority of cases are severe and 1–2% of patients die, usually from intracranial haemorrhage.

Chronic ITP is probably an autoimmune disorder. Bleeding is usually mild, and often confined to intermittent purpura, but can be severe and occasionally fatal. It is likely that a range of disorders hides under the diagnostic label. Antibodies are usually of IgG class but can be detected in plasma only in a minority of patients, though there is disagreement about the reliability of methodology. Platelet-associated IgG is present on normal platelets but in considerably greater amounts on platelets of patients with ITP, though there is not a direct correlation with platelet count. Antibodies have been characterized directed to the surface glycoproteins 1b and IIIa, others are directed to unknown antigen(s). Damaged platelets acquire increased concentrations of surface-associated IgG, raising the possibility that in some cases the immune reaction is in response to abnormalities on the platelets, rather than the initiator of injury. Some patients presenting with apparent ITP later develop systemic lupus erythematosus. Examination of bone marrow in ITP patients reveals normal or increased numbers of megakaryocytes and platelet survival is decreased. Accordingly, the mechanism of thrombocytopenia has been ascribed to accelerated removal of IgG-coated platelets by splenic macrophages. However, recent studies [10] indicate that platelet production is abnormal, and that treatment with steroids works by restoring more normal platelet production, so that circulating platelets survive longer.

At the onset of cardiopulmonary bypass, there is an abrupt fall in platelet count [11], due to a combination of haemodilution, removal of platelets from the circulation following adherence to components of the bypass circuit, and aggregate formation by surface-activated platelets. The platelet count remains depressed during the period of bypass, but usually rapidly returns to normal afterwards. Bleeding time, however, is prolonged to a greater extent than can be explained by the low platelet count, indicating that the function of circulating platelets is impaired. Two main mechanisms seem to be involved. Platelets are constantly activated by the exposure of blood to the bypass circuit and air in the oxygenator, and they undergo the release reaction, becoming depleted of dense and α-granule constituents. These depleted platelets are less reactive than normal and this is reflected in impaired tests of platelet aggregation *in vitro*. Platelets also lose surface membrane components, and loss of glycoprotein membrane receptors may impair both adhesion and aggregation. Mechanisms are thought to include mechanical trauma to the platelet surface, and proteolytic cleavage by proteinase enzymes generated by activation of the fibrinolytic mechanism and released from activated white blood cells. Recent studies have shown striking reductions in perioperative blood loss following the administration of the proteinase inhibitor, aprotinin, during bypass surgery and this may operate in part by limiting proteolytic damage to platelets.

Drug-induced thrombocytopenia can occasionally result in a fatal bleeding disorder. Some, for example cytotoxic agents, depress platelet synthesis by inhibiting megakaryocyte production and maturation in the bone marrow. Others induce an immune response which leads to increased immunoglobulin on the platelet surface, and accelerated removal of antibody-coated cells. Quinidine is probably the classic drug causing thrombocytopenia by this mechanism. Heparin, particularly when administered for longer than 3–4 days, is an important cause of immune-mediated platelet destruction which can lead to profound thrombocytopenia, though bleeding is uncommon. This complication is rarely seen in the UK due to the infrequent use of prolonged heparin therapy.

Severe bleeding, largely due to quantitative and qualitative platelet dysfunction, occasionally occurs after massive transfusion. Stored blood does not contain functioning platelets, so after more than 10 units have been replaced, significant thrombocytopenia can develop through haemodilution. Repeated transfusion can occasionally produce immune thrombocytopenia due to antibody production to platelet surface antigens.

Platelet interactions with blood coagulation and fibrinolysis

Platelets have complex interactions with the coagulation cascade and the fibrinolytic system, the details of which are not fully understood, but it is likely that impairment of the interplay between different arms of the haemostatic mechanism will come to be recognized as a significant cause of bleeding. For example, the bleeding time is prolonged during heparin therapy, probably because of weakening of platelet microthrombi formed without fibrin support, though heparin also has several direct effects on platelets. In patients with myeloproliferative disease the bleeding can be of a type more appropriate to a coagulation disorder, probably due to lack of platelet procoagulant activity. Inhibition of platelet activity may make fibrin clots more susceptible to thrombolysis, probably due to loss of platelet contractile activity in compacting platelet–fibrin clots, and possibly to reduction in plasminogen activator inhibitor derived from platelets.

Blood coagulation

The coagulation cascade is designed to amplify and control part of the response of blood exposed to injured tissues. It functions in two phases: (i) the (relatively) slow generation of trace amounts of thrombin; and (ii) the explosive reaction which then occurs due to multiple positive feedback interactions between thrombin and various points in the coagulation mechanism. Coagulation is controlled by several inhibitory mechanisms which can localize thrombin generation and fibrin formation appropriately to a site of injury. A glance at any outline of the biochemical pathways involved reveals the potential for breakdown in such a complex system. In fact, these pathways were mostly delineated by tracing the causes of the single-factor congenital deficiencies discussed in Chapter 2. Acquired coagulation disorders are rarely so specific, and more commonly multiple deficiencies coexist, making it difficult to apportion their relative significance.

Probably the commonest cause of bleeding due to an acquired disorder of plasma coagulation factors is therapeutic administration of oral anticoagulant drugs. Warfarin and its congeners are competitive inhibitors of vitamin K (Fig. 3.2) and disrupt the metabolic cycle through which vitamin K provides essential cofactor activity for hepatic synthesis of the vitamin K-dependent coagulation factors [13]. The activity of Factors II, VII, IX and X depends on their ability to bind calcium and, through calcium-dependent molecular interactions, form complexes on lipid surfaces. In the absence of vitamin K there is failure of carboxylation in hepatocytes of glutamic acid residues in these coagulation factors, and functionally inactive proteins are released. The effect of warfarin is progressive, depending on the rate of turnover of the factors, and takes about 10 days to become stable at therapeutic doses. During stable anticoagulant control, Factors II and X are depressed more than Factors VII and IX. Spontaneous bleeding is almost confined to patients who are over-anticoagulated (International Normalized Ratio, INR, >4.5) but as this includes about 5% of patients undergoing outpatient anticoagulant therapy in the UK, there is a significant morbidity and mortality.

Acute and chronic liver diseases account for some of the most severe acquired bleeding disorders [4,5], for the simple reason that coagulation factors are synthesized in the liver. Though there are some minor points of difference between acute and chronic hepatitis and cirrhosis and their effects on coagulation, they are not of clinical significance. Failure of normal coagulation protein synthesis is seen most conspicuously in the

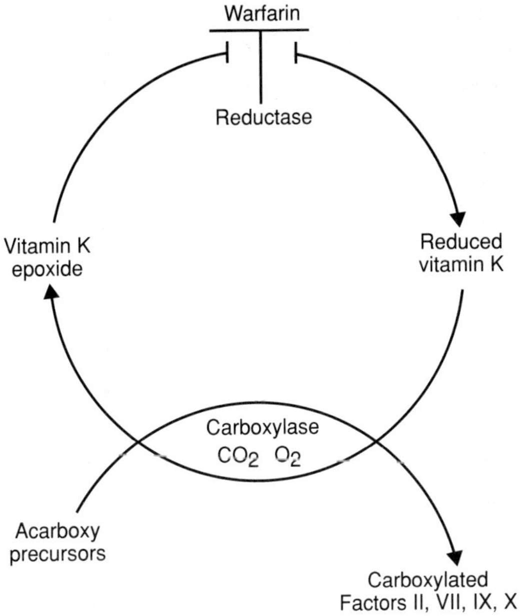

Fig. 3.2 Function is imparted to coagulation Factors II, VII, IX and X, which are produced in the liver by carboxylation of inactive acarboxy precursors. Carboxylation of glutamic acid residues enables the proteins to bind to cell surfaces in calcium-dependent reactions. Warfarin inhibits the recycling of reduced vitamin K, which is an essential cofactor for the carboxylase enzyme. It thereby indirectly inhibits synthesis of active proteins, though the inactive precursors can be detected immunologically in the circulation.

low plasma concentrations of Factors II, VII and X, three of the four vitamin K-dependent coagulation factors. The fourth, Factor IX, is usually not greatly reduced. The defect mainly involves a failure at some stage of primary protein synthesis. However, failure of posttranslational modifications also occurs with release into the circulation of functionally ineffective proteins, in which vitamin K-dependent carboxylation (which allows the proteins to bind to blood platelets for optimal efficiency) has not taken place [14]. These hypo- or acarboxylated forms are similar to the proteins produced in the presence of vitamin K antagonists such as warfarin. In patients with long-standing obstructive jaundice, failure of synthesis may be compounded by malabsorption of the fat-soluble vitamin K. In acute hepatitis plasma levels of Factor VII are the most sensitive harbinger of deteriorating function, as the half-life in plasma is only 6–7 h. A crude estimate of levels of coagulation Factors II, VII and X can be obtained by measuring prothrombin time and is adequate for clinical monitoring. Plasma concentrations of Factor V are usually also reduced, though the response is more variable. Because Factor V is an essential cofactor in thrombin generation, a low Factor V is likely to contribute significantly to any bleeding tendency. In contrast, Factor VIII, which has a very similar cofactor role in the generation of Factor Xa, is invariably markedly elevated in chronic liver failure, and often, though to a lesser degree, in acute disease. Factor VIII is synthesized mainly in the liver, though possibly to a small extent elsewhere, and why there should be this paradoxical response is not understood. Theories include reduced hepatic clearance from plasma of Factor VIII linked to its carrier protein, vWF, and increased synthesis or release in response to cytokines as part of the 'acute phase' reaction. How far the rise in Factor VIII might reverse the haemostatic effects of the fall in other coagulation factors is not clear. Plasma levels of coagulation Factors XI, XII and XIII tend to be reduced, though usually to a lesser extent than the vitamin K-dependent factors, particularly in chronic liver disease. Occasionally, fulminant hepatic failure will generate acute DIC, with consumption of coagulation and other plasma proteins, leading to very low levels of all the clotting factors. DIC is discussed in more detail later.

Plasma concentrations of fibrinogen are usually lower than normal due to the widespread impairment of protein synthesis, but rarely below the level needed for adequate haemostasis. Levels are significantly lower in most patients with acute hepatic failure, often below 1 g/l. Failure of fibrinogen synthesis due to destruction of hepatocytes is compensated, to a degree, in chronic liver disease by an acute-phase response affecting functioning hepatic cells which increases fibrinogen synthesis. Abnormal fibrinogens with an excess of sialic acid have been described, which are slow to polymerize following cleavage by thrombin or which result in structurally weakened fibrin. Profound hypofibrinogenaemia indicates development of DIC and accelerated consumption in intravascular thrombi.

Other acquired bleeding disorders can affect the coagulation mechanism through loss of coagulation factors by abnormal excretion, consumption in intravascular coagulation, or haemodilution induced by transfusion. Unless the liver is involved, synthesis is not impaired.

Patients with cancer can develop a marked bleeding tendency with a pattern, such as combined purpura and bruising, which suggests haemostasis is inhibited at several points [8]. As discussed earlier, impaired platelet function is likely to be the most significant factor, and major disturbances of coagulation are uncommon. Prolonged obstruction of the common bile duct by tumour leads to fat malabsorption and reduction in concentrations of the vitamin K-dependent coagulation Factors II, VII, IX and X, but is now rarely seen since the obstruction is usually promptly relieved. Secondary malignancy in the liver is a very rare cause of coagulation abnormality as sufficient hepatocytes remain for normal protein synthesis. Tumours, and cytokines associated with the inflammatory response, may release tissue factor into the circulation, activating the coagulation cascade and leading to DIC and consumption of coagulant proteins. In myeloma and the dysproteinaemias, the abnormal immunoglobulins, in addition to coating platelets, can interfere with fibrin polymerization resulting in delayed haemostasis, and an abnormally fragile coagulum leading to delayed bleeding at sites of injury. In systemic amyloidosis (sometimes associated with myeloma) specific reduction in plasma concentrations of Factor X may occur, it is thought because of binding to amyloid protein and accelerated clearance from the circulation.

Haemorrhagic disease of the newborn was recognized in the 19th century long before its basis was understood. The most important aetiological factors are immaturity of the infant liver and vitamin K deficiency. Plasma concentrations of the vitamin K-dependent coagulation Factors (II, VII, IX and X) range from 30 to 60% of adult levels in the normal newborn. This seems to be due largely to lack of primary synthesis which can take months to develop fully. Vitamin K deficiency is likely to exacerbate inadequate synthesis, since bleeding problems are extremely uncommon in infants given prophylactic vitamin K and tend to occur in the first 48 h after delivery when vitamin K intake is low. However, acarboxylated forms of the coagulation proteins, which indicate lack of vitamin K, have not been clearly demonstrated in the plasma of infants with haemorrhagic disease, and the precise mechanisms giving rise to the condition are not fully established.

Apart from the DIC syndromes discussed later, haemodilution is the other main mechanism which may affect coagulation tests, though it rarely leads to spontaneous bleeding. This is perhaps best illustrated by the fall in concentrations of coagulation factors during cardiopulmonary bypass, when haematocrit is reduced to 25–30% by transfusion, largely of plasma substitutes. In otherwise healthy patients, this rapidly reverses postoperatively and most serious bleeding problems during and after bypass are more probably related to surgical factors, thrombocytopenia, or difficulties with control of heparin therapy. Low levels of fibrinogen are partly due to fibrinogen deposition on the circuitry, and partly to a low-grade activation of coagulation which accompanies bypass surgery in spite of heparin treatment. In occasional patients, usually either very young, very old or very sick, there may be significant and more sustained falls in concentrations of Factors V and VIII through mechanisms which are unclear.

Similarly, reduction in coagulation Factors V and VIII can occur in patients who have been given massive blood transfusions exceeding 20 units. Stored blood has abnormally low levels of Factor VIII and to a lesser extent Factor V, but mechanisms other than simple haemodilution may be involved.

The bleeding of uraemia, as previously discussed, is due to defective activity of blood platelets. However, in a few patients levels of Factors V, VII, X and XIII have been found to be reduced, probably largely due to associated liver disease. In patients with nephrotic syndrome, concentrations of Factors XI and XII are lower than normal, probably because of activation of the kallikrein–kinin system, leading to consumption of the two contact-activated coagulation proteins. The changes do not significantly affect coagulation. In a few patients, plasma levels of Factor IX are low due to abnormal urinary loss in association with heavy proteinuria. Bleeding does not occur, perhaps partly because of concomitant loss of the anticoagulant protease inhibitor, antithrombin III.

Inhibitors of blood coagulation

Physiological inhibitors in the coagulation cascade retard coagulation, and reduced levels, whether acquired or inherited, consequently promote thrombosis rather than bleeding. The potential for bleeding induced by abnormal inhibition of coagulation is illustrated by the disorder α_1-antitrypsin Pittsburgh, in which a single amino acid substitution of arginine for methionine at position 358 altered the specificity of the plasma inhibitor from pancreatic elastase to thrombin. As a result of this potent circulating anticoagulant activity the patient had a serious life-long bleeding tendency and died aged 14 years. Similar cases, and other acquired antithrombins, have now been recorded.

Acquired inhibitors of coagulation Factor VIII are the most significant cause of bleeding disorders due to inhibition of the coagulation cascade, apart from anticoagulant drugs [12]. The pathogenesis is most easily understood in patients with haemophilia A, 5–15% of whom have circulating antibodies directed at a variety of epitopes on the Factor VIII molecule. Inhibitors are more likely to develop in severe haemophiliacs, probably because their immune systems more readily detect transfused Factor VIII molecules as foreign, whereas mild haemophiliacs may have sufficient circulating Factor VIII or a molecule with only minor structural change so that Factor VIII replacement does not elicit an antibody response. The pattern of antibody production is variable, though it usually develops in young patients soon after replacement therapy is started, and antibody titres to Factor VIII rise after Factor VIII infusions. Haemophiliacs with high levels of inhibitors to Factor VIII, particularly those which persist and do not fall away after treatment, present a difficult management problem.

IgG antibodies to Factor VIII develop spontaneously in some diseases in which other immunological manifestations occur, for example rheumatoid arthritis, systemic lupus erythematosus (SLE) and erythema multiforme. Although they prolong laboratory tests of intrinsic pathway coagulation, they do not usually result in a serious bleeding tendency. Why inhibitors should appear to Factor VIII and only very exceptionally to other coagulation proteins is unknown. Inhibitors to Factor VIII can also occur as a rare complication of pregnancy, typically developing 2–3 months after delivery and tending to disappear after 2 years. Some patients have died of uncontrollable haemorrhage, though in the majority the bleeding tendency has not been severe. The mechanism is unknown and in the few cases who have gone on to subsequent pregnancy, the antibody does not recur.

Acquired inhibitors, similar to the Factor VIII inhibitors which can occur in haemophilia A, have been described in patients with von Willebrand's disease (against vWF), with haemophilia B (against Factor IX) and with Factor XIII deficiency.

The lupus anticoagulant was first described in patients with SLE but about 50% of cases do not have SLE or other overt immune disease. The term describes a group of antibodies which are directed against phospholipids, and as a result, prolong laboratory tests of coagulation which are dependent on added phospholipid. The pattern of inhibitory activity is variable, but the kaolin clotting time is usually the most sensitive to the inhibitory activity. In spite of the action on coagulation *in vitro* the antibodies are not associated with a bleeding tendency, but paradoxically with thrombosis (as well as recurrent abortion). There are several aetiological theories to account for the clinical complications.

In clinical practice, bleeding due to inhibition of coagulation is most often due to heparin therapy. Heparin forms a complex in plasma with the physiological inhibitor antithrombin III, which normally inhibits activated coagulation Factors XII, XI, IX, X and thrombin (Factor II). In its complex with heparin, the rate at which antithrombin III inhibits coagulation reactions is variably accelerated between several hundredfold and several thousandfold. Accelerated inhibition of the activities of Factor X and thrombin is most important in clinical practice. Bleeding during heparin therapy is partly dose dependent but can occur spontaneously, even in patients well controlled in the target range of 1.5–2-fold control using laboratory tests of intrinsic coagulation time (activated partial thromboplastin time or kaolin cephalin clotting time). This is probably because heparin also affects blood platelets directly, and binds to endothelium where its activity will not be measurable in blood.

Low-molecular-weight and semisynthetic heparins are being introduced into clinical practice. Their precise effects depend on the molecular formulation, rendering them either more or less like unmodified heparin. In use their actions are likely to prove very similar to those of heparin and claims that they have greater antithrombotic activity with lower risk of bleeding have not yet been verified.

Direct inhibitors of thrombin are likely to be introduced shortly into therapeutics. Hirudin, the anticoagulant from leeches, can now be synthesized by recombinant technology, alleviating problems of supply. Because it inhibits thrombin specifically its activity is predictable, with a linear dose–response on coagulation times suggesting it might be more potent and safer in use than heparin.

Disseminated intravascular coagulation

Bleeding in DIC is less common than thrombosis. DIC is a complex disorder of haemostasis, also known by the terms consumptive coagulopathy or defibrination syndrome. It is usually secondary to one of a variety of systemic disorders including sepsis, obstetric complications and malignancy. Although the changes in platelet function, coagulation factors and fibrinolysis that occur have been well described, the precise aetiology of DIC is still not fully understood. In clinical practice, the development of DIC is commonly observed as a haematological diagnosis with no evidence of either systemic thrombosis or haemorrhage. While thrombosis is a more common manifestation of chronic DIC, for example associated with underlying cancer, bleeding is more likely to occur in acute conditions. This is perhaps most vividly illustrated by obstetric accidents in which torrential haemorrhage results from the consumption of blood platelets, coagulation factors and fibrinogen in microvascular thrombi, and from activation of the fibrinolytic system which degrades the few fibrin fragments which can still be generated.

Pathophysiology

For many years it was unclear whether the precipitating factor in DIC was activation of coagulation, with secondary fibrinolysis, or primary fibrinolysis followed by reactive changes in coagulation. It is now accepted that the primary event in DIC is the generation of excess thrombin which leads to clot formation, hypofibrinogenaemia, platelet aggregation and activation of coagulation and fibrinolysis [16,17]. Two principal mechanisms have been invoked to explain the initiation of this sequence of events. The presence in the circulation of endotoxins, viruses or antigen–antibody complexes damages endothelial cells and can lead to activation of Factor XII by the exposure of subendothelial collagen. This can initiate activity in the intrinsic coagulation pathway and the extrinsic fibrinolytic pathway. Endotoxins are lipopolysaccharide molecules produced by bacteria and released into the circulation during septicaemia. In experimental animals, two injections of endotoxin produce renal cortical necrosis and widespread fibrin deposition [17]. This response, seen in rabbits, is known as the Schwartzmann phenomenon. Evidence that other factors may play a role comes from the observations that only a single injection of endotoxin is required in pregnant animals, if fibrinolysis is inhibited, or if excess corticosteroids or adrenaline are present. Endotoxins have a number of pathological effects that tend to magnify the changes in haemostasis promoting fibrin deposition (Fig. 3.3). These include endothelial cell damage with release of tissue factor and other procoagulant molecules and activation of circulating monocytes with release of vasoactive cytokines such as interleukin-1 (IL-1) and tumour necrosis factor (TNF). *In vitro*, the presence of endotoxin has been shown to induce endothelial cell death in certain cell lines, indicating that endotoxin has direct effects. Alternatively, granulocytes exposed to endotoxin adhere to, and damage, endothelial cells, a process that is enhanced in the presence of complement and low-density lipoprotein. Endotoxin applied to endothelial cells causes a marked increase in tissue thromboplastin release, which would provide an immediate mechanism for cell-surface mediated activation of the extrinsic coagulation cascade. TNF and IL-1 have important effects on the cellular and fluid components of reactions accompanying DIC. Both cytokines are

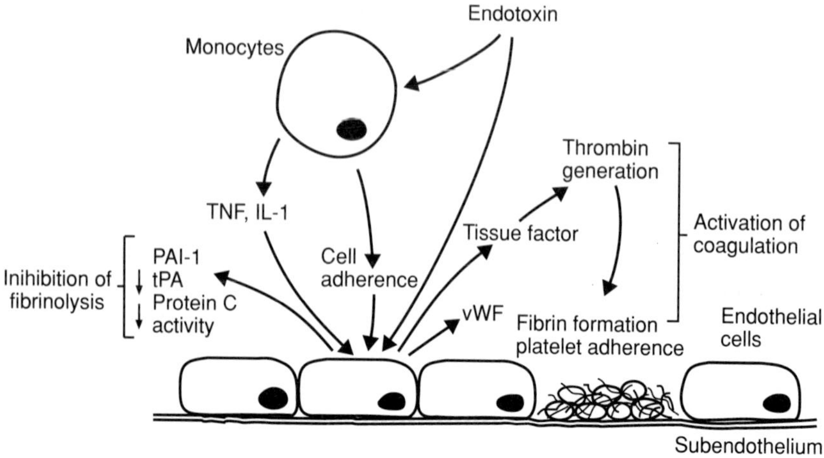

Fig. 3.3 Endotoxin triggers activation of coagulation and fibrinolysis in the pathogenesis of DIC. It can act directly on endothelial cells, and indirectly through stimulation of monocytes and release of cytokines.

released from monocytes following exposure to endotoxin. IL-1 promotes proliferation of activated T-lymphocytes and the adherence of lymphocytes to endothelial cells, and TNF enhances the binding of neutrophils to endothelium. Several studies have demonstrated that both TNF and IL-1 cause the expression of tissue factor activity on endothelial cells [18–20]. IL-1 decreases thrombin-mediated protein C activity and increases secretion of vWF. TNF and IL-1 cause depression of fibrinolysis *in vitro* by inducing transcription of the inhibitor, plasminogen activator inhibitor-1, whilst suppressing tissue plasminogen activator synthesis [21]. In man, infusion of TNF has produced increased levels of coagulation Factor xa, fibrinopeptide A and prothrombin fragments with no change in the intrinsic pathway. These results indicate that TNF activates the extrinsic pathway, probably through its effects on tissue factor expression. In some cancer patients the use of TNF has been associated with a fall in the platelet count, although this was not confirmed in infusion studies in healthy individuals. The pivotal role that TNF may have in the pathogenesis of DIC has been indicated by observations in animal models. Inoculation of animals with TNF antibodies prior to the introduction of experimental septicaemia greatly reduces the features of septic shock and mortality. Alternatively, it has been proposed that tissue damage may lead to the release of tissue factor and systemic activation of the extrinsic coagulation pathway. The continued stimulation of either pathway would lead to excess thrombin formation and the associated changes in haemostasis.

Coagulation factors

The activation of coagulation that occurs in relation to DIC is characterized by dramatic reductions in the circulating concentrations of most factors, with extensive microvascular fibrin deposition. Thrombin is initially generated in excess from its precursor, prothrombin, leading to an eventual deficiency of the latter. The production of a huge excess of thrombin leads to the conversion of fibrinogen to soluble fibrin, with lowering of fibrinogen levels and the release of two byproducts of this conversion, fibrinopeptides A and B, which are cleaved from the fibrinogen molecule. Thrombin also activates Factor XIII which functions to crosslink fibrin to form the basis of an established thrombus. The major serine protease inhibitor, antithrombin III, is also consumed in the presence of thrombin. In addition, free thrombin activates Factors VIIIC and V and there is commonly an initial increase in concentrations followed by a rapid fall as the coagulation cascade freewheels towards thrombin generation and fibrin formation. The fall in concentration of prothrombin is accompanied by a general decrease in the other vitamin K-dependent clotting Factors (VII, IX, X). vWF is reported to be increased in DIC, but this may be a non-specific change unrelated to the clinical course of the condition. Finally, increased circulating concentrations of the glycoprotein, fibronectin, have been described in association with DIC. Fibronectin can be incorporated in large molecular-weight aggregates and is thought to play an important role in wound healing and the control of inflammation. In the presence of activated Factor XIII, fibronectin binds to various macromolecules, including fibrin, and at high concentrations may interfere with fibrin structure.

The presumed key role of thrombin in the pathogenesis of DIC has encouraged the therapeutic use of anticoagulants, with the aim of disconnecting the cycle of thrombin generation and consumption of components of the haemostatic mechanism. Early studies with heparin were inconclusive, largely because of the very small numbers of patients studied. As heparin acts by accelerating inhibition of thrombin and other activated clotting factors by antithrombin III this approach was always suspect because of the low levels of antithrombin III in DIC. Low-molecular-weight heparins possess greater anti-Factor Xa activity and are reported to have a low incidence of bleeding compared with unmodified heparin. Other therapies which have been used in DIC include antithrombin III infusions and the use of the serine protease inhibitor gabexate mesilate. These can be relatively safe when haemorrhage, thrombocytopenia and antithrombin III deficiency coexist and emphasize the importance of activation of coagulation in the pathogenesis of DIC.

Fibrinolysis

The fibrinolytic pathway is a complex enzyme cascade that regulates the conversion of plasminogen to plasmin. When activated, the fibrinolytic system breaks down available fibrin and is thought to play an important role in maintaining vascular patency under normal conditions. DIC is associated with massive activation of fibrinolysis, as evidenced by the occurrence of high levels of fibrin breakdown products in plasma and urine. Most commonly plasminogen activator (PA) derived from endothelial cells, tissue type PA (tPA), is increased, although there are reports of increases in urokinase (uPA) in DIC associated with amyloidosis. *In vitro*, the increase in fibrinolytic activity can be demonstrated using the euglobulin clot lysis time, which is markedly shortened in patients with DIC. The production of excess tPA or uPA leads to the generation of the proteolytic enzyme plasmin from its precursor plasminogen. Levels of plasminogen in the circulation fall as this process continues and the production of free plasmin in the circulation can be inferred from an increase in circulating fibrinopeptide $B\beta_{15-42}$. DIC is one of the few conditions in which this occurs, as the presence of the plasmin inhibitor α_2-antiplasmin normally prevents the generation of significant quantities of free plasmin in the circulation. The increase in circulating plasmin in DIC leads to a fall in α_2-antiplasmin levels and measurement may be a relatively sensitive indicator of the extent of DIC and of the risk of haemorrhage. Unfortunately, the therapeutic use of fibrinolytic inhibitors, whilst reducing the bleeding tendency in such patients, has been associated with catastrophic organ failure, presumably because of an unopposed drive towards fibrin deposition.

The final result of the increased fibrinolytic activity seen in DIC is twofold. There is a generalized breakdown of both soluble and cross-linked fibrin to produce a wide variety of split products that are measurable in plasma and urine. In addition, because of similarities between fibrin and fibrinogen, fibrinogenolysis occurs, further reducing fibrinogen concentrations and increasing haemorrhagic risk.

Platelet function

Activation of platelets with associated thrombocytopenia is a common manifestation of DIC. Platelet aggregation probably occurs due to direct action of thrombin, and these platelets are either deposited in the fibrin meshwork produced by the activated coagulation cascade or they are scavenged by the reticuloendothelial system. Platelet release factors such as β-thromboglobulin and platelet factor 4 are often released into the circulation and high levels in plasma are taken as indicators of platelet activation. Thrombocytopenia in DIC is due to the consumption of platelets at a faster rate than the bone marrow can immediately replace.

Diagnosis

Clinically the diagnosis of DIC rests on producing evidence of ongoing coagulation and systemic fibrinolysis. Often, in a patient with systemic disease the first observation made will be the presence of thrombocytopenia, without clinical evidence of thrombosis or haemorrhage. The most useful tests to confirm the diagnosis under these circumstances are plasma fibrinogen levels, which will be low, the activated partial thromboplastin time, which is prolonged due to consumption of clotting factors, and plasma or urinary fibrinogen degradation products (FDPs), which are increased due to the systemic breakdown of fibrin and fibrinogen.

Fibrinolysis

Acquired bleeding disorders due to inappropriate activation of fibrinolysis do not occur other than as part of DIC syndromes or as a result of therapeutic administration of fibrinolytic drugs.

Streptokinase was discovered more than 50 years ago, but fibrinolytic therapy has been used relatively little until the last 10 years. Streptokinase activates plasminogen indirectly through an activator complex formed by streptokinase with plasminogen. Partly as a result, biological activity is unpredictable and streptokinase therapy is difficult to control. In the physiological activation of fibrinolysis, reactants are bound to fibrin in the clot as it develops, and activation of free plasmin in the circulation does not occur (other than in some DIC syndromes). This precision cannot be reproduced when a plasminogen activator is given therapeutically. Large doses need to be administered to overcome inhibitors in plasma and this can lead to proteolytic digestion of coagulation factor proteins and fibrinogen. Some of the degradation products of fibrin and fibrinogen can interfere with platelet function, inhibit thrombin, and disturb fibrin polymerization, adding to the bleeding risk. Finally, fibrinolytic agents obviously cannot be selective for a specific thrombus, and degrade all fibrin plugs equally, one of which may happen to be sealing a previously unsuspected lesion elsewhere. Accordingly, bleeding complicating thrombolytic therapy can be dramatic, difficult to treat, and fatal.

The advent of tPA, the natural activator, into therapeutics through genetic engineering, encouraged the prospect of enhanced 'natural' fibrinolysis, since tPA binds strongly to fibrin and unlike streptokinase, is much more active when fibrin-bound. In practice the theoretical benefits of tPA have been largely unrealized, and bleeding is still a hazard of treatment.

Conclusion

Acquired bleeding disorders by their very nature are heterogenous and resist neat classification, as Table 3.1 confirms. Many of the conditions described have a complex pathogenesis in which several elements of haemostasis are disturbed. Understanding has gradually improved in response to the clinical application of improved laboratory assay techniques, but the basis of the bleeding tendency in several relatively common disorders is not yet fully characterized.

References

1 Remuzzi, G. (1988) Bleeding in renal failure. *Lancet*, **i**, 1205–1208.

2 George, J.N. and Shatil, S.J. (1991) The clinical importance of acquired abnormalities of platelet function. *New Engl. J. Med.*, **324**, 27–39.

3 Harker, L.A. (1987) Acquired disorders of platelet function. *Ann. NY Acad. Sci.*, **509**, 188–204.

4 Boks, A.L., Brommer, E.J.P., Schalm, S.W. and Van Vliet, H.H.D.M. (1986) Hemostasis and fibrinolysis in severe liver failure and their relation to haemorrhage. *Hepatology*, **6**, 79–86.

5 Hughes, R.D., Lane, D.A., Ireland, H. *et al.* (1985) Fibrinogen derivatives and platelet activation products in acute and chronic liver disease. *Clin. Sci.*, **68**, 701–707.

6 Mikhailidis, D.P., Jenkins, W.J., Barradas, M.A. *et al.* (1986) Platelet function defects in chronic alcoholism. *Br. Med. J.*, **293**, 715–718.

7 Barrison, I.G., Knight, I.D., Viola, L. *et al.* (1981) Platelet associated immunoglobulins in chronic liver disease. *Br. J. Haematol.*, **48**, 347–350.

8 Ey, F.S. and Goodnight, S.H. (1990) Bleeding disorders in cancer. *Semin. Oncol.*, **17**, 187–197.

9 McMillan, R. (1981) Chronic idiopathic thrombocytopenic purpura. *New Engl. J. Med.*, **304**, 1135–1147.

10 Gernsheimer, T., Stratton, J., Ballem, P.J. and Slichter, S.J. (1989) Mechanisms of response to treatment in autoimmune thrombocytopenic purpura. *New Engl. J. Med.*, **320**, 974–980.

11 Holloway, D.S., Summaria, L., Sandesara, J. *et al.* (1988) Decreased platelet number and function and increased fibrinolysis contribute to postoperative bleeding in cardiopulmonary bypass patients. *Thromb. Haemost.*, **59**, 62–67.

12 Prentice, C.R.M. (1985) Acquired coagulation disorders. *Clin. Haematol.*, **14**, 413–442.

13 Bovill, E.G., Malhotra, O.P. and Mann, K.G. (1990) Mechanisms of vitamin K antagonism. *Baillière's Clin. Haematol.*, **3**, 555–581.

14 Blanchard, R.A., Furie, B.C., Jorgensen, M. *et al.* (1981) Acquired vitamin K dependent carboxylation deficiency in liver disease. *New Engl. J. Med.*, **305**, 242–248.

15 Jackson, C.M. (1990) Mechanisms of heparin action. *Baillière's Clin. Haematol.*, **3**, 483–504.

16 Lasch, H.G. and Oehler, G. Disseminated intravascular coagulation. In: *The Thromboembolic Disorders* (Eds van de Loo, J., Prentice, C.R.M. & Beller, F.K.), pp. 413–434. F.K. Schattauer Verlag, Stuttgart, New York (1983).

17 Bick, R.L. (1978) Disseminated intravascular coagulation and related syndromes: Etiology, pathophysiology, diagnosis and management. *Am. J. Hematol.*, **5**, 265–282.

18 Van der Poll, T., Buller, H.R. *et al.* (1990) Activation of coagulation after administration of tumour necrosis factor to normal subjects. *New Engl. J. Med.*, **322**, 1622–1627.

19 Bevilacqua, M.P., Pober, J.S., Majeau, G.R. *et al.* (1986) Recombinant tumour necrosis factor induces procoagulant activity in cultured human vascular endothelium: characterization and comparison with the actions of interleukin-1. *Proc. Natl. Acad. Sci. USA*, **83**, 4533–4537.

20 Tracey, K.J., Vlassara, H. and Cerami, A. (1989) Cachectin/tumour necrosis factor. *Lancet*, **i**, 1122–1125.

21 Schleef, R., Bevilacqua, R., Sawdey, M.P. *et al.* (1988) Cytokine activation of vascular endothelium. Effects on tissue-type plasminogen activator and type-1 plasminogen activator inhibitor. *J. Biol. Chem.*, **263**, 5797–5803.

22 Marder, V.J. and Sherry, S. (1988) Thrombolytic therapy: current status. *New Engl. J. Med.*, **318**, 1512–1520 and 1585–1595.

Chapter 4
Laboratory diagnosis of excess bleeding

MIN HONG SAW AND MICHAEL J. MACKIE

There are three situations in which a surgeon is interested in a haemostatic assessment of the patient.

1 The preoperative assessment of the likelihood of bleeding.

2 The management of a patient with a known bleeding disorder.

3 The evaluation and management of any patient bleeding postoperatively.

Most of this chapter will deal with the laboratory diagnosis of the patient bleeding postoperatively. The management of patients with a known bleeding disorder will be discussed in more detail in other chapters. There will be a discussion concerning preoperative haemostatic assessment.

Bleeding occurring in surgical patients carries an obvious urgency that requires rapid clinical assessment, choice of appropriate tests and close laboratory liaison. When bleeding occurs it is important to distinguish a systemic haemostatic defect from a bleed due to a local surgical cause. This may not be easy, in some cases, but when a patient has bruising or petechiae in addition to a local site of bleeding then a problem in the haemostatic mechanism rather than a surgical cause is more likely.

It is important to stress the relevance of a good history which will not only dictate which laboratory tests should be requested but also help to explain any abnormality found in the results. In the history the following points are important:

1 Previous history of significant bleeding—particularly spontaneous episodes and those associated with a need for blood transfusion.

2 A positive family history.

3 Drug history.

4 Information about underlying medical illnesses, particularly renal or liver disease.

Physical examination has a number of objectives in the bleeding patient. Quite apart from assessing that the patient is not hypoperfused due to the bleed, it is important to determine whether there is any evidence of more widespread bleeding, pointing to a systemic haemostatic defect. Signs on examination may help to identify an underlying cause. On initial inspection physical signs of abnormal bleeding are sought. Petechiae are small capillary haemorrhages. They are characteristic of platelet or vascular disorders and are more commonly found on the lower legs. Ecchymoses are larger areas of bruising and deep and spreading lesions are more characteristic of a coagulation disorder. Bleeding from previously intact venepuncture and line sites suggest the presence of disseminated intravascular coagulation (DIC). The other sites where abnormal bleeding may be found are the mouth and the fundi; in these situations haemorrhage is often due to thrombocytopenia. The presence of bruising and petechiae in addition to other manifestations such as epistaxis and haematuria make the possibility of abnormal haemostasis more likely.

Further examination should help delineate any underlying disease known to be associated with abnormal haemostasis. Liver and renal disease are common and have well-known associated physical signs. Evidence of diseases which can cause DIC should be sought. It is important to search for signs of systemic infection, or the patient may be known to have malignant disease. The presence of lymphadenopathy and hepatosplenomegaly point to lymphoma or leukaemia, but it is likely that these conditions would have been diagnosed preoperatively. Rare diseases associated with vascular disorders may have particular features, for instance hyperextensibility of the joints in Ehlers–Danlos syndrome.

When investigating a bleeding surgical patient screening tests are initially performed and depending on the results more specific assays requested. These tests can be divided into those that assess primary haemostasis and those that measure secondary haemostasis. The former process is mainly dependent on the platelets while the latter involves mainly clotting factors. Primary defects of fibrinolysis causing bleeding are rare but secondary activation of the fibrinolytic mechanism will be considered, particularly in the context of DIC. The following screening tests form the basis of the initial laboratory assessment:

1 Full blood count, which must include a platelet count.
2 The prothrombin time (PT).
3 The activated partial thromboplastin time (APTT).

These tests will be considered in the context of primary and secondary haemostasis.

Defects in primary haemostasis

The bleeding problem arising from defects in primary haemostasis is due mainly to either abnormalities in the platelet or the vascular endothelium, and in some cases both. This is characterized by signs of spontaneous mucous membrane and skin petechial type haemorrhage.

In a bleeding patient the platelet count can in fact be high, low or normal. While thrombocytosis is often secondary to bleeding itself or to some other underlying reactive cause, the possibility of a myeloproliferative disorder must be considered.

It may be difficult to diagnose essential thrombocythaemia in the immediate postoperative period. However, if other causes of a reactive thrombocytosis are not present and the patient has a palpable spleen, large platelets on the film, and a count which is in excess of $1000 \times 10^9/l$, then the diagnosis should be seriously considered. However, the most common numerical abnormality of platelets is thrombocytopenia.

Thrombocytopenia

Spontaneous bleeding is uncommon when the platelet count is above $50 \times 10^9/l$, provided the platelets are functioning normally. Serious spontaneous bleeding is usually seen when the platelet count falls to below $10\text{–}20 \times 10^9/l$. However, it is important to appreciate that erroneously low platelet counts may be found for the following reasons:

1 The presence of platelet clumps. This may be due to:

(a) Difficult venesection resulting in activation of clotting in the syringe.

(b) Poor mixing/loss of anticoagulant.

(c) The presence of an ethylenediaminetetra-acetic acid (EDTA)-dependent antibody.

2 The presence of unusually large platelets can give erroneous platelet counts.

Thus in patients with unexpected thrombocytopenia the sample tube should always be checked for the presence of small clots. The problem of an EDTA-dependent antibody can be circumvented by using another anticoagulant such as heparin. Alternatively, the blood can be taken using the finger-prick technique directly into platelet diluent, so that a manual platelet count can be performed. Many of the above problems can be diagnosed from inspection of the blood film. A list of abnormalities of cell morphology which may be found on the blood film

Table 4.1 Morphology of platelets, red cells and white cells

Platelet morphology
(a) An increase in the size of the platelet is seen in:
- increased platelet destruction (e.g. immune thrombocytopenia)
- myeloproliferative disease
- Bernard–Soulier syndrome

(b) Agranular platelets are found in grey platelet syndrome

Red-cell morphology
(a) The presence of red-cell fragments (schistocytes) may indicate microangiopathic haemolytic anaemia or thrombotic thrombocytopenic purpura. Fragments are also found in DIC
(b) Macrocytosis and target cells are suggestive of liver dysfunction
(c) Burr cells are found in uraemia
(d) Red-cell dysplasia suggests a possible primary marrow problem

White-cell morphology
(a) The presence of immature lymphoid or myeloid precursors would suggest malignancy of the haemopoietic cells
(b) Dysplasia involving the neutrophils may indicate a primary marrow disorder

and give a clue to the underlying disorder is shown in Table 4.1.

The causes of genuine thrombocytopenia can be divided into marrow and peripheral causes, as follows:

1 *Bone marrow defect.*
(a) Infiltration, e.g. leukaemia, lymphoma, secondary carcinoma.
(b) Hyperplasia, e.g. drugs or irradiation.
(c) Lack of vitamin B_{12} or folate.

2 *Peripheral.*
(a) Immune consumption, e.g. idiopathic immune thrombocytopenia (ITP), systemic lupus erythematosus, drugs.
(b) Other consumptive process, e.g. DIC and thrombotic thrombocytopenic purpura.
(c) Sepsis.
(d) Hypersplenism.

Thus in a patient with thrombocytopenia the examination of the bone marrow is a key investigation. It may show abnormalities which explain thrombocytopenia. However, if megakaryocytes are plentiful and the bone marrow is otherwise normal, then a peripheral cause should be considered. Abnormal clotting studies (see below) or the presence of an enlarged spleen may suggest the appropriate diagnosis. In immune thrombocytopenia none of these features are present but a platelet-associated antibody can be detected in the majority of cases.

Defects in secondary haemostasis

It would take too long and be too costly to measure all the potential coagulation factors that might be reduced in a patient who is bleeding. Thus tests which measure whole sections of the coagulation cascade are employed (Fig. 4.1). The two most frequently used of these global screening tests are:

1 The APTT.

2 The PT.

Coagulation samples are sent to the laboratory in the anticoagulant citrate. The screening tests by their nature are not specific and are only prolonged when there is a significant reduction in the activity of clotting factors. However, these may have to fall to around 30% of normal before the tests become prolonged. It is important to ensure that once a sample has been taken from the patient it is delivered to the laboratory

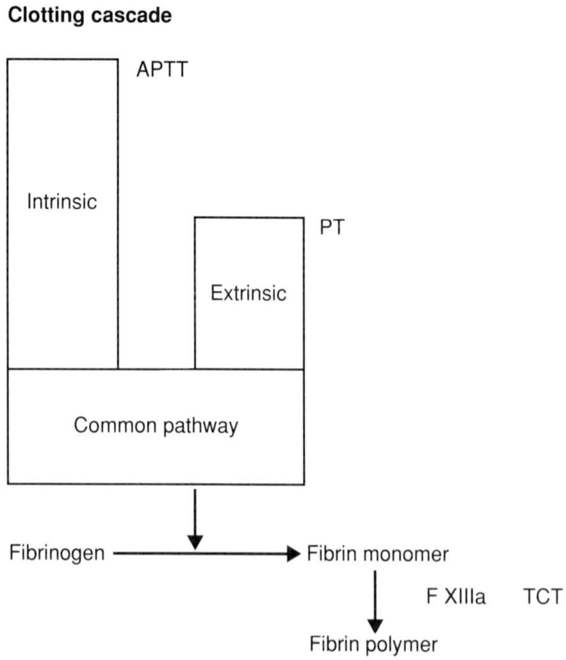

Fig. 4.1 Schematic diagram depicting the various laboratory tests in relation to the parts of the clotting cascade which they measure. APTT, activated partial thromboplastin time; PT, prothrombin time; TCT, thrombin clotting time.

as quickly as possible. Significant delays can result in an erroneously shortened time.

The activated partial thromboplastin time

This test measures the integrity of the intrinsic pathway (Fig. 4.2). A reduction of one or more of the factors in this part of the coagulation cascade may prolong the time. The assay is commenced by adding an activator of clotting such as kaolin. This results in changes of the conformation of Factor XII and initiates a series of positive feedback reactions involving other contact-phase factors. Once this is established, dilute thromboplastin is added. The test plasma is then recalcified and

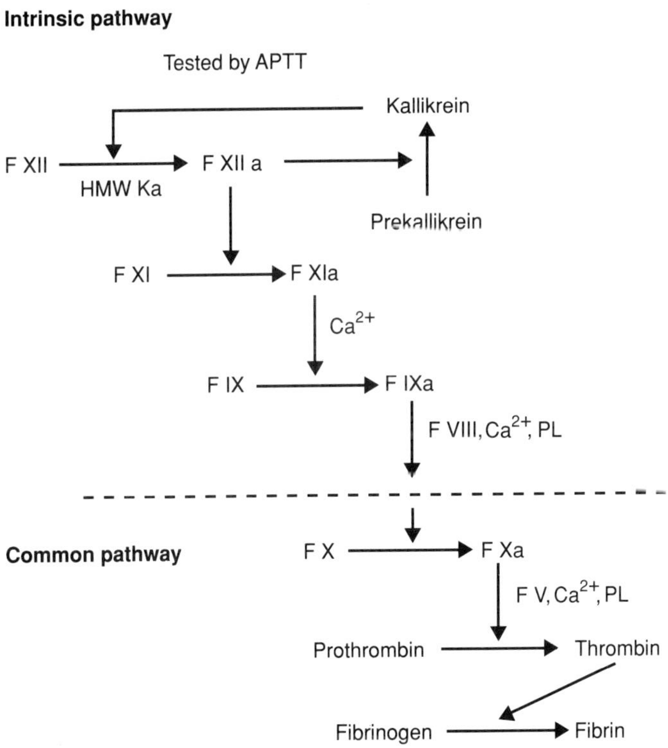

Fig. 4.2 Diagram showing the various clotting factors included in the intrinsic pathway of the clotting cascade. Activated partial thromboplastin time (APTT) is used as a responsive screening test to any changes in the pathway. Common causes of prolonged APTT are heparin therapy, advanced liver disease, Factor VIII deficiency (haemophilia A) and Factor IX deficiency (haemophilia B).

the time for clot formation measured. The normal range is 35–43 s. However, as with all laboratory assays, there is likely to be interlaboratory variation and the reference range of the laboratory actually doing the test should always be consulted. The result is sometimes expressed as a ratio using a control time.

Prolongation of the APTT may be caused by deficiency of Factors II, V, VIII, IX, X, XI, XII, kallikrein high-molecular-weight kininogen or fibrinogen. These deficiencies in turn can be caused by:

1 An inherited defect.

2 As an acquired abnormality secondary to DIC, liver disease, massive transfusion, vitamin K deficiency.

3 The presence of inhibitors: heparin, lupus anticoagulant, specific clotting factor inhibitor.

In order to determine the cause of a prolonged APTT test, plasma is mixed with normal plasma. The intention is to replace any deficient factor(s) thus causing the APTT to normalize. This will not be achieved if the prolongation is due to the presence of an inhibitor. Further studies are required to determine the nature of the inhibitor. Heparin may be detected using the reptilase time or by blocking its action with protamine sulphate. The lupus anticoagulant, which does not *per se* cause bleeding, may be demonstrated by ancillary tests such as the Russell viper venom time.

Shortening of the APTT usually reflects activation of the clotting factors in the patient's plasma prior to removal of the sample. This happens in many reactive conditions, particularly those in which there is elevation of Factor VIII. A similar result can be seen following a difficult venepuncture or be caused by poor technique during specimen collection.

Prothrombin time

This test is most sensitive to change in the extrinsic pathway (Fig. 4.3). The clotting time is disproportionately affected by low levels of Factor V, VII or X, being relatively less sensitive to decreased levels of prothrombin or fibrinogen. The test is usually prolonged when the former factors are reduced by at least 50%.

To perform the test, tissue thromboplastin is added. The time for clot formation is then measured once the test plasma has been recalcified. Thromboplastin complexes with Factor VII and then directly activates Factor X. This combines with Factor V and in the presence of calcium

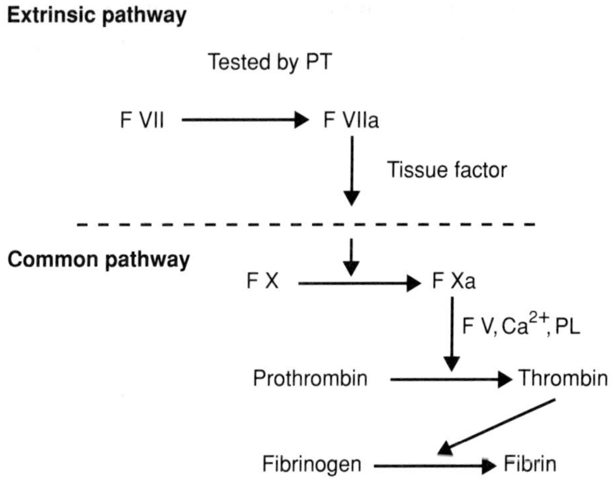

Fig. 4.3 Diagram showing the various clotting factors included in the extrinsic pathway of the clotting cascade. Prothrombin time (PT) is used as a responsive screening test to any changes in this pathway. Common causes of a prolonged PT are liver disease, warfarin therapy, vitamin-K deficiency and DIC.

and phospholipid, a prothrombin activator complex is formed. Thrombin is thus generated and coverts fibrinogen to fibrin. Because the number of reactions is reduced compared to those involved in the APTT, the clotting time is shorter. The normal time is 13–15 s, the result is usually expressed as a ratio compared to a normal control. Therefore the normal ratio is 1. In the past it was difficult to compare prothrombin ratios from different centres as different thromboplastins were used. Now individual laboratories present their results as the International Normalized Ratio (INR), which relates the performance of the locally used reagent to an international standard. The causes of prolonged prothrombin time are deficiency of Factors II, V, VII or X. This may be:

1 Inherited.
  (a) Quantitative deficiency.
  (b) Functional abnormality.

2 Acquired.
  (a) Consumption, e.g. DIC.
  (b) Failure of production, e.g. liver disease.
  (c) Massive transfusion.
  (d) Anticoagulation with coumarin derivatives.

3 The presence of inhibitors (high levels of heparin).

4 Very low levels of fibrinogen.

Bleeding in a patient with abnormal screening tests who is not known to have a congenital coagulation disorder

It is important to assess whether the defect in haemostasis indicated by the abnormal screening tests is severe enough to contribute to any haemorrhage. For example, a platelet count of $100 \times 10^9/l$ is certainly lower than normal but provided platelet function is satisfactory, it is unlikely that this mild thrombocytopenia is causing a problem. When the platelet count is $>50 \times 10^9/l$ and the prothrombin ratio is <1.5, then the surgeon can generally be reassured that any excess bleeding is unlikely to be due to an abnormality of haemostasis. As always it must be appreciated that there still may be a local cause for bleeding which may require surgery following correction of any significant haemostatic defect. Two particular acquired problems which may be associated with excessive haemorrhage will be considered. These are the massively transfused patient and DIC. Others will be considered elsewhere in this volume. However, it is pertinent at this point to review the roles of a number of other useful laboratory tests which have not been previously discussed.

Thrombin clotting time

In this simple test, commercial thrombin is added directly into the test plasma. Thus the patient's plasma is required only to provide functioning fibrinogen, which is cleaved by the thrombin to form the fibrin clot. The main use of the thrombin clotting time (TCT) is as a screening test which reflects the fibrinogen level. A normal TCT is 12–15 s.

Causes of a prolonged TCT are as follows:

1 A low level of fibrinogen caused by:
   (a) DIC.
   (b) Thrombolytic therapy.
   (c) Massive transfusion.
   (d) A failure of production due to severe liver disease.
2 Dysfibrinogenaemia.
3 The presence of an inhibitor: heparin or fibrin degradation products.

Fibrinogen assay

This is a direct measurement of the amount of fibrinogen present in the patient's plasma. The importance of a low level is obvious, both as regards *in vitro* and *in vivo* clotting.

The usual way to perform the test is to add an excess amount of thrombin. The similarity to the TCT is apparent except that in the fibrinogen assay there is quantification of the fibrin formed and hence the amount of fibrinogen present in plasma. The normal range is 1.5–4 g/l. Levels >1 g/l are usually sufficient for normal haemostasis. The causes of low fibrinogen encountered in clinical practice are few. The most important of these from the surgical viewpoint is increased consumption due to DIC. However, a failure of production is found in severe liver disease.

Dysfibrinogenaemia may be detected by measuring clottable and antigenic fibrinogen simultaneously. The diagnosis is suggested when antigenic fibrinogen is significantly increased relative to clottable fibrinogen.

Fibrin degradation products

Fibrin degradation product (FDP) measurement is used as a reflection of fibrinolytic activity. High levels are characteristic of DIC and this remains the main indication for the test. The active enzyme which cleaves both fibrinogen and fibrin is plasmin. This is produced by the action of plasminogen activators which convert inert plasminogen to plasmin. There are two types of activator—tissue plasminogen activator (tPA) and urokinase-like plasminogen activator (uPA).

The release of tPA is stimulated by thrombin, exercise and venostasis. Fibrinolysis is thus activated concurrently with the clotting system. There are also mechanisms to inhibit the process of fibrinolysis. Firstly, following the polymerization of fibrin, Factor XIII stabilizes the polymers by forming covalent bonds between the fibrin monomers. This cross-linked fibrin is more resistant to plasmin. There are also dedicated inhibitors of fibrinolysis. These are plasminogen activator inhibitors, α_2-antiplasmin and α_2-macroglobulin.

Plasmin can degrade fibrinogen and non-crosslinked fibrin as well as crosslinked fibrin. Progressively smaller fragments are formed, known as fragments X and Y, and later in the reaction fragments D and E are generated (Fig. 4.4). Fragment D remains crosslinked following the action of plasmin on crosslinked fibrin and is therefore specific to the lysis of fibrin clot. The measurement of this D–D fragment or D-dimer overcomes some of the problems inherent in the estimation of FDPs. Elevated levels of the latter could represent fibrinogen degradation which has occurred *in vitro* following specimen collection. Mildly elevated levels of both tests, however, do occur in most inflammatory and reactive

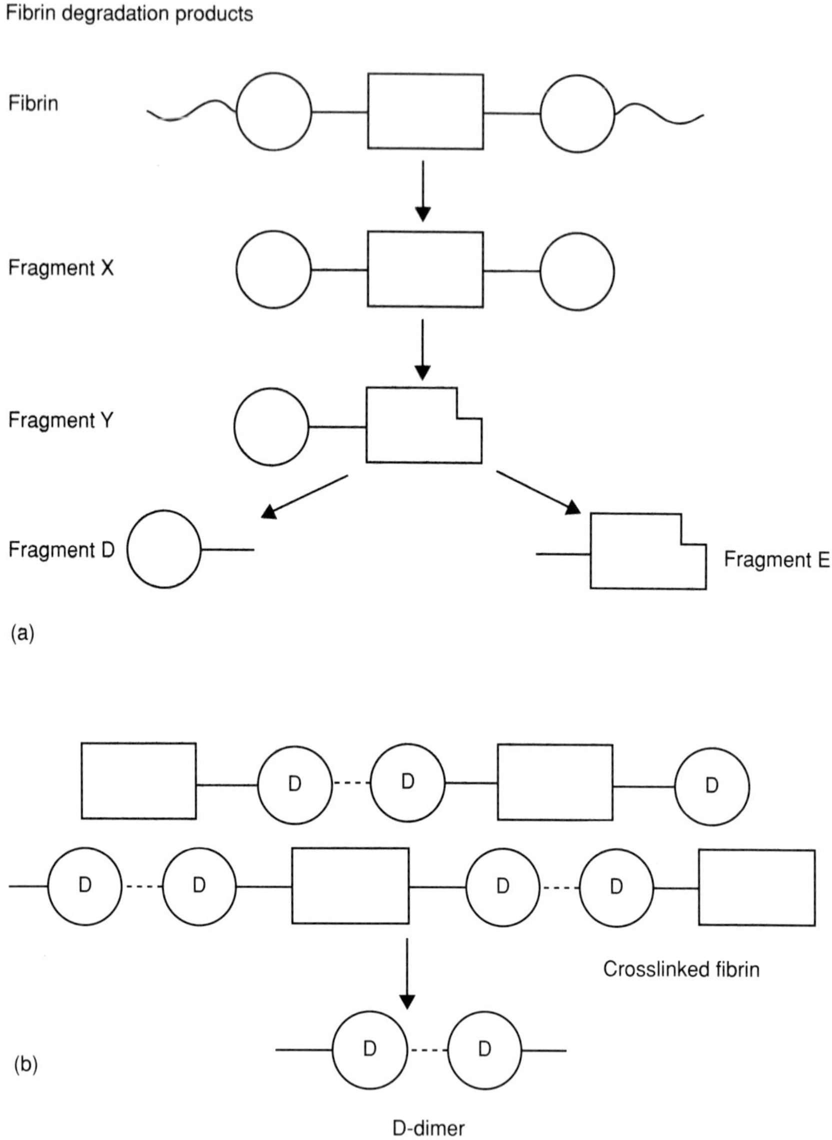

Fig. 4.4 (a) Stepwise fragmentation of the fibrin or fibrinogen by the action of plasmin. This action is non-specific; small quantities of the various fragments are found in normal plasma. The molecular weight of fragment X is 300 000, fragment Y is 150 000, fragment D is 94 000 and fragment E is 50 000. (b) A crosslinked fibrin is more resistant to the action of plasmin. Their formation is catalysed by Factor XIIIa, but if they are degraded, then D-dimer is the byproduct. It is therefore specific for the presence of fibrin clot.

states, many of which can be found postsurgery. Markedly elevated levels are characteristic of DIC.

D-dimer test

The advantages of this test compared to FDP estimation is that it can be estimated on a plasma sample and an elevated level only reflects fibrin degradation. It is most conveniently measured using a semiquantitative latex agglutination test. A more sensitive enzyme-linked immuno-adsorbent assay (ELISA) method is available but this is more time consuming. Elevated D-dimer levels in general parallel a rise in FDP. The normal range is usually below 0.25–0.5 mg/l when a semiquantitative latex agglutination test is used. Mildly elevated levels occur in inflammatory states and thromboembolic disease. Markedly raised levels of >2 mg/l are characteristic of DIC but may also be found in thrombo-embolic disorders.

Assay of individual coagulation factors

It is usually not necessary to measure individual coagulation factors in the surgical setting. An obvious exception involves the management of a patient with an individual factor deficiency (e.g. a haemophiliac) who is undergoing surgery. In this situation the amount of factor replacement is based on the plasma level. Factor assays are more technically demanding and time consuming than screening tests. An exception is the fibrinogen assay, which is often measured in patients with DIC, facilitating the replacement of this very important coagulation protein. Factor assays may also be required to elucidate the exact cause of abnormal screening tests if this is not apparent.

The results of the screening tests should be scrutinized to determine the nature of any abnormality. Table 4.2 provides a guide to common causes of various patterns of abnormal results.

Two conditions which are of particular importance to the surgeon are DIC and the massively transfused patient. These will now be discussed in further detail.

The massively transfused patient

This is defined as total replacement of the patient's blood volume by stored blood in <24 h. In practice this usually means 10–12 units of

Table 4.2 Patterns of test results and their causes

PT	Platelet count	APTT: Normal	APTT: Prolonged
Normal	Normal	See section on abnormal haemostasis with normal screening tests	Factor deficiency (VIII, IX, X, XI, XII) Heparin Specific clotting-factor inhibitor Lupus anticoagulant von Willebrand's disease
	Low	See causes of thrombocytopenia	von Willebrand's disease (a) Type IIb (b) Platelet type von Willebrand's disease Heparin-induced thrombocytopenia
Prolonged	Normal	Warfarin treatment Factor VII deficiency	Liver disease Heparin
	Low	DIC Liver disease Excess alcohol consumption	DIC Massive transfusion Cardiac bypass surgery Advanced liver disease

red-cell concentrate or 10 units of whole blood. This form of treatment has over the years caused many concerns but it is probably fair to say that any delay in transfusing, or undertransfusing, a patient who is hypotensive from blood loss is much more critical in deciding the morbidity and mortality of the patient than the problems that might arise from massive transfusion. Although there are a number of potential complications, in this chapter only those that cause abnormalities in the haemostatic mechanism will be discussed.

For many years, the predisposition to an increased bleeding tendency was largely thought to be related to dilution of platelets and coagulation factors by the large volume of blood transfused. In addition, stored blood is generally devoid of functioning platelets; furthermore, Factors V and VIII decline appreciably on storage. In actual fact, intravascular consumption is perhaps more relevant in most instances than the dilutional effect. This undoubtedly partly reflects the gravity of the underlying disease that has prompted massive transfusion. In some cases a combination of factors is responsible. In the more severe situation DIC certainly occurs and from the haemostatic viewpoint diffuse microvascular bleeding results. This is manifested quickly from diffuse oozing at the operation site or bleeding from the wound and venepuncture sites.

When investigating a massively transfused patient, the platelet count, the PT, the APTT and the fibrinogen level have been shown to be useful predictors. In studies a true bleeding tendency is much more likely if the platelet count is $<50 \times 10^9/l$, fibrinogen <0.5 g/l and the PT or partial thromboplastin time (PTT) ratio is >1.8.

In any circumstances when the patient is bleeding, the platelet count should be maintained at $>50 \times 10^9/l$ and possibly higher when there is evidence of platelet dysfunction, as may occur in renal failure or postcardiac bypass surgery. Routine use of coagulation factors is not recommended. It is much more sensible to perform the tests as indicated and only intervene when the results deviate from the figures quoted above. Mild abnormalities of clotting profiles are common and do not necessarily constitute an indication to intervene. Such action is largely dictated by the presence of microvascular haemorrhage.

Disseminated intravascular coagulation

Patients with DIC normally have an underlying disease that initiates and perpetuates this coagulation disorder. Common to all is an activation of the coagulation mechanism which may follow release of thromboplastic substances into the circulation or endothelial damage. More recently, monocytes and neutrophils have both been implicated in the process, especially when there is an underlying malignancy. DIC results in the formation of fibrin thrombi, with resultant reduction of platelets and clotting factors. It is the latter which results in bleeding.

DIC is a very heterogeneous process. Not all cases are disseminated and it may be chronic as well as acute. An important variable is the nature of the thromboplastin substance itself. The severity and tempo of the disease is determined by the amount and rate at which these thrombogenic substances are released into the circulation. The end result is excessive thrombin formation. This causes fibrin deposition resulting in tissue hypoperfusion, ischaemia or even infarction. Almost concurrently the fibrinolytic enzyme system is activated, causing lysis of fibrinogen and fibrin. In an individual patient, thrombotic or haemorrhagic sequelae may predominate, although both can occur simultaneously.

The three main laboratory findings that characterize DIC are:
1 Thrombocytopenia.
2 Reduction of clotting factors with prolongation of the screening tests.
3 Increased fibrinolysis.

The platelet count is $<50 \times 10^9/l$ in almost half the cases. The fibrinogen level is characteristically low but can be in the normal range, depending on the initial level. The prothrombin time is prolonged, mainly due to reduced levels of Factors X and V. In severe cases, the APTT and the TCT will also be prolonged.

The evidence of increased fibrinolysis is most conveniently provided by the presence of breakdown fragments of fibrinogen and fibrin. Increasingly laboratories are measuring D-dimer.

Lastly, physical damage to red cells may occur when they pass through the mesh of fibrin strands. This is seen on the blood film as red-cell fragmentation.

Causes

The causes of DIC are:
1 Sepsis.
2 Neoplasia.
3 Obstetric complications.
  (a) Pre-eclampsia/eclampsia.
  (b) Abruptio placentae.
  (c) Intrauterine death.
  (d) Amniotic fluid embolism.
  (e) Septic abortion.
4 Severe trauma.
5 Giant cavernous haemangioma.
6 Aortic aneurysm.

Patients with a known bleeding disorder

The general principles will be briefly discussed here as more detail will be found on the diagnosis and management elsewhere in this volume. The surgeon should normally have been alerted to the risk of bleeding and all efforts should have been made in the preoperative period to avoid excess bleeding. This really entails close liaison with the haematologist prior to surgery. This does not mean on the day before surgery but sufficient time should be given to assess the severity of the abnormality and look for complicating factors (e.g. the presence of inhibitor, HIV status). Then a programme can be agreed of appropriate blood product cover for the procedure and postoperative period so that excessive bleeding does not occur. Examples of disorders which should be diagnosed and assessed prior to surgery, and the appropriate laboratory tests for management and the requirements for adequate haemostasis are listed in Table 4.3.

Table 4.3 Laboratory tests for adequate haemostasis

Bleeding condition	Tests	Minimum requirement considered adequate for operation
Platelet disorders		
Qualitative:		
(i) Immune	Platelet count	$>50 \times 10^9/l$
(ii) Non-immune	Platelet count	$>100 \times 10^9/l$
Quantitative platelet defects:		
(i) Primary	Bleeding time	Good functional platelets are needed. Ideally the bleeding time should be near normal
(ii) Associated with systemic disease, e.g. renal failure	Platelet count Bleeding time	Near normalization of bleeding time. Haematocrit >0.30
(iii) Drug induced, e.g. aspirin	Platelet count	Do not normally present any haemostatic problem
Coagulation disorders		
Haemophilia A	APTT Factor VIII inhibitor assay	At least 30%. Higher if the operation is major or involves critical organ, e.g. CNS
Haemophilia B	APTT Factor IX assay Factor IX inhibitor	At least 30%. Higher if the operation involves critical areas, e.g. CNS. To maintain >30% during postoperative period
von Willebrand's disease	Bleeding time	Normalization of bleeding time and APTT. To maintain the same in the postoperative period
Liver disease	PT APTT Platelet count	PT ≤1.5 Platelets ≥80

Bleeding in a patient felt to have an underlying haemostatic problem but whose screening tests are normal

It is not uncommon to be faced with patients who are bleeding but have normal initial screening tests. In the surgical setting a local cause is likely to be related to the surgical procedure. However, if there are strong clues from the history and/or examination, the following should be considered:

1 Platelet function abnormality.
2 Factor XIII deficiency.
3 α_2-Antiplasmin deficiency.
4 A mild clotting-factor deficiency.
5 A vascular-wall abnormality.

Factor XIII and α_2-antiplasmin deficiencies are rare disorders which require specialist laboratory help for their diagnosis. A mild factor deficiency (e.g. a Factor VIII level of 25%) may well be associated with bleeding postsurgery in a patient who gives no history of spontaneous haemorrhage. It would be hoped that in the majority of laboratories the APTT would be sufficiently sensitive, but this may not always be the case. In order to diagnose a platelet function disorder, a bleeding time should be performed.

The bleeding time evaluates the overall competency of platelet plug formation. It reflects both platelet number and function. The only other bleeding disorder that is not strictly due to the platelet but which results in a prolonged bleeding time is von Willebrand's disease. Here there is deficiency of part of the Factor VIII molecule, which is important for platelet function. A prolonged bleeding time may be associated with certain rare disorders of connective tissue. A scheme for the investigation of a suspected platelet disorder is shown in Fig. 4.5.

For the test to be reliable careful attention must be paid to its performance. It is important that a standardized procedure is followed. The bleeding time measures the interval required for blood to stop flowing following a standard superficial incision (1 mm deep and 6 mm long) in the skin on the volar aspect of the forearm. The venous pressure is maintained at 40 mmHg by use of a sphygmomanometer cuff. Standardized template devices are commercially available which painlessly inflict the required incision. This has greatly facilitated the meaningfulness and reproducibility of the test. The normal range using the above system is 2–10 min.

The causes of a prolonged bleeding time are as follows:

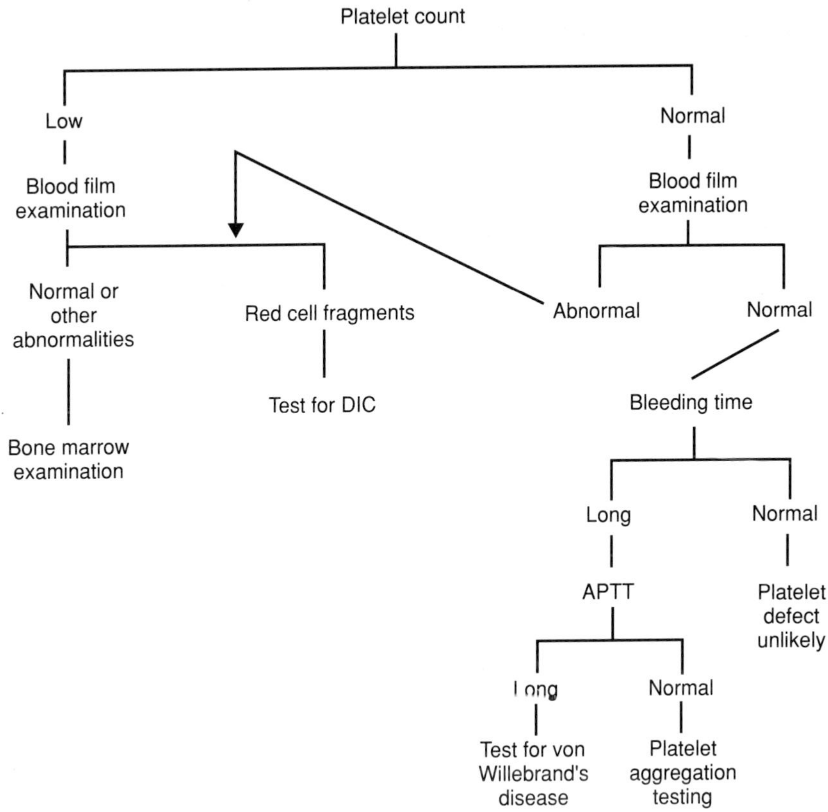

Fig. 4.5 Scheme for the investigation of a suspected platelet disorder.

1 Thrombocytopenia with a count $<100 \times 10^9/l$.

2 Platelet function defects.

(a) *Congenital*: Bernard–Soulier syndrome, Glanzmann's disease, grey platelet syndrome.

(b) *Acquired*: drug induced (e.g. aspirin, non-steroidal anti-inflammatory analgesics), renal failure, paraproteinaemia, myeloproliferative diseases.

3 von Willebrand's disease.

4 Vascular abnormalities.

Patients with a prolonged bleeding time as an isolated abnormality should have their platelet function further evaluated by platelet aggregometry. This type of testing is highly specialized and should be carried out only after consultation with the laboratory. The principle of this type of testing is that various agonists which are known to cause platelet agglutination/aggregation are added to the test plasma. Commonly used agonists are adenosine diphosphate, collagen, adrenaline and ristocetin. If the test plasma is placed in a machine which houses a light source and a photodetector cell, then following platelet aggregation there is increased light transmission. Typical traces are obtained using standard agonists. Failure to obtain these points to particular platelet abnormalities.

Preoperative haemostasis assessment

This should form a part of the routine preoperative assessment. The extent of investigation will depend on the history and examination. The other important consideration is the nature of the procedure. A major operation which would probably constitute a severe challenge to the competence of the haemostatic mechanism will require the system to be tested more rigorously.

Rappaport in 1983 proposed a practical scheme defining four categories with increasing risk of haemorrhage. In Level 1 the patient had a negative history; in Level 2 the history was negative but the patient was to have a major operation; in Level 3 the history raised a suspicion of haemostatic defect and the operation was major or in a sensitive area like the CNS; in Level 4 the history raised a serious suspicion or certainly of a generalized haemostatic defect. Obviously the first category of patient did not require any testing. All the others were felt in need of an increasing complexity of preoperative assessment. The system was devised on the basis of practice in the USA. In the UK it would not be the usual practice to test the coagulation system in patients with no history of bleeding. All patients undergoing surgery do have a full blood count which includes a platelet estimation. If there is a history of bleeding or the patient has a general condition known to impair haemostasis (e.g. liver or renal disease) then tests of haemostatic competency should be performed. In most cases a PT and a PTT will suffice. However, if the situation (e.g. presence of renal failure) suggests the probability of a platelet-function problem, then a bleeding time should be carried out. If the screening tests are prolonged, the laboratory will advise on the identification of the underlying abnormality. It is worthwhile emphasizing that the history and examination are of paramount importance in determining what is appropriate as far as laboratory diagnosis is concerned.

Further reading

Bloom, A.L. and Thomas, D.P. *Haemostasis and Thrombosis,* 2nd edn. Churchill Livingstone, Edinburgh (1987).

British Committee for Standardization in Haematology Blood Transfusion Task Force (1988) Guidelines for transfusion for massive blood loss. *Clin. Lab. Haemat.,* **10**, 265–273.

Chanarin, I. *Laboratory Haematology,* 1st edn. Churchill-Livingstone, Edinburgh (1989).

Ciavarella, D., Reed, R.L., Counts, R.B. *et al.* (1987) Clotting factor levels and the risk of diffuse microvascular bleeding in the massively transfused patient: *Br. J. Haematol.,* **67**, 365–368.

Colman, R.W., Hirsh, J., Marder, V.J. and Salzman, E.W. *Hemostasis and Thrombosis, Basic Principles and Clinical Practice,* 2nd edn. J.B. Lippincott, Philadelphia (1987).

Rappaport, S.I. (1983) Preoperative hemostatic evaluation: which tests, if any? *Blood,* **61**, 229–237.

Williams, W.J., Beutler, F., Erslev., A.J. and Lichtman, M.A. *Haematology,* 4th edn. McGraw-Hill, New York (1990).

Part 2
Particular Bleeding Problems

Chapter 5
Obstetrics and gynaecology

IAN A. GREER

The obstetrician and gynaecologist is regularly confronted with bleeding. This may be physiological, such as that encountered during the third stage of labour or menstruation. However, it is often pathological, related mainly to the complications of pregnancy. While such pathological bleeding may not always be life-threatening, it has the potential to present as, or to progress to, a clinical catastrophe. Indeed, in the UK, haemorrhage remains one of the five most common direct causes of maternal death [1]. This chapter aims to review the bleeding problems encountered in obstetric and gynaecological practice.

Abortion

The incidence of spontaneous abortion lies somewhere between 15 and 25% of all pregnancies. The precise incidence is difficult to define as an early spontaneous abortion may be mistaken for delayed menstruation, or vice versa. In addition, criminal abortion may be inadvertently classified as a spontaneous abortion due to the patient concealing the true aetiology of the problem.

The aetiology of spontaneous abortion is far from clear, but chromosomal abnormalities can be identified in around half the cases where the karyotype can be established. The most common chromosomal abnormalities are autosomal trisomies, 45X and triploidy [2]. Other causes include uterine abnormalities, cervical incompetence, infections, maternal disease such as systemic lupus erythematosus and immunological causes. Despite this wide range of possibilities, most spontaneous abortions remain unexplained although the risk is higher in women aged over 35 years, and in those having had a previous spontaneous abortion.

Traditionally, spontaneous abortions are divided clinically into three main categories:

1 Threatened abortion, where there is painless vaginal bleeding which may settle spontaneously with a continuing pregnancy, or progress to an inevitable abortion.

2 Inevitable abortion, where there is bleeding and pain associated with cervical dilatation.

3 (In)complete abortion, where part or all of the products of conception have been passed.

Ultrasound examination, however, will result in an alternative classification for spontaneous abortion [3]. These are blighted ovum, missed abortion and live abortion. 'Blighted ovum' (an anembryonic pregnancy) is where a gestation sac and placental tissue can be identified, but no fetus ever develops. Missed abortion is where the fetus is seen but the fetal heart is absent prior to abortion *per se* occurring. Live abortion is where the fetal heart may be identified shortly before expulsion of the products of conception, implying that the fetal loss is a consequence rather than the direct cause of the process.

The amount of bleeding associated with spontaneous abortion varies from minimal to massive. 'Live abortion' is usually regarded as the type associated with an increased risk of severe haemorrhage, although rarely a missed abortion retained for several weeks may result in a serious bleeding problem due to the development of disseminated intravascular coagulation (DIC). However, gestation is perhaps the factor most closely associated with the risk of haemorrhage, with bleeding risk increasing with advancing gestation during the first trimester. As abortion is usually complete when it occurs in the second trimester, serious haemorrhage is less common, although still a source of concern as two of the six deaths attributable to spontaneous abortion in the 1979–81 *Report on Confidential Enquiries into Maternal Deaths in England and Wales* [4] were due to haemorrhage and both were in the second trimester. However, in the most recent report into maternal deaths [1], which included four deaths following spontaneous abortion, none was a consequence of haemorrhage which, if continued in future reports, is an encouraging development.

The diagnosis of spontaneous abortion is usually straightforward although ectopic pregnancy may enter the differential diagnosis. History, clinical examination including pelvic examination to assess cervical state, uterine size and adnexal tenderness and ultrasound scan will usually resolve this. Clearly, particular attention should be paid to the patient's haemodynamic states. Blood loss may be greater than it seems as the vagina may balloon and contain a large volume of blood clot, while entrapment of products in a partially dilated cervix can lead to severe hypotension (and bradycardia) due to vagal stimulation. Thus, digital examination is mandatory. The usual measures to resuscitate the patient and manage major haemorrhage as discussed later will be required. In addition there is an urgent need to clear the cervix of any trapped products and arrest the bleeding. These measures will tend to occur concurrently with resuscitation. Ergometrine (0.25–0.5 mg) should be given intravenously if bleeding is continuing, and the patient prepared for theatre, where evacuation of the uterus will be performed. Evacuation is best performed digitally to avoid the risk of perforation, although a gentle curettage may be required to ensure that the uterus is empty. Intravenous oxytocin or ergometrine may be required intraoperatively to control bleeding.

Where the abortion has been complicated by sepsis, appropriate antibiotic therapy will be required and where possible evacuation should be delayed until sepsis has been controlled, usually after 24 h antibiotic therapy, to avoid the risk of disseminating the infection and provoking septicaemia.

Criminal abortion

Thankfully the incidence of criminal abortion and maternal death resulting from this procedure have fallen dramatically since the introduction in the UK of the Abortion Act 1967; the number of deaths attributable to illegal abortion having fallen from 37 in the triennium 1970–72 to none in the 1982–84 triennium in England and Wales [1]. The major complications of these procedures are trauma to the genital tract, haemorrhage and sepsis. Treatment will require resuscitation, antibiotic therapy and sometimes surgical repair of traumatic uterine damage. The hypovolaemia and sepsis which occurs may also result in further complications such as acute renal failure.

Therapeutic abortion

Using modern techniques, the risk of death following therapeutic abortion is very low in the UK. In Scotland in the quinquennium 1981–85, 44 235 abortions were carried out under the 1967 Abortion Act and no deaths followed these procedures [5]. In England and Wales, however, in the triennium 1982–84, there were seven direct and three indirect deaths associated with abortion, with three of the direct deaths resulting from haemorrhage. These figures, of course, take no account of the morbidity associated with non-fatal haemorrhagic complications of these procedures, and there is no room for complacency with regard to such procedures. It is important to be aware of the potentially large blood loss which may be concealed intra-abdominally following uterine trauma. In addition, it is important to procede to laparotomy sooner rather than later to deal with the problem. It is of course fundamental to the management of such haemorrhagic complications to maintain the intravascular volume and have blood readily available.

In the first trimester, most legal abortions will at present be carried out surgically by cervical dilatation and suction evacuation of the uterus, although surgical evacuation may also be performed. The risk of traumatic damage in this situation may be reduced by pretreatment with agents to promote cervical ripening, such as gemeprost (Cervagem, Rhone-Poulenc) and such agents will also act to significantly reduce blood loss [6,7]. Again the blood loss is likely to be proportional to gestational age due to the increased size of the uterus and time and difficulty to evacuate it. Perforation of the uterus during therapeutic abortion may occur and lead to massive intra-abdominal bleeding, especially if damage occurs at the isthmus, where uterine artery damage and torrential haemorrhage may ensue. In cases where perforation is suspected but not definite, laparoscopy should be performed to confirm the diagnosis. Laparotomy is usually required to control bleeding and repair the damage, and hysterectomy may be necessary.

Therapeutic abortion may also be obtained by medical means. This will usually require the administration of prostaglandins to induce cervical ripening and uterine activity, resulting in abortion. The use of antiprogestogens such as RU486 [7] can facilitate medical abortion and is highly successful both in the first and second trimesters, obviating the need for anaesthesia and surgical instrumentation of the uterus so minimizing the risk of traumatic bleeding. Where haemorrhage complicates medically induced abortion, the management is similar to that of haemorrhage complicating spontaneous abortion.

Ectopic pregnancy

Massive haemorrhage complicating ectopic pregnancy is a major cause of maternal mortality and morbidity. Despite a substantial reduction in deaths from 2.9 per 1000 ectopic pregnancies in the triennium 1970–72 to 0.7 per 1000 ectopic pregnancies in the triennium 1982–84 in England

and Wales, it remains the fourth most common cause of maternal mortality [1]. A similar pattern is seen in the USA where there has been a sevenfold decline in mortality from 3.52 per 1000 cases to 0.53 per 1000 over approximately the same time period [8], although in the USA it has become the second most common cause of maternal death, accounting for over 14% of maternal mortality, due to a reduction in deaths from other causes [9]. Haemorrhage is the most common mode of death, being responsible for 88% of fatal cases in the USA, with more than half the women dying prior to receiving any therapy [9]. This reflects the speed with which this catastrophe may develop. These changes in mortality are set against the rising incidence of ectopic pregnancy in the Western World, with a severalfold increase over the last 20 years. This has been due to factors such as a rising incidence of pelvic inflammatory disease and an increase in tubal surgery, including sterilization and its reversal. However, the rise in incidence reflects, at least in part, improvements in diagnosis due to increased use of laparoscopy, and high-quality ultrasound examination coupled with sensitive assays of the human chorionic gonadotrophin (hCG) which have allowed us to identify ectopic pregnancies which in the past may have resolved spontaneously before becoming a significant clinical problem. Such improvements in diagnosis along with greater clinical awareness have contributed to the improvement in mortality. In addition, the fertility prognosis is poor in this patient group and approximately two-thirds will never subsequently bear a live child and 12–18% will have a further ectopic pregnancy.

The most common ectopic implantation site is the fallopian tube, with >95% occurring in the tube *per se* and 2–4% in the interstitial portion; <1% will occur on the ovary and rarely it will occur on the cervix or in the abdominal cavity. The villous trophoblast rapidly invades the tubal mucosa with most of the growth occurring in the connective tissue between the endosalpinx and the serosa [10]. As the pregnancy grows, a haematoma may form at this site and eventually the tube may rupture and cause haemorrhage. However, in some instances the pregnancy will perish and be absorbed spontaneously, or may be aborted through the fimbrial end of the tube, thus resolving spontaneously. Histologically, chorionic villi will be seen within the tube and may show marked degeneration and hyalinization. Decidualization of the endometrium also occurs and the Arias–Stella reaction will be seen histologically. This consists of cellular enlargement, hyperchromatosis, pleomorphism and mitotic activity. The decidua will be shed if the embryo dies due to loss of hormonal support, presenting as vaginal bleeding.

The accurate diagnosis of ectopic pregnancy is an important clinical problem. The symptoms and signs may vary considerably depending on the site of implantation, the gestation and the viability of the ectopic pregnancy. The most common symptoms are abdominal pain and irregular, often scant, vaginal bleeding usually after a short period of amenorrhea or a mistimed or 'lighter than usual' last menstrual period [11]. Signs include abdominal tenderness often associated with rebound, and a tender mass in the adnexae. A normal-sized uterus may also be found. The patient may present with hypovolaemic shock. The condition is often misdiagnosed as pelvic inflammatory disease, threatened or incomplete abortion, ruptured ovarian cyst or corpus luteum or even dysfunctional uterine bleeding. A high degree of suspicion is required in all women presenting with gynaecological symptoms which could possibly be consistent with an ectopic pregnancy. It should be noted that women who have undergone surgical sterilization are not exempt from this condition and may even be at increased risk. The absence of chorionic villi and the presence of an Arias–Stella decidual reaction in 'products' obtained from women having uterine evacuation for presumed incomplete or inevitable abortion also suggests a misdiagnosis and the presence of ectopic pregnancy.

Modern assays for hCG or its β subunit in plasma or urine, provide a sensitive pregnancy test and can confirm the presence of trophoblast. Having biochemical confirmation of pregnancy, the differential diagnosis then lies between intra- and extrauterine pregnancy. Abdominal ultrasound scan will detect intrauterine pregnancy by the 7th week of amenorrhea. The presence of an intrauterine pregnancy virtually excludes ectopic pregnancy as heterotopic pregnancy (combined intra- and extrauterine pregnancy) is exceedingly rare in normal conceptions (1 : 30 000) [11]. Thus a positive pregnancy test coupled with an empty uterus on ultrasound implies ectopic pregnancy. A pseudosac formed from the decidualization of the endometrium may be misleading on ultrasound, but a mass or free fluid in the pelvis is highly suspicious. It is unusual for abdominal ultrasound to directly delineate the ectopic gestation. Transvaginal ultrasound provides a better image and the potential for the earlier detection of ectopic pregnancy. In a recent study of transvaginal ultrasound, a fetal heart beat was detected in eight out of 36 patients with ectopic pregnancy and this and the presence of other ultrasound signs of ectopic gestation provided a positive diagnosis in

80%; however, the false-negative rate in this study was 19% [12]. Ultrasound alone is not sufficiently sensitive or specific for diagnostic purposes, but abdominal sector scanning coupled with hCG estimation has a reported specificity of 98% and sensitivity of 95% [11].

In clinically stable women at early gestations, the combination of ultrasound and serial assay of hCG is reliable and may allow conservative management rather than proceeding directly to laparoscopy. The wide individual variation in hCG levels in pregnancy and the common uncertainty about the exact gestational age in these patients makes a single estimation of hCG of limited value. However, a discriminatory hCG level (6000–6500 iu/l) at which point an intrauterine gestational sac should be seen [13] is a useful tool. The doubling time of hCG in early pregnancy is also of value as hormone synthesis by the trophoblast is depressed in ectopic pregnancy [11]. In normal pregnancies, the rate of doubling of hCG is 1.4–2.1 days and is not influenced by the initial concentration of hCG [14].

While conservative management may have a place in the management of the unruptured or chronic ectopic, it has no place where serious haemorrhage is present; such patients should be resuscitated and taken for immediate laparotomy. Diagnostic tests are not required when the patient's condition necessitates laparotomy and will only delay the main objective of management, arrest of haemorrhage, while the patient rapidly deteriorates. The bleeding may be overwhelming from a ruptured ectopic and in such cases the control of haemorrhage by laparotomy and clamping of the tube is paramount. There is little point in delaying surgery while blood is crossmatched in these rapidly deteriorating situations, although several units of blood will be needed urgently, as resuscitation will fail unless the haemorrhage is stemmed; clearly, an experienced anaesthetist will be required in these situations to allow surgery and resuscitation to occur concurrently.

The classic treatment of ectopic pregnancy is laparotomy and salpingectomy to arrest or prevent haemorrhage. There is a case for less aggressive treatment and a number of methods have been described to remove the ectopic without sacrificing the tube. The aim of this more conservative surgery is to maintain tubal function and fertility while minimizing the risk of recurrent ectopic pregnancy. Salpingectomy and linear salpingostomy give similar live-birth and ectopic pregnancy recurrence rates, so that the case for conservative surgery, where the contralateral tube appears normal, is not particularly strong. Unruptured tubal pregnancies can sometimes be 'milked' out of the fimbrial end, so avoiding tubal surgery, but significant tubal damage may still result. Where it is essential to maintain tubal function the section containing the ectopic may be excised and the two adjacent ends of the tube sealed with sutures or even Filshie or Hulka–Clemens clips to minimize tubal damage with a view to subsequent tubal re-anastomoses. Other conservative approaches include laparoscopic surgery, direct injection of $PGF_{2\alpha}$ into the ectopic to stimulate contractions and provoke tubal abortion, chemotherapy with methotrexate to destroy trophoblast, which is highly sensitive to such chemotherapy, and antigestagens may also have a role.

Major obstetric haemorrhage

The causes of major obstetric haemorrhage are placental abruption, placenta praevia and postpartum haemorrhage. These constitute a significant problem in contemporary obstetric practice. Haemorrhage accounted for nine direct deaths, a rate of 4.8 per million pregnancies and the lowest ever reported, in the last triennium reviewed by the *Report on the Confidential Enquiries into Maternal Deaths in England and Wales* [1]. However, haemorrhage contributed to many deaths attributed to other causes and is a major source of morbidity. Despite the substantial improvement in deaths due to haemorrhage from a rate of 91.6 per million maternities in 1952–54 to 16.7 per million maternities in 1967–69, and a steady decline to current levels, there is no room for complacency as there is still room for improvement in the care of these patients [1].

There are common aspects to the management of all such major haemorrhages and guidelines have been issued with regard to the management of massive haemorrhage [1]. There is little time for thought and a planned protocol for the management of such patient is useful [26]:

1 Obstetric, anaesthetic and midwifery staff should be summoned urgently. Usually senior anaesthetists and obstetricians will be required. Haematologists and blood transfusion should be alerted.

2 Two peripheral lines (14 gauge) should be set up, and central venous monitoring carried out to guide therapy, ensuring adequate volume replacement while avoiding fluid overload. An arterial line, if available, is also extremely useful. A urinary catheter and hourly assessment of urinary output is essential.

3 Continuous monitoring of blood pressure, pulse and ECG should be performed. Blood gas and acid–base status require regular assessment.

4 A sample of venous blood, around 20 ml, is required for blood grouping and crossmatch, and assessment of coagulation status. At least 6 units of blood should be crossmatched initially; whole blood is preferable but if only packed cells are available. Additional plasma expansion with human albumin solution (4.5%) or artificial plasma expander such as polygeline (Haemaccel) will be needed. Dextran is contraindicated as not only does it interfere with crossmatching by causing pseudoagglutination, but it also interferes with coagulation by inhibiting platelet function and is associated with a risk of allergic and anaphylactic reactions. In very severe haemorrhage, uncrossmatched blood may be life-saving and it is useful to have two units of Group O Rh-negative blood kept on the labour ward at all times. Such unmatched Group O Rh-negative blood must not be given to patients with anti-c antibodies. Blood should be given rapidly using a pressure cuff, and via blood-warming equipment. A blood filter should not be used as it slows blood administration.

5 Haemoglobin concentration and coagulation status should be monitored regularly. Coagulation tests will include platelet count, prothrombin time and activated partial thromboplastin time to assess extrinsic and intrinsic coagulation pathways respectively, and thrombin time which measures thrombin clottable fibrinogen and fibrinogen. Fibrin degradation products (FDPs) should be measured to assess whether increased fibrinolysis is present. Restoration of normovolaemia is the first objective but fresh frozen plasma, cryoprecipitate or platelets may be required after rapid infusion of 5 units of stored blood, or where there is a significant coagulation defect, especially if bleeding is continuing and there is no clear surgically correctable source. The blood products required will be determined by the results of the coagulation studies. Platelet concentrate will not normally be required until the platelet count is $<20 \times 10^9/l$ with continuing bleeding.

6 Recourse to procedures such as internal iliac artery ligation or hysterectomy should not be left until the patient is moribund, and an experienced clinician is essential for such cases. Additional personnel such as vascular surgeons, if for example there is damage to a major vessel, should likewise be summoned sooner rather than later. If the abdomen is open, then even the most severe haemorrhage may be stemmed temporarily by aortic compression until the problem is corrected surgically.

7 Depending on staffing and resources in the labour ward and the patient's condition, the patient may be better transferred to an intensive care unit.

Placental abruption

Placental abruption is, by definition, premature separation of the normally implanted placenta from the uterine wall resulting in haemorrhage before the delivery of the fetus. Recent reports on frequency and perinatal mortality in abruption have estimated an incidence of between 1 per 77 and 1 per 89 deliveries, with between 30.5% and 36.5% perinatal mortality [15,16]. In the report by Abdella *et al.* [15], 14% of the surviving infants had significant neurological deficits which were apparent within the first year after delivery. The survival rate depends on the severity of the abruption, gestation, birthweight and the amount of concealed haemorrhage. Maternal mortality has improved considerably over the last few decades due to earlier diagnosis, intensive care and general improvements in health care, including the development of blood transfusion services. The *Report on The Confidential Enquiries into Maternal Deaths in England and Wales* reports a rate of 1.06 per million maternities in the triennium 1982–84 compared to a rare of 6.62 per million maternities in the triennium 1970–72 for direct deaths resulting from abruption [1]. Placental abruption is also a significant cause of maternal morbidity including postpartum anaemia and infection [16].

Placental abruption appears to be initiated by bleeding into the decidua basalis of the placenta which, due to the hydrostatic pressure and development of decidual haematoma, leads to separation of the adjacent placenta. As the uterus is still distended, it is unable to clamp down on the uterine vessels at the placental site, although there is increased resistance in both the maternal and fetal vessels [17] due to vasoconstriction. The expanding haematoma may dissect between the fetal membranes leading to vaginal bleeding; however, the bleeding may be in whole or in part concealed if the haematoma does not reach the margin of the placenta and the cervix, so that revealed blood loss *per se* is a poor guide to the degree of haemorrhage. The haematoma may also result in bleeding into the amniotic cavity, resulting in blood-stained liquor when the membranes rupture, or bleeding and haematoma may infiltrate the myometrium resulting in the so-called Couvelaire uterus. The infiltration into the myometrium is associated with sustained uterine contractions, resulting in labour and reduced uteroplacental blood flow, thus compromising the fetus.

The primary cause of placental abruption is usually unknown, but abnormal placentation is likely and may explain the necrosis of the decidua basalis and placental infarcts which are often seen in association with abruption. Risk factors which have been associated with placental abruption include sudden uterine decompression, external trauma, uterine anomaly, maternal age, parity, folate deficiency, socioeconomic status, smoking and an unexplained elevation of maternal serum α-fetoprotein in the second trimester [18,19]. Women who give up smoking in pregnancy reduce the incidence of abruption by 23% and stillbirth and neonatal deaths due to the abruption by 50% compared to women who continue smoking [20]. There is a relatively high rate of recurrence for abruption in subsequent pregnancies.

Although hypertension and placental abruption are frequently diagnosed together, the evidence for a causal relationship is controversial. The hypertension could result from sudden release of vasoactive substances such as thromboxane or endothelin into the maternal circulation from the disturbed placental bed. While some studies have not reported an increased frequency of pre-existing maternal hypertension in cases of abruption [20,21], a prospective study [15] has shown that patients with chronic hypertension have a ninefold risk of abruption and pre-eclamptic patients a twofold risk compared to normotensive patients. This study also found a high incidence in eclamptic patients (23.6%). This association would be in keeping with the theory of defective placentation, which may also be a factor in pre-eclampsia. Where hypertension and abruption coexist, the perinatal mortality is increased, with relative risks of 5.0 and 3.2 with chronic hypertension and pre-eclampsia, respectively [22].

The classic presentation of severe abruption is vaginal bleeding, uterine tenderness and irritability, and contractions or uterine hypertonus often resulting in premature labour. Fetal distress or intrauterine fetal death may be present. In more than half of patients the symptoms precede the onset of labour and in around 10% there is a history of vaginal bleeding up to 7 weeks earlier [23]. The diagnosis of placental abruption may not be obvious, with 22% of abruptions in a prospective study thought to be in idiopathic premature labour [16]; abruption should be considered in all patients presenting with unexplained vaginal bleeding, especially when associated with uterine pain or contractions and fetal distress. As discussed above, the amount of vaginal bleeding bears little relationship to the amount of blood loss or the extent of abruption, such that hypovolaemic shock may be present despite minimal or even absent vaginal bleeding. The degree of haemorrhage may be substantial, with a median blood loss of 2.5 litres in 24 severe cases studied by Pritchard and Brekken [19]. Feto-maternal haemorrhage can occur and may result in fetal anaemia and even death. Obviously anti-D immunoglobulin must be administered to all Rh-negative women who may have had a possible abruption.

Abruption is the most common cause of coagulation failure in pregnancy and usually correlates with the degree of abruption and blood loss. Haemostatic failure should be suspected if there is bleeding from puncture sites or mucous membranes. Platelet count will be reduced and fibrinogen will be low. The thrombin time and measures of the extrinsic and intrinsic pathways of coagulation such as the prothrombin and activated partial thromboplastin times, respectively, will be prolonged. Elevated levels of FDPs will also be found, reflecting the secondary activation of fibrinolysis stimulated by intravascular fibrin deposition. FDPs may also act as anticoagulants and it has been suggested that they may inhibit myometrial contractility, so predisposing to postpartum haemorrhage. Correction of hypovolaemia will maintain renal blood flow and allow clearance of these FDPs. The use of heparin and antifibrinolytics has also been advocated; while there is some logic in this to break the vicious circle of DIC, such treatment is potentially very hazardous in the dynamic and unstable coagulation problems seen in these patients. In the author's opinion there is no place for such therapy in routine practice and good results can be obtained using more conventional therapy.

The management of severe abruption aims to correct hypovolaemia, deliver the fetus and observe and correct any coagulopathy that may be present. All cases should be treated with the highest degree of care. Patients should be admitted to the labour ward where intensive monitoring of both mother and fetus can be adequately carried out. Resuscitation measures should follow the guidelines given above. Ultrasound scan is useful in the management of these patients to assess fetal viability and presentation, as clinical diagnosis is difficult due to uterine hypertonicity. Ultrasound is also useful in the differential diagnosis of placenta praevia.

In patients with severe abruption or in those who are clearly labouring, examination without anaesthesia, but with an anaesthetist present, in a theatre set for caesarean section should be performed, as the alternative or coexisting diagnosis of placenta praevia must be excluded. It is important that the examination should not be taken lightly and ultrasound examination excluding placenta praevia should not be totally relied on as it may be difficult to accurately delineate the relationship of the placenta to the lower uterine segment and exclude a succenturiate placenta. Amniotomy should be performed and fetal scalp electrodes applied for internal electronic monitoring of the fetal heart rate. In cases where fetal distress is present, caesarean section should be performed immediately as there is a close association between diagnosis to delivery time and perinatal mortality rate [19]. However, in the absence of fetal distress, labour, which is usually rapid in these cases, should be allowed to progress and an oxytocic to augment labour employed if required. By using continuous electronic cardiotocography and fetal blood sampling, where appropriate, to monitor fetal wellbeing, up to 50% may deliver vaginally. Vaginal delivery should also be anticipated where intrauterine death has occurred, but deterioration in maternal condition may still necessitate caesarean section. These patients are at high risk of post-partum haemorrhage.

Placenta praevia

Bleeding from placenta praevia is due to separation of the abnormally implanted placenta as a result of the cervix dilating. Placenta praevia is conventionally divided into grades of severity, but in the clinical situation it is adequate to consider the condition as major or minor placenta praevia. In major placenta praevia, the placenta covers the cervical os so that bleeding is inevitable as the lower segment forms and during labour. In minor degrees of placenta praevia, the placenta encroaches on the lower uterine segment, but successful vaginal delivery may still be possible as the placenta may be sufficiently clear of the cervix to allow labour without bleeding, or may 'move' clear of the cervix as the lower segment of the uterus forms and expands below the level of the placental implantation site. Although the placenta will be readily visualized with ultrasound, it can be difficult to accurately delineate the relationship of the placenta to the lower uterine segment and exclude a succenturiate placental lobe. The incidence of this condition is around 0.5%, but will be substantially higher than this if all placentae noted to be 'low lying' on ultrasound are included. It is associated with multiparity, high maternal age and previous caesarean section. Large placentae such as those associated with multiple pregnancy are clearly at increased risk of being praevia. Placenta accreta is also more common with placenta praevia. Just as with abruption, there has been a decline in direct deaths related to placenta praevia, with a rate of 1.06 per million maternities in the triennium 1982–84 compared to a rate of 6.62 per million maternities in the triennium 1970–72 [1].

The characteristic clinical presentation of placenta praevia is painless and often minor degrees of vaginal bleeding which settle spontaneously, at the time of formation of the lower segment in the first half of the third trimester. Such 'warning' haemorrhages heralding the diagnosis are common, but one study has shown that 34% of cases have no history of such warning haemorrhages [24] and the problem may only become apparent during labour. Malpresentations, unstable lie and high presenting parts are common as the lower pole of the uterus is occupied by the placenta and should raise suspicion as to the presence of placenta praevia. The uterus is usually soft and non-tender. Vaginal and speculum examination must be avoided in all cases of indeterminate vaginal bleeding until placenta praevia has been excluded, as in the case of placenta praevia this can initiate placental separation and provoke major haemorrhage.

The management of placenta praevia depends on the gestation at presentation, severity of bleeding and degree of praevia. Where bleeding is severe, delivery by caesarean section is required immediately in the maternal interest regardless of fetal maturity or condition. If placenta praevia first presents at 37 weeks' gestation or beyond, then the patient should be delivered. Where the fetus is preterm and the bleeding has been of a minor nature and stops spontaneously, then conservative management is warranted. In this situation the patient should remain in hospital with blood immediately available at all times in case of severe haemorrhage. Where the fetus is considered sufficiently mature, delivery by caesarean section is performed. This is usually around 37–38 weeks' gestation (before the onset of spontaneous labour, which would inevitably provoke bleeding). Minor degrees of placenta praevia may be managed conservatively with the possibility of subsequent vaginal delivery. Ultrasound can be used to monitor the placental site at fortnightly intervals. If the placenta is seen to 'move' well clear of the cervix as the lower segment forms and clinically there is no other contraindication, then vaginal delivery may be anticipated. In borderline and minor degrees of placenta praevia, examination in theatre set for section may be required to delineate whether the placenta is likely to be disturbed by, or to interfere with, delivery. A decision can then be made whether to proceed directly to section or whether to allow vaginal delivery. The latter can only be accomplished in the most minor degrees of placenta praevia. In any event, there should be early recourse to caesarean section if any bleeding occurs.

Caesarean section itself may be a hazardous procedure, especially in anterior placenta praevia, and an experienced operator is required. The fetus may be delivered through the placenta, in which case there is a risk of significant fetal blood loss, or round the placental edge. The placenta may be very adherent to the lower segment and may be accreta. This is thought to be due to the relative lack of decidua in the lower segment and can be a particular problem in women with a previous section scar on their uterus [25]. It may require to be removed piecemeal and substantial haemorrhage may be encountered. Major sinuses should be sutured and ligated; however, closure of the uterine wound may provide satisfactory haemostasis. Oxytocics may also be useful and should certainly be tried, but further surgical manoeuvres such as ligating the uterine arteries, performing a hysterectomy or ligating the internal iliac arteries should be considered in the face of intractable haemorrhage. The important factor here is that such procedures are not delayed until the patient is in extremis. With continued blood loss, a coagulopathy will develop and concurrent monitoring of haemodynamic condition and coagulation status is required, with adequate volume replacement and correction of coagulopathy. Following delivery the patient remains at increased risk of postpartum haemorrhage. Four to 6 units of blood and good venous access should be available for such deliveries.

Postpartum haemorrhage

Primary postpartum haemorrhage (PPH) is conventionally defined as blood loss exceeding 500 ml during the first 24 h following delivery of the baby and can be subdivided into third-stage haemorrhage and true postplacental postpartum haemorrhage. Secondary PPH is excessive blood loss in the puerperium after the first 24 h.

The blood loss resulting from uncomplicated vaginal delivery and caesarean section is frequently >500 ml and visual estimations are notoriously inaccurate [27,28], so that blood loss >500 ml is not necessarily abnormal. Estimates of incidence between 3.9% and 8.6% have been quoted for primary PPH [29]. One study put the incidence at 11% [30]; however, of the 86 patients with PPH, only eight required a blood transfusion although 'varying degrees of anaemia' were more common. Because of these problems in definition, the incidence of postpartum haemorrhage which constitutes a clinical problem is hard to define. The maternal mortality rate from PPH continues to decline from 7.86 per million maternities in 1970–72 to 1.6 per million maternities in 1984–86 [1]. PPH is usually the result of uterine atony or trauma to the genital tract and may be compounded by coagulation failure.

Uterine atony accounts for the majority of serious postpartum haemorrhage. There are a number of antenatal and intrapartum risk factors associated with it, although it can also occur after a normal pregnancy and delivery. Following delivery of the placenta, bleeding from the placental bed is halted by vasoconstriction *per se* and by external compression by the criss-cross latticework of myometrial fibres as the uterus contracts and retracts, so providing a natural 'ligature' for the vessels in the placental bed. Uterine atony results in failure of this mechanism and PPH may result. Uterine atony may occur in the absence of any predisposing factor, but many risk factors have been identified which should alert the obstetrician to the possibility of PPH. These risk factors include operative intervention, high parity, overdistension of the uterus such as in multiple pregnancy and polyhydramnios, retained placenta and morbidly adherent placenta (placenta accreta), multiple fibroids which may interfere with contraction and retraction, prolonged and precipitate labour and previous atonic PPH. Primary PPH also appears more common in primigravidae even allowing for their higher incidence of forceps deliveries [30]. Induction of labour by amniotomy and oxytocin infusion is more likely to result in PPH compared to prostaglandin-induced labours. The best way to minimize the risk of PPH is to correctly and actively manage the third stage of labour with an oxytocic agent, usually Syntometrine (Sandoz) and controlled cord traction, a process which has become routine in most obstetric units.

Two oxytocic agents are commonly employed in the third stage of labour, oxytocin and ergometrine: Syntocinon (synthetic oxytocin) takes effect rapidly when administered intravenously but has a short duration of action, while ergometrine is a powerful oxytocic with a long duration of action. The combination of Syntocinon with ergometrine (Syntometrine), is valuable due to the rapid onset of action of the Syntocinon and the sustained action of ergometrine [31]. Ergometrine has a powerful vasoconstrictor action and should be avoided or administered with extreme caution in patients with conditions such as hypertension and heart disease, as it may provoke serious hypertensive problems especially in patients with pre-eclampsia. Ergometrine also commonly provokes nausea. An overview of nine published controlled trials on the effects of routine oxytocic administration compared to placebo or to no prophylactic oxytocic, concluded that routine administration of oxytocics appeared to reduce the risk of postpartum haemorrhage by about 40% [32]. A similar review of trials has also been performed with regard to the choice of oxytocic, and Syntometrine appeared to be the safest and most effective, but the authors commented that there was still scope for a controlled trial comparing Syntometrine with oxytocin alone, which may have a better side-effect profile [33]. The Bristol third-stage trial [34] compared the neonatal and maternal morbidity of routine active management of the third stage of labour to physiological management. The study was halted following an interim analysis as active management significantly reduced the incidence of postpartum haemorrhage (5.9% vs. 17.9%), shortened the third stage (median time 5 min vs. 15 min) and also resulted in reduced neonatal packed-cell volume. The need for therapeutic oxytocics was also greater in the physiological management group (29.7% vs. 6.4%).

Prostaglandin analogues, which are potent stimulants of the myometrium, have also been used successfully in the active management of the third stage of labour, comparing favourably with ergotamine-treated patients [35]. However, the expense of prostaglandins compared to oxytocin and ergometrine is such that they are unlikely to replace conventional oxytocic treatment.

Management of postpartum haemorrhage

Despite the benefit of active management of the third stage of labour, PPH remains a problem. It should be anticipated where risk factors are present and crossmatched blood should be immediately available for such cases. The diagnosis of PPH is usually clear but the problem may be partly concealed in terms of overt haemorrhage, as intrauterine or intravaginal accumulation of blood may occur. The distinction between uterine atony and trauma is based on the state of the uterus. Bleeding despite a firm well contracted uterus is suggestive of trauma while a large, soft uterus suggests atony. Resuscitation measures as discussed above will be required. A thorough and well-illuminated examination of the cervix, vagina and perineum is essential to identify the bleeding source and the possibility of intra-abdominal bleeding or retroperitoneal bleeding must be borne in mind. Trauma to the birth canal can occur at any site although uterine and cervical damage is probably the least common. The damage should be efficiently repaired by an experienced operator and appropriate resuscitation measures including assessment of the coagulation system made. Again recourse to internal iliac artery ligation or hysterectomy if the bleeding is not controllable should not be delayed until the patient is in extremis. If the placenta is retained the uterus must be explored and emptied under anaesthesia. Infusion of

Syntocinon (20–40 iu/500 ml crystalloid) and transabdominal uterine massage is the conventional method to correct atony. Ergometrine and Syntometrine are also useful.

It is becoming clear that prostaglandins have a significant role in the management of atonic postpartum haemorrhage. They were first used by direct injection into the myometrium, either abdominally or vaginally [36]. Since then, intravenous and intramuscular routes using a variety of prostaglandins and prostaglandin analogues have been used successfully, often in patients who were unresponsive to conventional therapy and often avoiding surgery such as caesarean hysterectomy [37]. Hayashi, reviewing this topic [37], found a failure rate of 15% in 143 patients reported in five publications, with infection being associated with many of the failures. Hayashi *et al.* [38] have also reported a good outcome in 51 patients with PPH using the 15-methyl analogue of $PGF_{2\alpha}$ (carboprost) with 86% being successfully controlled. When carboprost (0.25 mg) was administered by intramuscular injections, 68% responded to a single dose, 20% required a second injection and 7% required multiple injections. Several further patients received intramyometrial injection after a single intramuscular injection with good response. The incidence of 'mild' side-effects, nausea, vomiting and diarrhoea was <10%. The intramyometrial route may be valuable when tissue perfusion is compromised due to hypovolaemic shock. Other studies have supported the efficacy and safety of this agent in both intramuscular and intramyometrial administration [39,40]; these included a multicentre study which obtained satisfactory control of bleeding in 208 out of 237 patients (87.8%) with refractory atonic postpartum haemorrhage after a single dose of carboprost, and an additional 17 successful outcomes were obtained after further administration of oxytocics. Thus the use of carboprost by intramuscular route in a dose of 0.25 mg, repeated as necessary every 1.5 h, appears an effective and safe treatment for atonic PPH. Other techniques such as intravenous infusion of $PGF_{2\alpha}$ and vaginal administration of PGE_2 pessaries have also been reported, but the experience is limited and carboprost would appear to be a more convenient preparation.

Conclusion

Haemorrhage constitutes a major problem in obstetric and gynaecological practice and appropriate and intensive care is required for these patients, involving not only the obstetrician and gynaecologist, but also the anaesthetist, haematologist and blood transfusion staff. Despite the encouraging reduction in deaths from major obstetric and gynaecological haemorrhage in recent years, there is no room for complacency in this potentially ever-present and catastrophic situation. An alertness and awareness to the possibility and extent of haemorrhage—the latter often being at least partly concealed by intra-abdominal or intrauterine bleeding, and the complications which may ensue, not least coagulation and renal failure—is important if we wish to maintain and further reduce the morbidity and mortality from this problem.

References

1 Department of Health. *Report on The Confidential Enquiries into Maternal Deaths in England and Wales.* HMSO, London (1989).

2 Huisjes, H.J. Spontaneous abortion. *Current Reviews in Obstetrics and Gynaecology* (Series Ed. Lind, T.). Churchill Livingstone, Edinburgh (1984).

3 Robinson, H.P. (1975) The diagnosis of early pregnancy failure by sonar. *Br. J. Obstet. Gynaecol.*, **82**, 849–857.

4 Department of Health and Social Security. *Report on Confidential Enquiries into Maternal deaths in England and Wales 1979–81.* HMSO, London (1986).

5 Scottish Home and Health Department. *Report on Maternal and Perinatal Deaths in Scotland 1981–85.* HMSO, London (1989).

6 Elder, M.G. Pre-operative cervical dilatation by vaginal pessaries containing a prostaglandin E_1 analogue. In: *Cervagem—a new Prostaglandin in Obstetrics and Gynaecology* (Ed. Karim, S.M.M.), (1983) pp. 134–138. MTP Press, Lancaster.

7 Calder, A.A. and Greer, I.A. Pharmacological modulation of cervical compliance in the first and second trimesters of pregnancy. In: *Seminars in Perinatology* (Ed. Huszar, G.), pp. 162–172. W.B. Saunders, Philadelphia (1991).

8 Centers for Disease Control: Ectopic Pregnancy in the United States 1970–83. CDC Surveillance Summaries (1986) *Morbidity and Mortality Weekly Report*, **35**, 29.

9 Atrash, H.K., Friede, A. and Hogue, C. (1987) Ectopic pregnancy mortality in the United States. *Obstet. Gynecol.*, **70**, 817–822.

10 Budowick, M., Johnson, T.R. and Genadry, R. (1980) The histopathology of the developing tubal ectopic pregnancy. *Fertil. Steril.*, **34**, 169–171.

11 Stabile, I. and Grudzinskas, J.G. (1990) Ectopic pregnancy: a review of incidence etiology and diagnostic aspects. *Obstet. Gynecol. Surv.*, **45**, 335–347.

12 de Crespigny, L.Ch. (1988) Demonstration of ectopic pregnancy by vaginal ultrasound. *Br. J. Obstet. Gynaecol.*, **95**, 1253–1256.

13 Kader, N. and Romero, R. (1981) Discriminatory hCG zone: its use in the sonographic evaluation for ectopic pregnancy. *Obstet. Gynecol.*, **58**, 156–161.

14 Kader, N. and Romero, R. (1987) Observation on the log hCG–time relationship in early pregnancy. *Am. J. Obstet. Gynecol.*, **157**, 73–76.

15 Abdella, T.N., Sibai, B.M., Hays, J.M. and Anderson, G.D. (1984) Perinatal outcome in abruptio placentae. *Obstet. Gynecol.*, **63**, 365–370.
16 Hurd, W.W., Midovovnik, M., Hertzberg, V. and Lavin, J.P. (1983) Selective management of abruptio placentae: A prospective study. *Obstet. Gynecol.*, **61**, 467–473.
17 Morrow, R.J. and Ritchie, J.W.K. (1988) Uteroplacental and umbilical artery blood velocity waveforms in placental abruption assessed by Doppler ultrasound. *Br. J. Obstet. Gynaecol.*, **95**, 723–724.
18 Egley, C. and Cefalo, R.C. Abruptio placentae. In: *Progress in Obstetrics and Gynaecology* (Ed. Studd, J.), Vol. 5 pp. 108–120. Churchill Livingstone, London (1985).
19 Pritchard, J.A. and Brekken, A.L. (1967) Clinical and laboratory studies on severe abruptio placentae. *Am. J. Obstet. Gynecol.*, **97**, 681–700.
20 Naeye, R.L. (1980) Abruptio placentae and placenta previa: frequency perinatal mortality and cigarette smoking. *Obstet. Gynecol.*, **55**, 701–704.
21 Paterson, M.E.L. (1979) The aetiology and outcome of abruptio placentae. *Acta Obstet. Gynecol. Scand.*, **58**, 31–35.
22 Krohn, M., Voigt, L., McKnight, B. *et al.* (1987) Correlates of placental abruption. *Br. J. Obstet. Gynaecol.*, **94**, 333–340.
23 Paintin, D.B. (1962) The epidemiology of antepartum haemorrhage. *J. Obstet. Gynaecol. Br. Commonw.*, **69**, 614–624.
24 Hill, D.J. and Beischer, N.E. (1981) Placenta praevia without antepartum haemorrhage. *Aust. NZ J. Obstet. Gynaecol.*, **20**, 21–24.
25 Clarke, S.L., Koonings, P. and Phelan, J.P. (1985) Placenta praevia/accreta and prior caesarean section. *Obstet. Gynecol.*, **66**, 89–93.
26 Letsky, E.A. *Coagulation Problems During Pregnancy.* Churchill Livingstone, Edinburgh (1985).
27 Newton, M. (1966) Post-partum haemorrhage. *Am. J. Obstet. Gynecol.*, **94**, 711–717.
28 Pritchard, J.A., Baldwin, R.M., Dickey, J.C. and Wiggins, K.M. (1962) Blood volume changes in pregnancy and puerperium. *Am. J. Obstet. Gynecol.*, **83**, 890–898.
29 Knott, P.D. (1990) The current problem of postpartum haemorrhage. *J. Obstet. Gynaecol.*, **10** (Suppl. 2), S4–S6.
30 Gilbert, L., Porter, W. and Brown, V.A. (1987) Postpartum haemorrhage—a continuing problem. *Br. J. Obstet. Gynaecol.*, **94**, 67–71.
31 Embrey, M.P., Barber, D.T.C. and Scudamore, J.M. (1963) Use of Syntometrine in prevention of postpartum haemorrhage. *Br. Med. J.*, **i**, 1387–1389.
32 Prendiville, W., Elbourne, D. and Chalmers, I. (1988) The effects of routine oxytocic administration in the management of the third stage of labour: an overview of the evidence from controlled trials. *Br. J. Obstet. Gynaecol.*, **95**, 3–16.
33 Elbourne, D., Prendiville, W. and Chalmers, I. (1988) Choice of oxytocic preparation for routine use in the management of the third stage of labour: an overview of the evidence from controlled trials. *Br. J. Obstet. Gynaecol.*, **95**, 17–30.
34 Prendiville, W.J., Harding, J.E., Elbourne, D. and Stirrat, G.M. (1988) The Bristol third stage trial: active versus physiological management of third stage of labour. *Br. Med. J.*, **297**, 1295–1300.

35 Bhattacharya, P., Devi, P.K., Jain, S. *et al.* (1988) Prophylactic use of 15(*S*), 15-methyl $PGF_{2\alpha}$ by intramuscular route for control of postpartum bleeding—A comparative trial with methylergometrine. *Acta. Obstet. Gynaecol. Scand.* (Suppl. 145), 13–16.

36 Takagi, S., Yoshida, T. and Togo, Y. (1976) The effects of intramyometrial injection of prostaglandin $F_{2\alpha}$ on severe postpartum haemorrhage. *Prostaglandins*, **12**, 565–579.

37 Hayashi, R.H. (1990) The role of prostaglandins in the treatment of postpartum haemorrhage. *J. Obstet. Gynaecol.*, **10** (Suppl. 2), S21–S24.

38 Hayashi, R.H., Castillo, M.S. and Noah, M.L. (1984) Management of severe postpartum haemorrhage with a prostaglandin $F_{2\alpha}$ analogue. *Obstet. Gynecol.*, **63**, 806–808.

39 Thiery, M. and Parewijck, W. (1985) Local administration of (15*S*), 15-methyl $PGF_{2\alpha}$ for management of hypotonic postpartum haemorrhage. *Z. Geburtshilfe Perinatol.*, **189**, 179–180.

40 Oleen, M.A. and Mariano J.P. (1989) Controlling refractory atonic postpartum haemorrhage with Hemabate sterile solution. *Am. J. Obstet. Gynecol.*, **162**, 205–208.

Chapter 6
Newborn and paediatric bleeding

RICHARD SOUTAR AND BRENDA GIBSON

The physiology and regulation of haemostasis in the adult has been discussed in Chapter 1. The haemostatic mechanism in the older child is similar to that of the adult. However, like many physiological systems, haemostasis is not fully mature in the neonate, and is further impaired in the preterm infant [1]. In addition, considerable differences exist in the clinical setting and aetiology of haemorrhagic problems in the neonate compared to the older child. They will therefore be considered separately.

Normal haemostasis in the neonate

Many of the procoagulants, natural anticoagulants and fibrinolytic proteins are gestation dependent and only reach adult values by 6 months of age (Table. 6.1), by which time coagulation parameters should be within the adult range. For the healthy term baby, this is of no clinical significance but if the neonate is premature and/or unwell there may be serious haemostatic problems contributing to morbidity, mortality and management difficulties.

Procoagulants

Coagulation factors do not cross the placenta in any significant degree [2]. Factors I (fibrinogen), V, VIII:C and von Willebrand factor (vWF) reach normal adult levels by the beginning of the third trimester [3]. Fetal fibrinogen, however, differs from adult fibrinogen, containing more sialic acid residues [4]. Although this may be regarded as a form of 'dysfibrinogenaemia' which may prolong *in vitro* tests of coagulation, it does not seem to have any adverse affect *in vivo* [5]. A fibrinogen level of <1.5 g/l should be considered abnormal in both the term and preterm neonate [6]. All other procoagulants are reduced at birth and are dependent upon gestational age (Table. 6.1). The vitamin K-dependent Factors (II, VII, IX, X)

Table 6.1 Procoagulant and anticoagulant values by gestational age**

		Weeks of gestation			
Procoagulant/anticoagulant*	Adult	37–41	33–36	25–32	≃20
Procoagulants					
I (g/l)	3.40	2.40	3.00	2.50	0.96
Cofactors (iu/ml)					
V	1.00	1.00	0.82	0.80	0.70
VIII : C	1.00	1.50	0.93	0.75	0.50
vWF : Ag	1.00	1.60	1.66	1.50	0.65
Vitamin K-dependent factors (iu/ml)					
II	1.00	0.52	0.45	0.32	0.16
VII	1.00	0.57	0.59	0.37	0.21
IX	1.00	0.35	0.41	0.22	0.10
X	1.00	0.45	0.44	0.38	0.19
Contact factors (iu/ml)					
XI	1.00	0.42	–	0.20	–
XII	1.00	0.44	0.25	0.22	–
PK	1.00	0.35	0.33	0.26	–
HMWK	1.00	0.64	–	0.28	–
XIII	1.00	0.61	–	0.11–0.40	0.30
Anticoagulants (iu/ml)					
AT-III	1.00	0.56	0.40	0.35	0.23
α_2-antiplasmin	1.00	0.78	–	–	–
C_1 inhibitor	1.00	1.00	–	–	–
α_2-macroglobulin	1.00	1.80	1.29	1.58	–
Plasminogen	1.00	0.49	0.38	0.35	–
Protein C : Ag	1.00	0.50†	0.38	0.29	0.10
Protein S . Ag	1.00	0.24†	–	–	–

* 1 unit is the amount of factor in 1 ml of normal plasma; means stated.
All values (except†) are venous and for the first 24 h of life.
All subjects received vitamin K at birth.
† Cord blood.
** Adapted from McDonald and Hathaway [36] with kind permission of Grune and Stratton Inc, and from Hathaway and Bonnar [35] with kind permission of Elsevier Science Publishing Company Inc.

are approximately 25% of adult values at 24 weeks' gestation and 50% by term [6]. The 'contact' Factors (XI, XII, prekallikrein (PK), high-molecular-weight kininogen (HMWK)) are 20–30% of adult values in the preterm and 30–50% in the term neonate [7,8].

Table 6.2 Reference ranges for the PT, APTT, and TCT in the neonate and infant [10,12]

Parameter(s)	30–36 weeks	Term	6 months	Adult
PT	13 ± 3	13 ± 3	12 ± 2	12 ± 2
APTT	54 ± 25	43 ± 12	36 ± 7	34 ± 7
TCT	25 ± 5	24 ± 5	26 ± 6	25 ± 5

The net effect is a reduced ability to generate thrombin and laboratory tests of clotting reflect this. The 'normal' values for the commonly used coagulation screening tests—prothrombin time (PT), thrombin clotting time (TCT), activated partial thromboplastin time (APTT)—may be prolonged at birth, especially the APTT, reflecting low levels of vitamin K-dependent and contact factors. Deficiency of the contact factors usually results in a greater prolongation of the APTT than a corresponding deficiency of Factor VIII : C or Factor IX : C [6].

Levels of Factor XIII in the term infant are about 50–70% of adult values [9]. As only small quantities are required for clot stabilization, this minor decrease in activity has no clinical significance.

The variety of 'normal' ranges quoted in the literature reflects differences in sample type (venous vs. capillary blood, cord vs. fetal blood), ethnic group and reagents used. Table 6.2 is derived from the results of Andrew *et al.* [10,12] who use calcium buffering to correct for the prolongation in TCT induced by fetal fibrinogen, and ellagic acid as an activating agent in the APTT system, thereby narrowing the normal range and increasing the usefulness of the APTT as a screening test in the newborn.

Natural anticoagulants

The naturally occurring anticoagulants antithrombin III (AT-III), protein C and protein S are gestation dependent (proteins C and S are also vitamin K requiring). At birth, the levels of these inhibitors are in the range at which thrombotic disorders occur in heterozygote deficient adults (AT-III 50–60% and protein C <60% of adult levels, respectively [11]. However, the combination of reduced levels of procoagulants, the presence of protein S principally in the unbound, active form and elevated levels of other inhibitors including C_1-esterase and α_2-macroglobulin appears to protect the healthy neonate from spontaneous thrombosis during the first few months of life [6].

Fibrinolysis and platelets

The fibrinolytic system is also immature at term with decreased plasmin generation in infants [12], although this does not appear to be of major clinical importance.

Platelets and the vessel wall

The neonate's platelet count is in the normal adult range, $>150 \times 10^9/l$ from the second trimester onwards [13]. Although formal platelet function tests (e.g. aggregation studies) may be impaired in the newborn, the neonatal bleeding time, probably the best test of platelet function and vessel wall integrity, is similar to (or shorter than) adult values [12].

The bleeding neonate

Although such infants present specific problems the approach to the bleeding neonate is no different, in principle, from any other clinical problem: history, examination, laboratory investigation, interpretation and diagnosis.

History

This should include that of the family, i.e. hereditary bleeding disorders, the sex of the child, the obstetric history (e.g. of maternal idiopathic thrombocytic purpura (ITP)), intrauterine infection or drug ingestion, problems during delivery and whether or not vitamin K was administered at birth.

Examination

The most important finding is whether the neonate is well or unwell. Bleeding in an otherwise healthy neonate suggests immune-mediated or inherited thrombocytopenia, a hereditary bleeding disorder or vitamin K deficiency. Bleeding in a sick neonate is usually due to disseminated intravascular coagulation (DIC) and may be associated with jaundice and pyrexia.

Acquired disorders, such as DIC, tend to present with generalized bleeding, whilst inherited disorders are usually localized (e.g. uncontrolled or excessive umbilical stump bleeding in Factor VIII : C or Factor XIII deficiency). The nature of the bleeding may also identify the problem, i.e. haemorrhage from the skin and mucous membranes suggests a platelet disorder, whilst deep-seated haematomas (haemarthroses in the older child) are characteristic of severe clotting-factor deficiencies. Purpura fulminans (overwhelming subcutaneous and submucosal haemorrhage) can be precipitated by acute infections [14] but is also characteristic of homozygous protein C deficiency [15]. The presence of petechiae solely over the presenting part postdelivery is normal and does not require investigation [16].

Laboratory investigation

This usually involves a full blood count with platelet number, blood film and baseline tests of the coagulation system. The PT principally tests the extrinsic coagulation pathway (Factors I, II, V, VII, and X), the APTT assesses the intrinsic pathway (Factors I, II, V, VIII, IX, X, XI, XII, PK, HMWK) and the TCT measures the conversion of fibrinogen to fibrin and is prolonged in hypofibrinogenaemia, and by heparin and fibrin degradation products (FDPs) (see below). Other routine tests include measurement of the fibrinogen level and a simple test to detect fibrinolysis (e.g. FDPs, generated by the lysis of fibrinogen and non-crosslinked fibrin) or D-dimers (generated by the lysis of crosslinked fibrin).

Interpretation may be difficult, not only because of the differing 'normal' range in the preterm and term neonate (see Table 6.2), but also because of problems with small samples (requiring the use of microtechniques), heparin contamination from lines (usually detected by prolongation of the TCT) and the necessity for anticoagulant ratios to be based on plasma, rather than whole blood, volume. Abnormal results which are not in keeping with the clinical picture should be repeated in the first instance.

Most bleeding neonates, and unfortunately particularly those the surgeon is likely to encounter, are unwell with an acquired coagulopathy, usually a combination of low birthweight, congenital or acquired infection and hypoxia. The less common situation where the bleeding neonate appears well will be discussed first.

Bleeding in the apparently well neonate

Neonatal thrombocytopenia

Thrombocytopenia (platelet count $<150 \times 10^9/l$) is perhaps the most common haemostatic abnormality in newborns, with approximately

20% of neonates admitted to one tertiary-care intensive therapy unit developing this problem [17]. Serious bleeding is a risk when the platelet count falls to $<30 \times 10^9/l$ [18] and active intervention should be considered. Although specific management depends upon the underlying cause, in the presence of active bleeding a trial of platelet concentrate (10–15 ml/kg) should be given.

In the healthy neonate, thrombocytopenia is usually due to immune destruction, either (i) autoimmune (secondary to maternal ITP) or (ii) alloimmune.

Autoimmune neonatal thrombocytopenia

Thrombocytopenia secondary to maternal ITP is caused by the passage of antiplatelet antibodies across the placenta leading to immune-mediated platelet destruction in the neonate. The diagnosis is confirmed by the maternal history and platelet count. The degree of maternal thrombocytopenia does not, however, correlate with the risk of neonatal thrombocytopenia, especially if the mother has undergone splenectomy [19]. Neither does the level of maternal platelet-associated IgG nor free antiplatelet antibodies in the maternal serum provide an accurate prediction of thrombocytopenia in the infant. Following birth the platelet count may continue to fall and may remain depressed for the first few months of life [20].

The main cause of morbidity and mortality is CNS haemorrhage. Management of both the mother and child is complex and outwith the scope of this chapter (for a useful review see [12]). If surgery is imperative, treatment is with steroids or intravenous immunoglobulin and haematological consultation is required. Infused platelets are rapidly destroyed and do not produce detectable increments but may lessen, or terminate, bleeding and should not be withheld in the face of haemorrhage.

Alloimmune neonatal thrombocytopenia

This has a frequency of 1 : 2000 births [12] and runs a more severe course than the autoimmune form above, from which it is distinguished by a normal maternal platelet count. The aetiology is similar to rhesus disease: a fetal platelet antigen (usually PL^{A1} (platelet antigen), present on the platelets of 98% of the general population) derived from the father, and absent on the maternal platelets, stimulates production of maternal alloantibody. The latter crosses the placenta leading to platelet destruction. There is a high probability of subsequent siblings being affected. CNS haemorrhage is again the main risk, may occur in up to 15% of infants and can be an antenatal event [12].

Except in an emergency, surgery should be delayed. The most effective therapy is transfusion with PL^{A1}-negative platelets. PL^{A1}-negative platelets may be available from a donor panel, or mother's platelets, washed to remove alloantibody, are an alternative, readily accessible source. In an emergency, random platelets should be given until compatible platelets are available.

Although congenital syndromes associated with thrombocytopenia due to failure of production are rare (e.g. thrombocytopenia with absent radii (TAR) syndrome [21], Fanconi's anaemia and Wiskott–Aldrich syndrome [22]), they frequently have associated cardiac or orthopaedic defects requiring surgery. The platelet count in infants with TAR syndrome will rise spontaneously with time and surgery should simply be delayed. For infants with other conditions, the necessity for surgery should be weighed against the risk and the anticipated life expectancy from the underlying disorder. If surgery is to proceed, platelet infusions will be required.

Platelet function may additionally be impaired by drugs (e.g. non-steroidal anti-inflammatories given therapeutically) to close the ductus, in neonates whose mothers have received aspirin [23], and in rare syndromes associated with impaired platelet function (e.g. Bernard–Soulier and Glanzmann syndromes).

Hereditary bleeding disorders

Haemophilias A and B, and von Willebrand's disease account for >90% of inherited bleeding disorders. All other bleeding disorders are rare. Haemophilia A has a frequency of 1 : 10 000 in the general population [24]; 30–40% of severely affected haemophiliacs (Factor VIII : C or IX : C, <2%) present in the newborn period [5], usually with bleeding at needle puncture sites, at the Guthrie test site, from circumcision wounds, or less commonly from the umbilical stump. Moderate (2–10%), mild (>10–40%) and the remaining 60–70% of severely affected haemophiliacs do not present until older when crawling and walking leads to self injury, or at the time of surgery. Diagnosis and treatment are discussed below.

Congenital Factor XIII (fibrin stabilizing factor) deficiency merits brief mention as it is an important cause of prolonged umbilical stump haemorrhage (80% of cases present in this way [25]). Routine coagulation tests are not affected. The diagnosis is made by demonstrating increased clot solubility in 1% monochloracetic acid or 5 M urea, and by a high index of clinical suspicion.

Haemorrhagic disease of the newborn

This condition, recognized in 1894 by Townsend [26], classically presents in the second or third day of life with bleeding from the gastrointestinal tract. Three patterns of clinical presentation are recognized based on the timing of bleeding complications and each is associated with a propensity for different sites of bleeding. However, all may be complicated by severe and even fatal haemorrhage. Vitamin K is required for the post-translational carboxylation of glutamic acid residues on the vitamin K-dependent coagulation Factors (II, VII, IX and X), and it is deficiency of these carboxylated factors which leads to prolongation of the PT and APTT and subsequent haemorrhage.

Classic haemorrhagic disease of the newborn (HDN) is readily preventable by administration of 1 mg vitamin K intramuscularly at delivery, or 2–4 mg orally. This should be routine practice in all neonatal units. Much controversy presently surrounds the need for subsequent doses of vitamin K to prevent late-onset HDN in exclusively breast-fed babies.

Treatment of HDN is by slow (to avoid anaphylaxis) intravenous administration of 1 mg vitamin K (intramuscular injections will lead to haematomas) together with fresh frozen plasma (FFP), 10–15 ml/kg in the presence of bleeding.

Bleeding in the sick neonate

The principal cause of bleeding in the sick neonate is DIC, which has been discussed elsewhere (Chapters 3 and 11). Similar mechanisms and complications occur in the neonate. Uncontrolled activation of the coagulation cascade leads to consumption of clotting factors and platelets, activation of fibrinolysis and fibrin deposition in vital organs and small vessels. The result is haemorrhage, organ ischaemia and microangiopathic haemolytic anaemia. The causes of DIC in the neonate are listed in Table 6.3. Laboratory manifestations include a prolonged PT, APTT, TCT, reduced fibrinogen, thrombocytopenia, elevated FDPs and possible evidence of red-cell fragmentation on the blood film. AT-III levels fall from an already low baseline predisposing to thrombosis, especially in the presence of indwelling catheters.

Table 6.3 Causes of DIC in the neonate

Fetal disorders	Maternal disorders
Infection: bacterial, viral, protozoal (toxoplasma)	Associated with:
Severe asphyxia/acidosis	Placental abruption
Giant haemangioma (Kasabach–Merritt syndrome)	Eclampsia
Hypothermia	Placenta praevia
Homozygous protein C deficiency	Dead fetal twin syndrome
	Amniotic fluid embolism

Therapy must primarily be directed at reversing the underlying cause: treating sepsis, restoring blood pressure, correcting acidosis and hypoxia. Treating the coagulopathy is purely supportive. The mainstay of treatment is with FFP (10–15 ml/kg), providing procoagulants and anticoagulants infused rapidly (over 30–45 min) for maximum benefit. If the platelet count falls to $<20 \times 10^9/l$ (higher if invasive procedures or surgery are planned) platelet concentrate should be considered: 1 iu/5 kg. Cryoprecipitate (10 ml/kg) will correct hypofibrinogenaemia (<1.5 g/l). Blood products will be rapidly consumed, requiring frequent laboratory monitoring and replacement therapy. Treatment should, however, be based on clinical rather than laboratory indicators. The neonate's small blood volume may limit or produce problems with replacement therapy, and exchange transfusion may be necessary to allow adequate volumes of red cells, platelets, FFP and cryoprecipitate to be given.

Bleeding in the older child

The approach to the bleeding child is similar to the bleeding neonate: history, examination, laboratory investigation.

History

This has been discussed above. The older child may present with bleeding or bruising after surgery (e.g. tonsillectomy, dental extraction, mild trauma or intramuscular immunization). There may be prolonged or recurrent epistaxis presenting to the ear–nose–throat surgeon. Confusion with non-accidental injury (NAI) may arise.

Examination

The nature of the bleeding may help to distinguish the underlying disorder. Haemorrhage from the skin and mucous membranes suggests a platelet disorder, while deep-seated haematomas and haemarthroses are characteristic of severe clotting-factor deficiencies.

Laboratory investigation

This follows the scheme previously outlined.

Inherited abnormalities

Haemophilia

Of cases of haemophilia 30% arise from new mutations [6], with no prior family history. In a previously undiagnosed child with postoperative haemorrhage, the laboratory diagnosis is straightforward and characterized by a normal platelet count and bleeding time, normal PT and isolated prolonged APTT. Although the APTT should be standardized to detect Factor VIII : c levels <30%, it may fail to identify mild forms of haemophilia and a factor assay may be appropriate despite a normal coagulation screen. Direct measurement of Factor VIII : c or Factor IX : c is necessary to confirm the diagnosis and to differentiate Factor VIII deficiency (haemophilia A) from Factor IX deficiency (Christmas disease, haemophilia B). Both behave identically clinically and are inherited in an X-linked manner.

The principle of treatment of bleeding episodes in haemophilia is the infusion of an appropriate blood product in sufficient quantity to raise the deficient factor to a haemostatic level. The risk of viral transmission with blood products should always be borne in mind and virucidally treated blood products or non-plasma-derived treatment given whenever possible. Therefore patients who can be managed without blood products, e.g. desmopressin (deamino-D-arginine vasopressin (DDAVP)) in mild haemophilia (see below), should be. With a combined surgical/haematological approach, surgery in the haemophiliac child should not present undue difficulty; in fact, these children often bleed less than their normal peers. Children treated with blood products before 1985 may be HIV-positive. Surgery, including dental extraction, should be performed as an inpatient procedure and only in an institution where there is adequate clinical and laboratory support available. Nursing, medical and anaesthetic staff should be aware that aspirin and intramuscular injections are contraindicated. The factor concentrate used should be the safest available and have undergone virucidal treatment.

Haemophilia A

The appropriate Factor VIII : c level depends upon the invasiveness of the surgery (see Chapter 2). Although formulae exist for calculating the desired dose, i.e.

$$\frac{\%\ \text{increment required} \times \text{weight (kg)}}{2}$$

the response can be unpredictable and hence for major surgery a test dose must be given preoperatively and the increment in Factor VIII : c should be measured. Failure to achieve a predicted rise suggests an inhibitor (allo-antibody) to Factor VIII : c and surgery in such situations is contraindicated, except in life-threatening circumstances: expert haematological advice must be sought. From the test dose, the factor half-life can be determined and this is the most sensitive means of detecting low levels of inhibitor.

The normal half-life of Factor VIII : c is 8–12 h; therefore initial therapy will be twice or thrice daily, with a possible postoperative 'boost'. Replacement therapy should begin 1 h preoperatively in a dose sufficient to raise the Factor VIII : c level to 80–100% and continued for 10–14 days to maintain Factor VIII : c levels of 50% for the first 4–5 days and thereafter to >30%. Factor VIII : c levels require monitoring pre- and posttreatment to determine the frequency of subsequent therapy. Purification using ion exchange or monoclonal antibodies produces a very concentrated, pure product, minimizing the volume to be infused, which may be critical in the young child and may have additional advantages of further reducing the risk of viral transmission and immunosuppression.

For dental extraction, a single dose of concentrate (20–25 iu/kg) may be satisfactory. Haemostasis, however, should be augmented by the administration of tranexamic acid (a fibrinolytic inhibitor) at 25 mg/kg, every 8 h for 5 days, with the first dose given preoperatively. Tranexamic acid is strictly contraindicated in the presence of haematuria as it can precipitate unlysable clot formation in the ureters; the urine should be tested prior to treatment. Local anaesthesia may be given by papillary infiltration [27] but nerve block requires replacement therapy

(40–50 iu/kg) and carries the risk of bleeding. Unlike dental extraction, fillings can be performed as an outpatient procedure. Preventive dental care is imperative.

For children with mild and moderate haemophilia, treatment with DDAVP is an attractive alternative avoiding the need for blood products. DDAVP, administered at a dose of 0.3 μg/kg in 20 ml saline over 20 min, acts by releasing stored Factor VIII : c (and vW Factor) from vascular endothelium. Side-effects, including transient facial flushing and, rarely, hypotension, do not usually limit therapy. Tranexamic acid can be given concurrently as DDAVP also stimulates fibrinolysis by releasing endothelial tissue plasminogen activator. Prior to surgery, a test DDAVP infusion must be given and factor increments checked to ensure an adequate response. The principal drawback to DDAVP is the phenomenon known as 'tachyphylaxis': repeated infusions lead to diminishing responses as endothelial stores become depleted [28], therefore DDAVP can only be used for approximately 3 days and is not suitable for major surgery.

Haemophilia B (Christmas disease)

Similar principles to the above apply for surgery in haemophilia B. Factor IX : c has a longer half life (18–24 h) than Factor VIII : c and once daily administration may be satisfactory. Pure Factor IX concentrates are now available but many concentrates still in use contain Factors II, X and protein C, and are thrombogenic, meriting the use of concurrent prophylactic subcutaneous heparin, and contraindicating simultaneous tranexamic acid. Antibodies to Factor IX : c are rare in haemophilia B [6]. The approximate dose of Factor IX concentrate can be calculated by the formula:

$$\frac{\%\ \text{increment} \times \text{weight (kg)}}{0.9}$$

For surgery, an initial Factor IX : c level of 60% should be achieved, followed by a level of 40% for several days and then >20% for a total of 7–10 days.

von Willebrand's disease

This complex disease (three major types and numerous subvariants [29]) is probably the commonest bleeding disorder, with mild forms having a prevalence estimated as high as 1% of the population [30].

Similar principles to haemophilia A apply: DDAVP is used where possible, together with tranexamic acid. For severely affected children who do not respond to DDAVP, for those in whom DDAVP is contra-indicated (e.g. type IIb) and for major surgery, replacement therapy is necessary. A factor concentrate rich in high-molecular-weight von Willebrand multimers will temporarily correct the bleeding time and these have recently been reviewed [31]. If haemostasis is not achieved with concentrate, cryoprecipitate can be used but this carries the risk of viral transmission if not virucidally treated. The frequency of treatment is guided by clinical bleeding, the bleeding time and laboratory coagulation tests.

Acquired abnormalities

Most of the acquired abnormalities of haemostasis are discussed in other chapters: renal disease (Chapter 8), liver and biliary disease (Chapter 7), neoplasia (Chapter 3) and infection and DIC (Chapter 11). Similar complications occur in paediatric and adult populations and do not merit reiterating. Many of these conditions require a tissue biopsy for diagnosis. Prior to organ biopsy the coagulation screen and bleeding time should be checked and abnormalities corrected, as far as possible.

Congenital heart disease (CHD) does, however, present specific problems. CHD is readily divided into cyanotic and acyanotic forms. Although impaired platelet function is recognized in both conditions most haemostatic problems arise with cyanotic CHD, principally thrombocytopenia and fibrinolytic activation [32].

Thrombocytopenia is usually mild ($<50 \times 10^9/l$) but can be severe, is related to the severity of hypoxia, worsens as the child ages and occurs in 40–50% of cases [32]. Fibrinolytic activation leads to hypofibrinogenaemia and elevated FDPs which impair platelet function and the conversion of fibrinogen to fibrin. The commonest 'coagulopathy' in cyanotic CHD is, however, artefactual: the raised haematocrit leads to overcitration of the plasma in the sample and spurious results.

The above abnormalities usually only produce minimal symptoms, e.g. easy bruising, until the time of corrective cardiac surgery when the combination of cyanotic CHD, cardiopulmonary bypass, infection, etc. may lead to haemostatic failure. Treatment, as before, is directed at correcting precipitating factors, e.g. hypoxia, sepsis, heparin reversal with protamine and supportive treatment with platelets, FFP and possibly cryoprecipitate.

Thrombosis and thromboembolism in childhood

Thromboembolic disease is common in the newborn period, predominantly in the presence of vascular catheters. Severe vessel obstruction has been reported to occur in 1% of neonates with umbilical artery catheters [33]. The incidence then declines until the second decade and thereafter rises to adult levels. Table 6.4 lists some of the inherited and acquired conditions associated with thrombosis and thromboembolism. Detection is along adult lines, i.e. ultrasound and radionuclide scanning.

Treatment

Treatment is directed at removing the thrombus, either medically (thrombolytic therapy) or surgically (thrombectomy and embolectomy) and at inhibiting propagation of the clot by anticoagulation, initially by heparin and then with warfarin if recurrence is a possible or likely event.

Thrombolytic experience is limited in children and adapted from adult practice. Both streptokinase and urokinase have been used and carry the same risks and contraindications as in adults. Suitable doses

Table 6.4 Causes of thrombosis in the neonate and child

Venous thrombosis	Arterial thrombosis
Acquired	*Acquired*
Vascular trauma	Vascular trauma
Vascular stasis	Arteritis
Dehydration	Thrombotic thrombocytopenic purpura
DIC	Tranexamic acid
Raised haematocrit	Prothrombin concentrates
Nephrotic syndrome	Kawasaki disease
Prothrombin concentrates	DIC
Tranexamic acid	
Liver disease	
Inherited	*Inherited*
AT-III deficiency	Congenital heart disease
Protein C deficiency	Familial hypercholesterolaemia
Protein S deficiency	Homocystinuria
Plasminogen deficiency	
Dysfibrinogenaemia	
Congenital heart disease	
Sickle-cell disease	

and a discussion of the careful laboratory monitoring required are given by Corrigan [34]. Heparin is given intravenously, initially as a bolus injection of 50–75 iu/kg followed by a continuous infusion at 15–25 iu/kg/h. The APTT should probably be maintained at 1.5–2.5-fold the patient's own preheparin control time [34], provided this was not prolonged. Warfarin can initially be given in a dose of 0.1 mg/kg/day and the dose altered according to the PT ratio (International Normalized Ratio).

Conclusion

Haemorrhagic and thrombotic disorders are common in childhood. They present additional problems during surgery. With surgical and haematological liaison, together with laboratory and blood-bank support, they should not, however, present unsurmountable difficulties.

References

1 Corrigan, J.J. *Haemorrhagic and Thrombotic Diseases in Childhood and Adolescence*, pp. 1–16. Churchill Livingstone, Edinburgh (1985).

2 Gitlin, D., Kumate, J., Urresti, J. *et al.* (1964) The selectivity of the human placenta in the transfer of plasma proteins from mother to fetus. *J. Clin. Invest.*, **43**, 1938–1951.

3 Bell, E.J. and Corrigan, J.J. (1973) Platelet counts, fibrinogen concentrations and Factor VIII levels in healthy infants according to gestational age. *J. Paediatr.*, **82**, 1029–1032.

4 Galankis, D.K. (1984) Dysfibrinogenaemia: a current perspective. *Clin. Lab. Med.*, **4**, 295–418.

5 Donaldson, V.H. Hemorrhagic disorders of neonates. In: *Disorders of Haemostasis* (Eds Ratnoff, O.D. & Forbes, C.D.), 2nd edn, pp. 423–458. W.B. Saunders, Philadelphia (1991).

6 Gibson, B.E.S. Haemostasis. In: *Paediatric Haematology* (Eds Lilleyman, J.S. & Hann, I.M.). Churchill Livingstone, Edinburgh (1992).

7 Gordon, E.M., Ratnoff, O.D., Saito, H. *et al.* (1980) Studies on some coagulation factors in the newborn. *Am. J. Pediatr. Hematol. Oncol.*, **2**, 213–216.

8 Barnard, D.R., Simmons, M.A., Hathaway, R.E. (1979) Coagulation studies on extremely premature infants. *Pediatrics*, **13**, 1330–1335.

9 Henriksson, P., Hedner, U., Nilsson, I.M. *et al.* (1974) Fibrin stabilising factor (Factor XIII) in the fetus and newborn infant. *Pediatr. Res.*, **8**, 789–791.

10 Andrew, M., Paes, B., Johnston, M. *et al.* (1990) Development of the hemostatic system in the neonate and young infant. *Am. J. Pediatr. Hematol. Oncol.*, **12**, 95–104.

11 Andersson, T.R., Bangstad, J. and Lassen, M.C. (1988) Heparin cofactor II, anti-

thrombin III and Protein C in plasma from term and preterm infants. *Acta Paediatr Scand.*, **12**, 485–488.

12 Andrew, M. (1991) An approach to the management of infants with impaired haemostasis. In: *Pediatric hematology* (Eds Hann, I.M. & Gibson, B.E.S.), *Baillière's Clin. Haematol.*, **4**(2), 254–260.

13 Ablin, A.R., Kushner, J.H., Murphy, A. *et al.* (1961) Platelet enumeration in the neonatal period. *Pediatrics*, **28**, 822–824.

14 Corrigan, J.J. *Haemorrhagic and Thrombotic Disease in Childhood and Adolescence*, pp. 177–206. Churchill Livingstone, Edinburgh (1985).

15 Branson, H.E., Katz, J., Marble, R. *et al.* (1983) Inherited Protein C deficiency and chronic relapsing purpura fulminans in a newborn infant. *Lancet*, **ii**, 1165–1168.

16 Poley, J.R. and Stickler, G.B. (1961) Petechiae in the newborn infant. *Am. J. Dis. Child.*, **102**, 111–114.

17 Castle, V., Andrew, M., Kelton, J. *et al.* (1986) Frequency and mechanism of neonatal thrombocytopenia. *J. Pediatr.*, **108**, 749–755.

18 Hedge, U.M. (1985) Immune thrombocytopenia in pregnancy and the newborn. *Br. J. Obstet. Gynaecol.*, **92**, 657–659.

19 Epstein, R.D., Lozner, E.L., Cobbey, T.S. *et al.* (1950) Congenital thrombocytopenic purpura; purpura haemorrhagica in pregnancy and in the newborn. *Am. J. Med.*, **9**, 44–56.

20 Karpatkin, M., Porges, R.F., Karpatkin, S. (1981) Platelet counts in women with autoimmune thrombocytopenia: Effects of steroid administration to the mother. *New Engl. J. Med.*, **305**, 936–939.

21 Emery, T.L., Gordon, R.R., Rendle-Short, J. *et al.* (1957) Congenital amegakaryocytic thrombocytopenia with congenital deformities and a leukaemoid blood picture in the newborn. *Blood*, **12**, 567–576.

22 Aldrich, R.A., Steinberg, A.G. and Campbell, D.C. (1954) Pedigree demonstrating a sex-linked recessive condition characterised by draining ears, eczematoid dermatitis, and bloody diarrhea. *Pediatrics*, **13**, 133–139.

23 Bleyer, W.A. and Breckenridge, R.T. (1970) Studies in the detection of adverse drug reactions in the newborn. II. The effect of prenatal aspirin on newborn haemostasis. *JAMA*, **213**, 2049–2053.

24 Levine, P.H.P. Clinical manifestations and therapy of haemophilia A and B. In: *Haemostasis and Thrombosis* (Eds Coleman, R.W., Hirsh, J., Marder, V.J. & Salzman, E.W.), Vol. 6, 2nd edn. pp. 97–111. J.B. Lippincott, Philadelphia (1987).

25 Losowsky, M.S. and Miloszewski, K.J. (1977) Annotation: Factor XIII. *Br. J. Haematol.*, **37**, 1–5.

26 Townsend, C.W. (1984) The haemorrhagic disease of the newborn. *Arch. Paediatr.*, **11**, 559–565.

27 Ah Pin, P.J. (1987) The use of intraligamental injections in haemophiliacs. *Br. Dent. J.*, **162**, 151–152.

28 Isola, L., Forster, A. and Aledort, L.M. (1984) Desamino-D-arginine vasopressin and bleeding time in von Willebrand's disease. *Ann. Intern. Med.*, **101**, 719–720.

29 Tuddenham, G.D. Inherited bleeding disorders. In: *Postgraduate Haematology* (Eds Hoffbrand, A.V. & Lewis, S.M.), Vol. 23, 3rd edn, pp. 627–654. Heinemann, Oxford (1989).

30 Rodeghiero, F., Castaman, G. and Dini, E. (1987) Epidemiological investigation of the prevalence of von Willebrand's disease. *Blood*, **69**, 454–459.

31 Fricke, W.A. and Wong, M.-Y. (1989) Characterization of von Willebrand factor in Factor VIII concentrates. *Am. J. Hematol.*, **31**, 41–45.

32 Corrigan, J.J. *Haemorrhagic and Thrombotic Disease in Childhood and Adolescence*, pp. 110–112. Churchill Livingstone, Edinburgh (1985).

33 O'Neill, J.A., Neblett, W.W. and Born, M.L. (1981) Management of major thromboembolic complications of umbilical complications of umbilical artery catheters. *J. Paediatr. Surg.*, **16**, 972–978.

34 Corrigan, J.J. *Haemorrhagic and Thrombotic Diseases in Childhood and Adolescence*, pp. 163–171. Churchill Livingstone, Edinburgh (1985).

35 Hathaway, W.E. and Bonnar, J. *Hemostasic Disorders of the Pregnant Woman and Newborn Infant*. Elsevier, New York (1987).

36 McDonald, M.M. and Hathaway, W.E. (1983) Neonatal haemorrhage and thrombosis. *Sem. Perinatol.*, **7**, 213–225.

Chapter 7
Liver and biliary tract

PAUL McMASTER AND MARK DEAKIN

Patients with hepatic dysfunction, obstructive jaundice and endotoxaemia associated with hepatobiliary sepsis, can readily develop acquired coagulation disorders. In addition the liver receives 300–800 ml of blood via the hepatic artery and 1–2 litres of blood through the portal vein every minute. It is not surprising therefore that hepatic and biliary problems (Table 7.1) can present the general surgeon with significant bleeding problems.

There are specific clinical problems associated with liver disease, portal hypertension, hepatic resection, trauma, transplantation and bleeding from the biliary tree, yet increasingly approaches are available which can reduce these risks and help avoid problems. These approaches will be described and a brief review of specific clinical problems outlined.

General principles and measures to prevent bleeding when operating on the liver and biliary tree

Preoperative clotting abnormality

The cause of bleeding in liver dysfunction and disease is multifactorial. Malabsorption of fat-soluble vitamin K in obstructive jaundice as well

Table 7.1 Hepatic and biliary problems associated with bleeding

Hepatic 'dysfunction'	Obstructive jaundice Cirrhosis—portal hypertension Varices—hypersplenism Coagulopathy
Normal liver	Surgical resection Trauma
Hepatic	Transplantation

Table 7.2 Preoperative clotting abnormalities in obstructive jaundice or hepatic dysfunction

Haemoglobin	Decreased
Platelets	Decreased
Factors II, VII, IX, X (vitamin K)	Decreased
PT	Increased
PTT	Increased
Fibrinogen, fibrin degradation products (DIC)	Increased

as in hepatic dysfunction leads to impaired hepatic synthesis of clotting Factors II, VII, IX and X. In more severe liver disease, levels of Factor V are also reduced and as the severity increases fibrinogen deficiency develops. Factor VIII synthesis is usually preserved. Activated clotting factors are normally removed by the hepatic reticuloendothelial system, and in endotoxaemia an acute, subacute or chronic consumptive coagulopathy may develop. Anaemia and thrombocytopenia commonly occur, especially when portal hypertension leads to hypersplenism.

Factor VII has a short half-life (4–5 h) and therefore the prothrombin time (PT) is a sensitive index of liver synthetic function. The partial thromboplastin time (PTT) is also prolonged and low levels of fibrinogen, increased levels of fibrin degradation products and short clot lysis time may suggest disseminated intravascular coagulation (DIC) (Table 7.2).

Preoperative and intraoperative monitoring of PT and PTT are required at intervals. Levels of fibrinogen degradation products (FDPs) warn of DIC and the thromboelastograph which produces a visual interpretation of clot formation and lysis can be a valuable aid to the early identification of clotting abnormality. Platelet count should be maintained above 80×10^9/l. Levels of clotting factors can be maintained by the infusion of fresh frozen plasma (FFP), which contains all clotting factors, but when fibrinogen levels and Factor VIII levels fall, then cryoprecipitate, which contains approximately 12-fold the concentration of Factor VIII than FFP, is required.

Surgical exposure

The key to surgery of the liver and biliary tree is abdominal exposure. Good exposure can be achieved with an upper abdominal curved transverse incision with a vertical midline extension if necessary—the so-

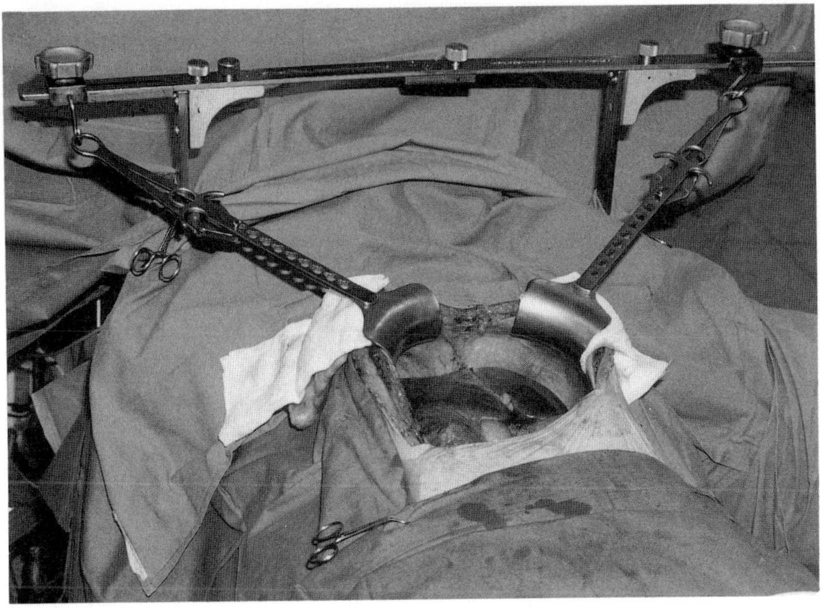

Fig. 7.1 Upper abdominal self-retaining retractor and exposure used for hepatobiliary surgery.

called Mercedes incision. Retraction is vital and can be best achieved with an overtable bar with two extensions to retract each costal margin (Fig. 7.1).

Dissection techniques

In the patient with hepatic impairment, especially portal hypertension, haemostasis must be maintained throughout the dissection. This often entails dissection with diathermy (bipolar in children) and coagulating current. Small vessels that are prone to later ooze, especially around the porta hepatis, are divided between ligatures. In this way, the dissection is slow but the anatomy is accurately defined and should a coagulopathy subsequently develop, oozing surfaces are minimized. In extended complex surgery lasting many hours it is not unusual for coagulation to deteriorate due to dilution/consumption of clotting factors. Areas of dissection, initially 'dry', may begin to bleed rapidly: thus meticulous haemostasis must be the rule.

During the anhepatic phase of liver transplantation veno-venous bypass between the portal vein and axillary vein decreases portal pressure and thereby reduces bleeding and progressive oedema of the small bowel. This technique can also be used during operative surgery on patients with severe portal hypertension and in complex hepatic surgery. In this situation, if the portal vein is to be left undivided, bypass can be established using the inferior mesenteric vein.

Achieving haemostasis

If dissection has proceeded with care, then ooze from cut surfaces should not be a problem. There are those instances, however, where large raw areas exist after dissection where complete haemostasis may be difficult to achieve. These areas are the diaphragmatic bare area behind the liver, the area around the retrohepatic cava and the divided liver parenchyma. In these circumstances, systematic under-running with a 4/0 prolene stitch and the application of haemostatic foams or fibrin glue coat (Tisseal, Immuno Ltd, Vienna) are often successful (Table 7.3). In addition, there are several ways to apply a diathermy current: the sapphire coagulator is slow and the tip may adhere to tissue, spray diathermy is available and the argon beam coagulator (Baird) has been the most significant advance. This machine enables a coagulating diathermy current to be conducted along a jet of argon gas. This results in surface blood being blown away leaving the diathermy current to produce a superficial char over an area of $0.5\,cm^2$. This device when used as a 'paintbrush' over raw areas rapidly stops oozing.

Liver packing may rarely be needed but, in the presence of a coagulopathy and physically uncontrollable ooze, it is unwise to persist with local measures. Large abdominal rolls are used to pack around the liver but can be wrapped in Op-site or other plastic material to aid removal.

Table 7.3 Techniques to control 'oozing'

Improve coagulation
Platelets
Suture
Diathermy coagulation
Bipolar
Argon beam coagulation
Topical haemostatic agents
Fibrin glue spray — Tisseal spray

The patient is returned to the intensive care unit where the coagulation defect is controlled and packs are removed within 48 h. External abdominal binders are an alternative but both packing and binders cause a rise in intra-abdominal pressure, which in turn leads to respiratory embarrassment. A rise in intra-abdominal pressure >25 mmHg may result in renal shutdown and re-exploration may be required.

The cirrhotic liver with portal hypertension

Bleeding varices

The general surgeon may be presented with a complex problem. Patients with known portal hypertension are sometimes referred for the following:

1 Treatment to 'prevent' variceal bleeding.
2 During an episode of acute bleeding.
3 Following an acute bleed to prevent recurrence.
4 For consideration of hepatic transplantation.

Treatment to 'prevent' variceal bleeding

Of patients with cirrhosis, 50% will die during their first episode of variceal bleeding, although variceal bleeding only occurs in approximately 30% of all cirrhotics. Prophylactic sclerotherapy has been advocated but even in groups with a high risk of bleeding there is no convincing benefit [1]. Shunt surgery has no role in the prevention of the first bleed, as results are worse than in controls [2–5]. This is mainly because of the low incidence of bleeding in controls and the availability of successful treatment of the first bleed when it occurs.

The best hope for the future lies with pharmacological manipulation of portal pressure, although trials with propranolol have thus far shown only marginal benefit.

During an episode of acute bleeding

A patient-management plan involves a careful assessment of the cause of portal hypertension and the prognosis of underlying liver disease. The site of bleeding should be determined and it should be remembered that there is an increased incidence of bleeding from gastric and duodenal ulcers in cirrhotic patients. Gastric varices, hypertensive gastropathy and, rarely, duodenal varices pose difficult clinical problems.

Primary care

All patients should be resuscitated ideally in an intensive care or high dependency unit with full monitoring. Encephalopathic patients and those at risk of aspiration may need elective ventilation. Careful endoscopy with airway protection should provide a diagnosis of the site of bleeding and sclerotherapy at the first endoscopy will control bleeding in the majority of patients. Where initial sclerotherapy does not control bleeding, then a combination of vasopressin and nitroglycerin infusions, with or without balloon tamponade, may help. Thus sclerotherapy in experienced hands has largely replaced prolonged pharmacological/balloon initial management techniques.

Full evaluation of each patient may take 3–4 days. The aetiology of portal hypertension and the severity of underlying liver disease influences the outcome. Standard work-up includes a full history, blood count and film, liver-function tests, full clotting studies, α-fetoprotein estimation, α_1-antitrypsin levels, autoantibodies and hepatitis virology. Further investigation may need specialized hepatological and liver-unit support and includes transjugular liver biopsy, Doppler portal assessment and angiography.

Many cirrhotic patients will decompensate following intestinal bleeding and full intensive support will be needed to support the liver. This will usually include glucose monitoring, vitamin K plus clotting factors, lactulose/neomycin, frequent blood cultures and culture of ascitic fluid.

The role for oesophageal transection

Should bleeding continue following two episodes of sclerotherapy, repeating sclerotherapy is less effective and surgical intervention may be needed. In this situation, the advantage of oesophageal transection is that it has no effect on background encephalopathy. Oesophageal staple gun transection can also be used as an alternative to sclerotherapy in acute bleeding, with no adverse effects on outcome and a lower incidence in rebleeding [5]. Whether more extensive devascularization should also be performed is controversial. The upper half of the stomach can be devascularized abdominally with delayed recurrence of varices [6]. Extensive abdominothoracic devascularization in addition to transection is used in Japan with good results [7] but in Western patients, where the disease pattern is different, its use has not been supported [8]. However, it should clearly be borne in mind that in the non-alcoholic patient in whom further hepatic deterioration occurs, hepatic transplantation will usually now be considered. Surgical intervention should be considered with care and ideally discussed with colleagues in specialized liver units to minimize the problems which may occur later.

The role for emergency shunting

Encephalopathy following portosystemic shunts is unpredictable in onset and can be severely incapacitating. Shunts are associated with an unacceptably high rate of hepatic failure but appear to be better tolerated by patients with alcoholic cirrhosis [9]. The important variables when considering the place of emergency shunting are the cause and degree of liver dysfunction and the site of pathology, hepatic or extrahepatic. The patient with well-preserved liver function may be a shunt candidate but if hepatic reserve is limited, transplantation is a better option.

The role for emergency liver transplantation

Survival of variceal bleeding is more related to the underlying disease and Child's classification than to successful treatment. In patients who are candidates for liver transplantation (see below), then transplantation in the acute bleeding phase may be necessary to control both portal hypertension and underlying liver disease. Early discussion with a transplant centre is recommended.

Following an acute bleed

Long-term management depends on the risk of rebleeding and development of liver failure. Our current management scheme is to continue sclerotherapy at weekly or 2-weekly intervals until varices are obliterated. Patients then enter a surveillance programme. Shunt surgery may have a place in patients with well-preserved hepatic function and frequent uncontrolled bleeds.

Distal shunting has come to be preferred over portacaval shunts. Portacaval shunts may complicate liver transplantation, whereas distal shunts do not directly interfere with transplantation [10] unless the shunt clots, with subsequent portal vein thrombosis. The incidence of rebleeding may be greater following distal shunts, however [11]. The earlier distal splenorenal shunt consisted of splenectomy followed by end-to-side anastomosis of the splenic and renal vein. The distal splenorenal or Warren shunt without splenectomy [12] has the theoretical advantage of selective left-sided shunting without diminishing portal flow. Trials have, however, described conflicting results when the incidence of encephalopathy is compared to standard shunts, and even in Warren's group [12] longer-term results have not been as good as in patients treated initially by sclerotherapy [13]. The best results are seen in the group of patients treated primarily by sclerotherapy with splenorenal shunts being performed if bleeding recurs, despite the sclerotherapy programme. This is our current policy in patients who are not transplant candidates.

Extrahepatic (portal or splenic vein thrombosis)

These patients form a special group. In Western society, prehepatic obstruction comprises 5–10% of all patients with portal hypertension but in developing countries this proportion may reach 40%. Extrahepatic obstruction is the most commonly encountered cause of variceal bleeding in childhood. Diagnosis is made on clinical presentation and visceral angiography.

Patients with extrahepatic obstruction often present with well-tolerated episodes of massive haematemesis without encephalopathy. On clinical examination, the spleen is enlarged but the liver is normal sized and liver-function tests are normal. Ascites is uncommon. The diagnosis is confirmed by ultrasound of the portal and splenic veins and venous phase visceral angiography. As previously, the initial treatment is directed towards blood replacement and controlling bleeding with sclerotherapy. Since hepatic reserve is undiminished, this group of patients are good candidates for shunt surgery rather than repeated sclerotherapy if control is not readily achieved.

Budd–Chiari syndrome

The features of this syndrome follow hepatic vein thrombosis or vena caval obstruction, but can occasionally be due to central hepatic veno-occlusive disease. The prognosis of this group of patients is variable as the majority of patients are eventually shown to have underlying myeloproliferative disease, but the condition can occur in pregnancy, in association with the oral contraceptive pill, in association with hepatic, renal or adrenal carcinomas or occasionally in association with inferior vena caval webs. There is a spectrum of presentations, from a chronic picture often presenting with bleeding oesophageal varices to patients with rapidly deteriorating liver function.

Variceal bleeds can usually be controlled by injection sclerotherapy. In the absence of a caval web or thrombosis, then a portacaval shunt can be formed. Where the inferior vena cava is occluded or there is a significant pressure gradient, the results of mesoatrial shunts using reinforced PTFE (polytetrafluoroethylene) have been encouraging [14,15]. In patients with rapidly deteriorating liver function, shunting alone may produce an improvement but liver transplantation may be necessary.

Consideration of hepatic transplantation

It is important now to be aware that hepatic replacement is increasingly seen as the logical treatment of portal hypertension when hepatic function deteriorates. While liver replacement would rarely be recommended for portal hypertension itself, it is important to remember that portal hypertension is merely a symptom, usually of profound underlying disease. Its treatment has little impact on overall survival if the underlying liver disease progresses!

If the patient's prognosis is limited by hepatic failure and decompensation, then transplantation is a better option than repeated sclerotherapy or even shunt surgery.

Indications

The main indications for liver transplantation are:

- *In adults*: chronic liver disease; acute liver failure (excluding active alcoholics).
- *In children*: biliary atresia; inborn errors of metabolism and acute liver failure.

Contraindications

The following are considered absolute contraindications for transplantation:

- Active sepsis outside the liver.
- HIV antibody positivity.
- Metastatic malignancy.

Relative contraindications are:

- Previous upper abdominal surgery.
- Hepatitis B or delta hepatitis.
- Hyponatraemia.
- Pulmonary hypertension.
- Alcoholism.

Some of the above relative contraindications may be corrected before transplantation, while others which cannot be corrected will increase the risk of transplantation. It is important not to allow the patient's condition to deteriorate to a state which may prejudice the chance of a successful transplant, yet transplantation with its risks should not be offered to patients whose predicted survival without transplantation is in years. Careful specialized evaluation may be needed.

Liver trauma

The liver, the largest abdominal organ, is frequently injured in road-traffic accidents and is involved in 30% of patients undergoing laparotomy for penetrating abdominal injury and around 20% for blunt abdominal trauma. The majority of hepatic lesions are managed without difficulty and bleeding ceases, but treatment of major injuries such as to the porta, retrohepatic cava and extensive hepatic disruption is more difficult [16].

Diagnosis

Liver injuries are rarely isolated and should be suspected in any patient with multiple injury. Tenderness or bruising of the upper abdomen, particularly with seat-belt marks and fractured lower ribs following road accidents should arouse suspicion. In penetrating trauma, the entry and exit wounds are important but the intra-abdominal track of missiles can be variable. Peritoneal lavage and laparoscopy are useful aids but in stable patients computed axial tomography is the mainstay of diagnosis, particularly in blunt trauma. The recognition of hepatic injury in a stable patient with lacerations or subcapsular haematomas requires complete patient monitoring, with the need for surgical intervention being repeatedly reassessed. In this way approximately 80% of patients, and particularly children, with hepatic injury can be treated conservatively.

Operative options

The key to management of the majority of patients is rapid resuscitation, assessment and control of simultaneous injuries, early diagnosis of liver injury and in case of haemodynamic instability the recognition of the need for operation (Fig. 7.2).

The surgeon faced with an unstable patient needs carefully to plan the intervention following full evaluation and resuscitation. While the majority of liver injuries are minor/moderate capsular and parenchymal tears easily controlled by simple sutures, few younger surgeons will forget the experience of finding *major damage* for whom inadequate resuscitation/anaesthesia/blood-bank support is available. Now is not the time *to begin* to think through surgical options! Time spent in recovery/planning is never wasted.

Wide exposure is required for all operative treatment, with an upper abdominal self-retaining retractor such as is used for resectional liver surgery.

The description of, and comparison of, results from different centres has been delayed by the failure to adopt a classification of liver injury. A simple grading has much to recommend it, being related both to treatment and eventual outcome (Table 7.4).

Grade 1 *Injuries may not need surgical intervention in the absence of continued bleeding,* if it is identified on a CT scan. If discovered at laparotomy, then superficial suture or the application of haemostatic foams is all that is required.

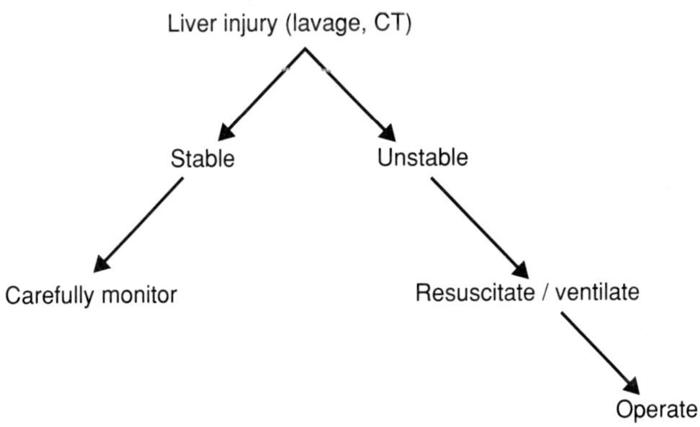

Fig. 7.2 Management and diagnosis of liver injury.

Table 7.4 Grading of severity of hepatic trauma (modified from [17]). See text

Grade 1:	Simple superficial laceration
Grade 2:	Major parenchymal injury
Grade 3:	Major complex injury, massive bleeding or extensive parenchymal destruction
Grade 4:	Hepatic venous injury

Grade 2 *Blunt trauma resulting in significant parenchymal disruption.* This can be successfully treated non-operatively particularly in children [18]. Biliary leaks and abscess formation are a surprisingly infrequent complication and can be treated by percutaneous placement of pig-tail drains under ultrasound guidance. However, meticulous continuous monitoring is needed and this conservative approach in adults remains controversial.

Grade 3 *Major complex injury with massive bleeding or extensive parenchymal destruction.* This requires laparotomy. Following assessment of other intra-abdominal injuries, the sequence of events should be first, local compression, then the Pringle manoeuvre (compression of the portal structures), followed by finger fracture of the liver to provide adequate exposure of the bleeding area. Haemostasis is best achieved by individual suture ligation of lacerated vessels and bile ducts followed by debridement of non-viable hepatic parenchyma. Any dead space can be filled with an omental pedicle based on the right or left gastroepiploic vessels, held in place by interrupted sutures. Using such an approach it is possible to achieve a mortality rate of around 5% [17]. Formal lobectomies are rarely indicated except in complete lobar destruction, and carry an excessive mortality rate of >30% in some series.

In the face of major bleeding, the Pringle manoeuvre is safe for times at least up to 1 h [19]. Hepatic artery ligation is an alternative to local suture ligation but fails to control bleeding from hepatic veins: haemorrhage continues in around 15% of patients and there is a 25% incidence of early rebleeding [20,21]. In this situation, coagulation is frequently deteriorating because of clotting-factor dilution and rather than embark on complex surgery, direct packing of the injury site may gain temporary control.

The abdomen is then closed and the patient monitored continuously in intensive therapy unit on ventilation with strenuous efforts to improve clotting (*Note*: exclude DIC, see Chapters 3 and 11).

Pack removal should be performed within 48–72 h of injury following correction of the clotting abnormality [22,23].

Once under control by packing, if there is more extensive hepatic or biliary injury than can be dealt with locally, then transfer to a specialist centre is an option [24].

Grade 4 *Hepatic venous injury.* When the inferior vena cava is injured this occurs most commonly below the liver. In 1983 Millikan *et al.* [25] reported a series of 58 cases of caval injury. Only 12 of these involved the retrohepatic cava although 16 others involved the suprarenal cava; 10 of the 12 patients with retrohepatic injuries died. In this situation, patients commonly have multiple venous and portal injuries. For retrohepatic caval injuries, rapid vascular isolation of the liver is possible [26].

The infrahepatic cava is approached by reflecting the right colon towards the left upper quadrant and the suprahepatic cava by median sternotomy. Once isolation has been successfully accomplished, then a variety of atriocaval shunts have been devised but with only limited success [25–28]. However, direct approach to the injury using fracture of the injured liver is normally possible without shunting.

Hepatic resection

Haemorrhage is the main complication of liver resection, but it is preventable with careful preparation and technique. The key to uncomplicated liver surgery is a clear understanding of the anatomy of the liver, preoperative assessment as to the resectability of the lesion to be removed and an estimation of hepatic reserve following resection.

The functional anatomical model is now well established [29] and can be understood simply with regard to the position of the three main hepatic veins (left, right and middle) (Fig. 7.3). The middle hepatic vein is seen to divide the liver into halves, the functional right and left lobes, each supplied by the right or left branches of the hepatic artery and portal vein. The right and left hepatic veins run along the right and left portal scissura dividing each half liver into two sectors, each supplied by individual branches of the hepatic artery and portal vein. The left liver further consists of segments 1–4 and the right of segments 5–8, segment 1 being the caudate lobe. The ligamentum teres runs directly into the left anterior sector, appearing to divide the liver into two; however, this is in fact an artificial division. The surface marking of the division between the functional left and right lobes runs from the left side of the vena cava posteriorly to the middle of the gall-bladder bed

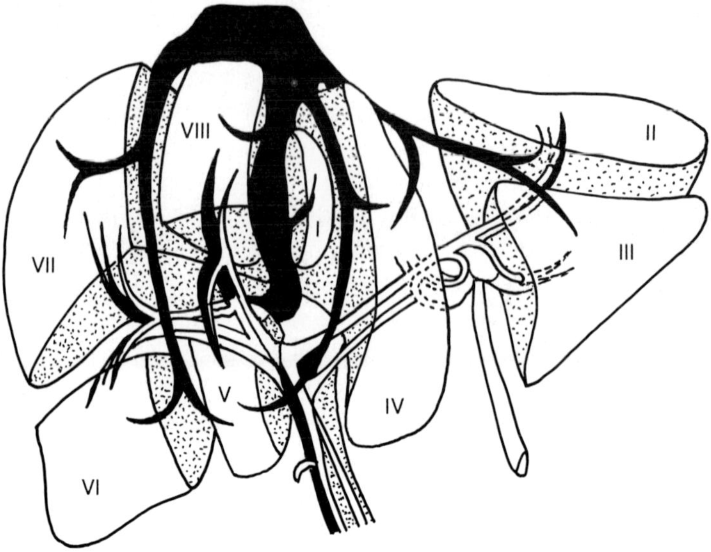

Fig. 7.3 The functional division of the liver and the segments according to Couinaud's nomenclature [34].

anteriorly. The main hepatic veins can be easily identified using intra-operative ultrasound (Fig. 7.4).

Operative technique

The key to safe liver resection is initial vascular control of the liver. For vascular control the dissection begins by identification of the portal vein and is followed by lifting the hepatic plate until the division into left and right branches is identified. The hepatic artery is dealt with in a similar manner and in left or right hepatectomy each portal and hepatic division may be divided between vascular clamps. The supra-hepatic cava is approached with care and individual hepatic veins can be identified.

Following a decision on the line of resection, the hepatic parenchyma is fractured, traditionally with the finger although a small haemostat is more accurate. Division of the hepatic parenchyma in this way leaves smaller portal arterial branches and bile radicles to be individually suture ligated. Using an ultrasonic dissector (cavitron-ultrasonic surgical aspirator) preserves the smaller structures more accurately.

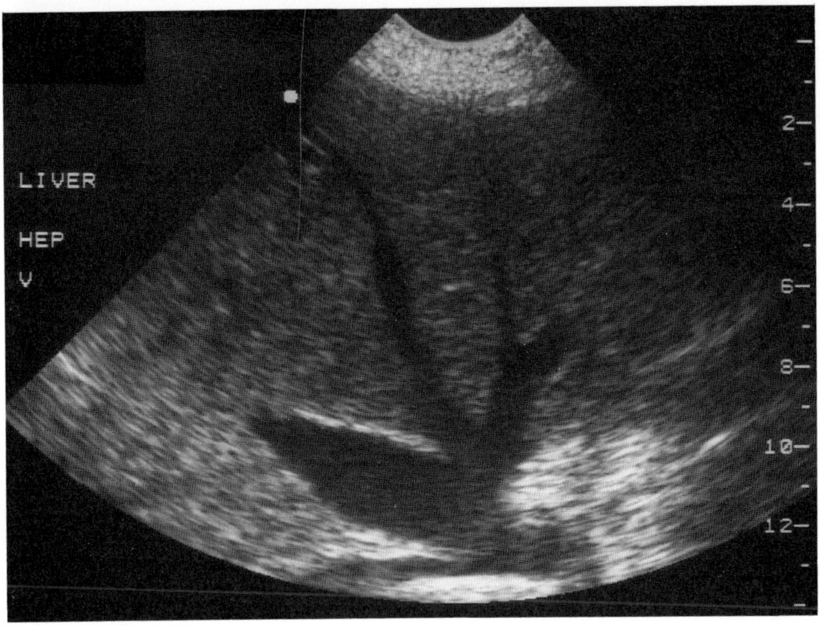

Fig. 7.4 Intraoperative ultrasound showing the confluence of the hepatic veins.

Ex-situ liver surgery and surgery on the in-situ perfused liver

A further option in circumstances where tumours are too large to be removed by conventional techniques because of the proximity of major structures is that of bench procedure liver surgery, or alternatively of surgery on the *in-situ* perfused liver [30]. The aims of this type of surgery are to increase the resectability rate in patients with large intrahepatic tumours.

The *ex-situ* technique is particularly applicable to hepatocellular tumours or metastases in patients who do not have seriously impaired liver function [31].

Surgery on the *ex-situ* or *in-situ* perfused liver proceeds as for conventional resections following the segmental structure of the liver. Care should of course be directed to the preservation of all arterial branches to the liver parenchyma that will remain. The particular advantage of this approach is that segmental resection lines can be extended by dissecting along the wall of major veins where segmental boundaries are not always readily definable, and following resection, perfusion of the portal vein and artery identifies leaks which can be dealt with by oversewing or Ligaclips. The application of fibrin glue over the cut surface then seals smaller vessels.

Hepatic replacement

Bleeding and consequent blood usage was one of the major problems encountered during orthotopic liver transplantation in the early years and difficulties can still be encountered.

Our own transfusion requirements in over 400 cases have fallen but have now plateaued at a median of 7 units per adult (Fig. 7.5). In our earliest patients haemostasis was often difficult to control [32] using standard surgical techniques and this problem was addressed by using diathermy for all dissection during the recipient hepatectomy, the increased use of veno-venous bypass [33] and advanced coagulation techniques such as an argon beam coagulator (Baird). The cell-saver (Haemonetic Corp., Braintree, Boston, MA, USA) was used during the early phase of the programme but is now rarely needed.

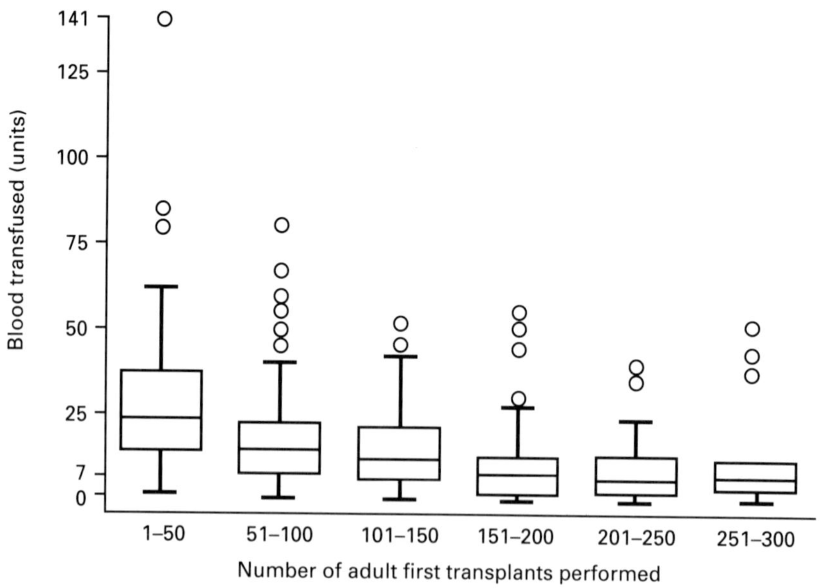

Fig. 7.5 Blood-transfusion requirement in each 50 cases of adult first liver transplants performed in Birmingham from 1982 to 1990. (Box whisker plots show medians, interquartile range, upper and lower adjacent values and outside values.)

Bleeding occurs (i) in high-risk patients, (ii) during dissection due to technical problems and (iii) following graft reperfusion. It is possible to identify factors that are associated with above average blood use. Transfusion requirements are related to ultimate survival and the individually significant risk factors are preoperative low platelet count or haemoglobin, the presence of ascites, previous encephalopathy, previous variceal bleeding, previous upper abdominal surgery, the patient's weight and hyponatraemia. With the exception of previous surgery almost all the factors are indicative of advanced hepatic disease. Following reperfusion there may be loss of platelets and a decrease in all clotting factors, suggesting a consumptive coagulopathy. While poor initial graft function is one factor, DIC remains an unsolved problem which infrequently requires intensive transfusion supervision.

Bleeding from the biliary tree

Haemobilia is an infrequent cause of gastrointestinal bleeding but does occur following trauma, endoscopic cannulation of the papilla of Vater (ERCP), and more recently, biliary lithotripsy.

The diagnosis is often obvious from the history but in obscure cases of gastrointestinal bleeding, a fortunate endoscopy may detect blood leaving the papilla of Vater but angiography, repeat angiography and ^{99m}Tc-labelled red-cell scanning may be required to make a diagnosis.

Associated with hepatic trauma haemobilia occurs by two mechanisms:

1 Due to incomplete debridement and haemostasis of hepatic rupture (e.g. closing the exit sites with the development of an intrahepatic haematoma which then ruptures into the biliary tree).

2 A false aneurysm may rupture. The clinical picture is that of bouts of cholangitis associated with bleeding, and treatment consists of repeat debridement and suture haemostasis.

Following biliary lithotripsy, minor episodes of haemobilia are not uncommon and almost invariably self-limiting but, following ERCP and sphincterotomy, the surgeon may be presented with uncontrolled bleeding. Management lies initially with prevention. The majority of sphincterotomies are performed in jaundiced patients so care should be taken to ensure that preoperative platelet count is normal, and any coagulation defect is corrected by vitamin K administration or fresh frozen plasma if necessary. The sphincterotomy itself should be performed with a blended current. When bleeding does occur, most commonly either the posterior or anterior superior pancreaticoduodenal artery will have been divided running adjacent to the lower end of the common bile duct within the duodenal loop. These arteries are branches of the gastroduodenal artery. Bleeding will often stop following transfusion, but vasopressin as an infusion may be a useful adjunct. In the presence of exsanguinating haemorrhage, then surgical intervention will be necessary and consists of taking interrupted sutures to join the biliary epithelium to duodenal mucosa following duodenotomy. It is rarely necessary to ligate the gastroduodenal artery.

Conclusions

The early biliary surgeons in the 1880s quickly realized the problems associated with bleeding in jaundiced patients. Current knowledge allows a planned management schedule to be instituted which combines the optimum timing of haematological control with meticulous surgical techniques. Even the most complex hepatic procedures in critically ill individuals can often now be undertaken with success.

References

1 DeFranchis, R. (1989) Prophylactic sclerotherapy in high risk cirrhotics selected by endoscopic criteria: interim report of a multicenter randomized controlled trial. *J. Hepatol.*, **9**(Suppl.), S23 (Abstract).

2 Jackson, E.C., Perrin, E.B., Smith, A.G. *et al.* (1968) A clinical investigation of the portacaval shunt. II. Survival analysis of the prophylactic operation. *Am. J. Surg.*, **11**, 22–42.

3 Resnick, R.H., Chalmers, T.C., Ishihara, A.M. *et al.* (1969) A controlled study of the prophylactic portacaval shunt. A final report. *Ann. Intern. Med.*, **70**, 675–688.

4 Conn, H.O., Lindenmuth, W.W., May, C.J. and Rambsy, G.R. (1972) Prophylactic portacaval anastomosis. A tale of two studies. *Medicine*, **51**, 27–40.

5 Burroughs, A.K., Hamilton, G., Phillips, A. *et al.* (1989) A comparison of sclerotherapy with staple transection of the esophagus for the emergency control of bleeding from esophageal varices. *New Engl. J. Med.*, **321**, 857–862.

6 Hoskins, S.W. and Johnson, A.G. (1987) What happens to esophageal varices after transection and devascularisation. *Surgery*, **101**, 531–534.

7 Sugiura, M. and Futagawa, S. (1984) Results of six hundred and thirty six esophageal transections with paraesophagogastric devascularisation in the treatment of esophageal varices. *J. Vasc. Surg.*, **1**, 254–260.

8 Gouge, T.H. and Ranson, J.H.C. (1986) Esophageal transection and paraesophagogastric devascularisation for bleeding oesophageal varices. *Am. J. Surg.*, **151**, 47–54.

9 Henderson, J.M. (1986) Variceal bleeding: which shunt? *Gastroenterology*, **91**, 1021–1023.

10 Esquivel, C.O., Klintmalm, G., Kwatsuki, S. *et al.* (1987) Liver transplantation in patients with patent splenorenal shunts. *Surgery*, **101**, 430–432.

11 Burroughs, A.K. and McKormick, P.A. Variceal bleeding: acute and long term management. In: *Therapy of Liver Disease, Clinical Gastroenterology* (Ed. Davis, M.), Vol. 3, pp. 131–163. Baillière Tindall, London (1989).

12 Warren, W.D., Zeppa, R. and Fomon, J.J. (1967) Selective transsplenic decompression of gastroesophageal varices by distal splenorenal shunt. *Ann. Surg.*, **137**, 437–455.

13 Warren, W.D., Henderson, J.M., Millikan, W.J. *et al.* (1986) Distal splenorenal shunt versus endoscopic sclerotherapy for long term management of variceal bleeding. Preliminary report of a prospective randomized trial. *Ann. Surg.*, **203**, 454–462.

14 Cameron, J.L., Herlong, H.F., Slanfey, H. *et al.* (1983) The Budd–Chiari syndrome. Treatment of mesenteric systemic shunts. *Ann. Surg.*, **198**, 335–346.

15 Stringer, M.D., Howard, E.R., Green, D.W. *et al.* (1989) Mesoatrial shunt: a surgical option in the management of the Budd–Chiari syndrome. *Br. J. Surg.*, **76**, 474–478.

16 Trukie, D.D., Shires, G.T. and McLelland, R. (1974) Management of liver trauma in 811 consecutive patients. *Ann. Surg.*, **179**, 722–728.

17 Patcher, H.L., Spencer, F.C., Hofstetter, S.R. and Coppra, G.F. (1983) Experience with the finger fracture technique to achieve intra-hepatic haemostasis in 75 patients with severe injuries of the liver. *Ann. Surg.*, **197**, 771–778.

18 Oldham, K.T., Guice, K.S. & Ryckman, F. (1986) Blunt liver injury in childhood: Evolution of therapy and current perspectives. *Surgery*, **100**, 542–549.

19 Huguet, C., Nordlinger, B., Gallopin, J.J. *et al.* (1978) Normothermic hepatic vascular occlusion for extensive hepatectomy. *Surg. Gynecol. Obstet.*, **147**, 689–693.

20 Lucas, C.E. and Ledgerwood, A.M. (1976) Prospective evaluation of haemostatic techniques for liver injuries. *J. Trauma*, **16**, 442–451.

21 Flint, L.M. and Polk, H.C. (1979) Selective hepatic artery ligation: limitations and failures. *J. Trauma*, **19**, 319–323.

22 Feliciano, D.V., Mattox, K.L., Burch, J.M. *et al.* (1986) Packing for the control of hepatic haemorrhage. *J. Trauma*, **26**, 738–743.

23 Feliciano, D.V., Jordan, G., Bilando, C.G. *et al.* (1986) Management of 1000 consecutive cases of hepatic trauma (1979–1984). *Ann. Surg.*, **204**, 438–445.

24 Calne, R.Y., McMaster, P. and Pentlow, B.D. (1979) The treatment of major liver trauma by primary packing and transfer of the patient for definitive treatment. *Br. J. Surg.*, **66**, 338–339.

25 Millikan, J.S., Moore, E.E., Cogbill, J.H. and Kashuk, J.L. (1983) Inferior vena caval injuries. A continuing challenge. *J. Trauma*, **23**, 207–212.

26 McMaster, P. and Tolley, M. (1977) Management of inferior vena caval injury in liver trauma. *Ann. R. Coll. Surg. Engl.*, **59**, 502–506.

27 Kudsk, K.A., Sheldon, G.F. and Lim, R.C. (1982) Atrial-caval shunting (ACS) after trauma. *J. Trauma*, **22**, 81–85.

28 Rovito, P.F. (1987) Atrial caval shunting in blunt hepatic trauma. *Ann. Surg.*, **205**, 318–321.

29 Couinaud, C. Le foie. In: *Études anatomiques et Chirurgicales*. Masson, Paris (1957).

30 Fortner, J.G., Shiu, M.H. and Kinne, D.W. (1974) Major hepatic resection using vascular isolation and hypothermic perfusion. *Ann. Surg.*, **180**, 644–552.
31 Pichlmayer, R., Grosse, H. and Hauss, J. (1990) Technique and preliminary results of extracorporeal liver surgery (bench procedure) and of surgery on the *in situ* perfused liver. *Br. J. Surg.*, **77**, 21–26.
32 Kirby, R.M., McMaster, P., Clements, D. *et al.* (1987) Orthotopic liver transplantation: postoperative complications and their management. *Br. J. Surg.*, **74**, 3–11.
33 Shaw, B.W., Martin, D.J., Marqez, J.M. *et al.* (1984) Venous bypass in clinical liver transplantation. *Ann. Surg.*, **200**, 524–534.
34 Bismuth, H. (1982) Surgical anatomy and anatomical surgery of the liver. *World J. Surg.*, **6**, 3–9.

Chapter 8
Renal disease and urology

VILMA E. QUIJADA AND JAMES F. WINCHESTER

Bleeding abnormalities are common in patients with renal disease. The causes are multiple and for diagnostic purposes and classification they can be divided into coagulation abnormalities associated with the following:

1 Chronic nephropathies with uraemia, nephrotic syndrome or nephritis.

2 Acute renal failure.

3 Urogenital neoplasms.

4 Transplantation.

The manifestations and mechanisms of coagulation disturbances in genitourinary diseases are outlined in Tables 8.1 and 8.2, respectively.

Chronic nephropathies

Chronic renal insufficiency

Coagulation abnormalities in the uraemic syndrome have been extensively studied since this association was first recognized by Bright in 1827 [1]. Although severe thrombocytopenia is not frequently reported, a decrease in platelet count may be found in chronic uraemia, probably as a result of impaired thrombopoiesis [2]; increased platelet turnover, particularly in patients on haemodialysis and also in those who may develop heparin-induced thrombocytopenia [3]. Uraemic patients usually exhibit abnormalities in platelet function, vessel-wall coagulation and plasma coagulation factors, which makes renal biopsy procedures hazardous. In uraemia, different abnormalities of platelet function such as decreased aggregability in response to epinephrine, adenosine diphosphate (ADP) and collagen have been extensively described [4–6]. In non-dialysed patients, a strong correlation between serum creatinine concentrations and severity of bleeding abnormalities is apparent, particularly when serum creatinine is above 500 mmol/l (6 mg/dl) [7] with normal

Table 8.1 Major manifestations of coagulation disturbances in genitourinary diseases*

Chronic renal failure	Acute renal failure	Nephrotic syndrome	Urogenital neoplasia	Renal transplant
Bleeding disorders				
Bruising				
Prolonged bleeding time	GI bleeding		Local bleeding (prostate cancer)	DIC (rejection)
	Intracranial bleeding			
GI bleeding	DIC		DIC	
Haemorrhagic pericarditis	HUS			
Subdural haematoma, etc.	TTP			
Thrombosis				
	Extrarenal thrombosis (10%)	Extremity thrombosis	Renal-vein/IVC thrombosis (renal-cell cancer)	Local renal vessel thrombosis (mechanical)
		Renal-vein thrombosis (membranous glomerulonephritis)	Vascular thrombosis (Wilms' tumour, prostatic cancer)	Vascular thrombosis (rejection and cyclosporin)
		Pulmonary embolism		

* DIC, disseminated intravascular coagulation; HUS, haemolytic uraemic syndrome; IVC, inferior vena cava; TTP, thrombotic thrombocytopenic purpura.

Table 8.2 Major mechanisms of coagulation disturbances in genitourinary diseases*

Chronic renal failure	Acute renal failure	Nephrotic syndrome	Urogenital neoplasia	Renal transplant
Bleeding disorders				
Impaired platelet function Increased PGI_2 activity	Impaired platelet function Thrombocytopenia (DIC, HUS, TTP)		Thrombocytopenia related to therapy Increased fibrinolysis (prostate renal-cell cancer) Local urokinase (prostate)	Renal platelet consumption
Defective vWF and Factor VIII activity	Circulating polymers of vWF/Factor VIII *E. coli* verocytotoxin		Increased thrombin and reptilase time	
Thrombosis				
	Decreased fibrinolysis 'Slow' antiplasmin Hyperfibrinogenaemia	Increased platelet activity Increased PF_4, β-TG Increased Factors II, V, VII, VIII: Ag, X Increased α_2-MG Decreased plasminogen activators	Elevated fibrinogen Increased sialic acid Increased FDP Decreased AT-III (oestrogens)	Thromboxane genesis
			Increased hyaluronic acid hyperviscosity (Wilms' tumour)	Cyclosporin

* α_2-MG, macroglobulin; AT-III, antithrombin III; BTG, β-thromboglobulin; DIC, disseminated intravascular coagulation; FDP, fibrin degradation products; HUS, haemolytic uraemic syndrome; IVC. inferior vena cava; PF_4, platelet factor 4; PGI_2, prostacyclin; TTP, thrombotic thrombocytopenic purpura; vWF, von Willebrand factor.

platelet function below this concentration. Decreased platelet aggregation has been suggested to relate to phenolic compounds [8], guanidinosuccinic acid [9], 24 h after infusion of urea [10], or uraemic 'middle molecules' [11].

Decreased thromboxane A_2 production in response to collagen, epinephrine or ADP, but normal response to administered exogenous arachidonic acid [12,13] suggests a defect in platelet formation or release of arachidonic acid from phospholipids. An increase in plasma β-thromboglobulin and thrombospondin, two platelet-specific proteins stored in the α-granules but released when platelets are disrupted or aggregated, is seen in severe renal insufficiency, probably reflecting an increased breakdown of platelets (as seen in patients in haemodialysis) [14,15]. Intracellular calcium concentration fails to rise after a stimulus (ADP, and arachidonic acid) [16], probably accounting for the platelet aggregation abnormalities and the abnormal bleeding time seen in uraemia [17]. Qualitative improvement in bleeding time is seen with correction of the anaemia [18] and prolonged haemodialysis time [7], although a maximal improvement is seen in patients on continuous ambulatory peritoneal dialysis, probably due to differences in solutes transferred through the peritoneal membrane compared to standard membranes for haemodialysis [7].

Vascular factors also have been implicated in the pathogenesis of bleeding disturbances in chronic renal insufficiency [19]. A potent platelet aggregation inhibitor, a prostacyclin (PGI_2, epoprostenol)-like substance produced by venous tissue has been found to be increased in the vessel wall of uraemic patients [20], although the exact effect on bleeding abnormalities has not yet been established.

Some coagulation factors and profibrinolytic plasma proteins have been found to be abnormal in uraemic patients. The von Willebrand Factor (vWF) and Factor VIII, both requiring platelet binding to subendothelial collagen, have been reported to be elevated in uraemic patients [21–23], although they exhibit deficient biological activity, as measured by ristocetin cofactor activity. Ristocetin cofactor activity and Factor VIII coagulant activity increase with cryoprecipitate infusion (fibronectin, fibrinogen and Factor VIII enriched) [24], and desmopressin (deamino-D-arginine vasopressin (DDAVP)). The latter promotes von Willebrand factor release [25], and is associated with shortening of the bleeding time. Protein C activity, a vitamin K-dependent profibrinolytic activated plasma protein, is decreased in uraemic patients [26,27]; this abnormality can be corrected by haemodialysis, suggesting the presence of a dialysable inhibitor. Patients with end-stage renal disease, particularly on chronic haemodialysis, can also exhibit lupus-like anticoagulant activity, as has been found by some workers [28], but these findings are not related to an increased bleeding tendency since the incidence of haemorrhagic episodes is not higher in these patients when they are compared to those with no lupus-like anticoagulant activity. In addition, the presence of a circulating lupus-like anticoagulant is an *in vitro* phenomenon and its presence is more likely to be associated with extrarenal and intrarenal thrombosis [29]. Also described in uraemia are the high plasma concentrations of fibrinogen and the decreased activity [15] of antithrombin III (AT-III) [30]. These findings may be consistent with simultaneous activation of opposing compensatory mechanisms, since a correlation exists between the depression of protein C activity and the severity of uraemia [15,27,31].

All these laboratory abnormalities are consistent with the high incidence of bruising, ecchymosis, purpura, prolonged bleeding from venepuncture sites, and gastrointestinal-tract bleeding frequently seen in uraemic patients [32]. More severe complications have also been described, such as haemorrhagic pericarditis with or without cardiac tamponade [33], haemorrhagic pleural effusion, spontaneous subcapsular and retroperitoneal haematomas, and subdural haematomas, the latter with a mortality rate reported to be as high as 90% [34–36].

Different approaches to the treatment of chronic uraemic patients with bleeding diathesis have been proposed. The selection of any particular treatment or drug will depend, for instance, on the rapidity of correction of an abnormal bleeding time in a patient who may potentially undergo a surgical procedure. Whole blood or packed red-cell transfusion is known to decrease the bleeding time [38]. Increased haematocrit is probably the cause for this finding, since the administration of erythropoietin has recently been shown to normalize the bleeding time in uraemia [39]. All dialysis modalities are associated with improvement in the bleeding time, particularly with prolonged haemodialysis and peritoneal dialysis [40]. Infusion of cryoprecipitate, rich in Factor VIII, fibrinogen and fibronectin, will correct the bleeding tendency 1 h after infusion, and the maximum effect may last for 4–12 h, while improvement in bleeding time may last up to 24–36 h after infusion [25]. Administration of DDAVP (0.3 μg/kg intravenously) will maximally correct the bleeding time 1–2 h after the infusion but no effect is noticed when given over a prolonged period of time, probably due to temporary exhaustion of vWF and Factor VIII from the endothelium, since some effect is noticed when some time has elapsed between doses [25]. Different conjugated oestrogens also have been advocated to correct the bleeding time, and may be given intravenously at a rate of 3 mg/kg for 5 days [41]. The effect requires several hours to become apparent, but may last for up to 14 days. A significant decrease in the bleeding time is noticed from the 2nd day after beginning therapy with oestrogens. More recently a β-resorcyclic acid lactone, a compound structurally very close to oestrogens, but without their side-effects, has been tested in uraemic rats, with significant and protracted shortening of the bleeding time [42]. Clinical studies have not yet been performed in uraemic patients to determine the efficacy of this product.

Finally, it should be remembered that the dialysis patient may be at risk of bleeding related to anticoagulation (regional—anticoagulation of the dialysis apparatus alone—or systemic) required for haemodialysis. Anticoagulants used for haemodialysis include regional and systemic heparin, regional sodium citrate, and regional prostacyclin infusions.

Nephrotic syndrome

That there is an increased thrombotic tendency in nephrotic syndrome has been known since the descriptions by Osborne and by Rayer [43] in the 19th century. These reports were largely overlooked until 1948 when Addis [44] reported an increased tendency to venous thrombosis in the extremities of patients with nephrotic syndrome. The overall incidence of thromboembolic episodes ranges from 8.5 to 44% [45] and the incidence of renal-vein thrombosis ranges from 5 to 62% in different series [46,47]. Pulmonary embolism, the most serious complication, accounts for up to 11.9% of these episodes [48]. Membranous glomerulonephritis, primary or secondary, is the nephropathy most frequently associated with these thrombotic tendencies in adults as described in most large series in the UK and USA. Patients with membranoproliferative glomerulonephritis may also be at higher risk [49], and in the paediatric age the congenital nephrotic syndrome (Finnish type) is most frequently associated with renal-vein thrombosis [50].

As in uraemia, platelet and coagulation factor abnormalities have been described. Regardless of the presence of the nephrotic syndrome, platelets are known to be activated in all forms of glomerulonephritis [51], platelet turnover seems to be accelerated and the presence of platelets and fibrin is a common finding on histology of the glomerular lesion [52–55]. The presence in plasma of β-thromboglobulin and platelet Factor IV is indicative of this excessive platelet degradation, and so is the detection of platelets in circulating macroaggregates [56–59]. Most of the reports suggest an increase in the number of platelets [60,61]. In addition, several abnormalities have been identified in these platelets, such as depletion of serotonin and ADP [62], suboptimal aggregation in buffer when compared to the serum of patients with nephrotic syndrome [63], and hyperaggregability to ADP *in vitro* [64]. These hyperaggregability states seem to correlate very well with the severity of the proteinuria and the serum albumin and fibrinogen concentrations [65,66], with serum albumin concentration probably being the most important. As the carrier for fatty acids (including arachidonic acid, precursor of thromboxane A_2 and PGI_2), the absence of albumin will provide more free arachidonic acid available to platelets and account for the consequent hyperaggregability phenomenon. This is supported by recent findings that in relapses in minimal-change nephrotic syndrome, urinary thromboxane B_2 is significantly higher than in controls or in the same patients during remission [67]. This effect is noticed when serum albumin concentrations are <3 g/dl, but is more prominent when serum albumin falls <2 g/dl. If albumin is added to nephrotic blood, the arachidonic acid-induced aggregation is completely inhibited.

Synthesis, turnover and loss in urine of several coagulation factors and fibrinolytic proteins have been reported in the nephrotic syndrome. The vast majority of patients with nephrotic syndrome tend to hypercoagulability. Coagulation Factors VII, IX [68], prothrombin [69] and fibrinogen may be abnormally high in urine, while the decreased levels of some other factors such as XI and XII, also could be the result of urinary losses [70–72]. Increased plasma levels of Factors II, VII and X as well as cofactors V and VIII: antigen (FVIII Ag), have also been reported [73]. In the fibrinolytic pathway, increases in α_2-macroglobulin [74–76] an antiplasmin factor [77], have been reported along with decreases in plasminogen and plasminogen activators such as fibrin [78], antithrombin III, plasminogen, α_2-antiplasmin [79] and α_1-antitrypsin. Also described is the increased synthesis rate and the differential losses in urine of low-molecular-weight coagulation proteins and increased consumption of Factors XI and XII. Prolongation of fibrin polymerization time, frequently seen in these patients, has suggested the presence of an abnormal fibrinogen molecule [53]. The presence of fibrin degradation products (FDPs) in urine is believed to be the consequence of fibrinogen degradation and not fibrin degradation and is due to the effects of urokinase on the filtered fibrinogen [53]. Protein C and the cofactor protein S, identified as potent inhibitors of coagulation [80] through the inactivation of Factors V and VIII, have been proposed as potential causes for the increased coagulation state of these patients. Protein C concentrations of <50% are associated with thrombosis but there is insufficient evidence to support that either a defect or low biological activity of any of these proteins in nephrotic patients plays a role in the abnormalities described [81].

Clotting studies in nephrotic patients are usually normal. Bleeding time and prothrombin time (PT) is usually in the normal range, although partial thromboplastin time (PTT), reptilase and thrombin times may be prolonged [82].

In a review of coagulation disturbances in the nephrotic syndrome, Cameron suggested that determination of the AT-III : α_2-macroglobulin ratio could be a useful marker to assess the thrombotic tendency, based on their opposing actions, and the association of thrombotic tendency in plasminogen insufficiency [83] and in AT-III deficiency. Although attractive, there is yet no proof that such a ratio is predictive of the thrombotic tendency, since different antiplasmin agonist substances exist, and some patients may have changes in this ratio without thromboembolic complications [84]. Also well known is the correction of these abnormalities when remission of the nephrotic syndrome occurs [85].

Particular caution should be taken in patients with nephrotic syndrome receiving diuretic therapy, since the hyperviscosity induced by volume depletion predisposes to thrombotic events [86]. Steroid usage in some of these patients is also associated with an increased tendency to the hypercoagulable state, probably because of the well-known increase of Factor VIII concentration and the inhibition of neutrophil–plasminogen activator secretion observed in these patients [87,88]. Decrease in PT, whole-blood clotting time and PTT have been observed in steroid-treated patients.

Prevention and therapeutic use of several anticoagulants, antiplatelet and fibrinolytic agents is still highly controversial. Heparins exert their action through AT-III, making it more active on thrombin and Factor Xa [89]. When low concentrations of AT-III are present, as may occur in patients with nephrotic syndrome, a reduced sensitivity to heparin is reported [90], expressed in a higher mean concentration of heparin required to achieve anticoagulation. Warfarin is largely bound to serum albumin, and therefore in nephrotic patients the free concentration can reach high levels. There is no conclusive clinical proof of anti-platelet drug efficacy in the correction of the hypercoagulable state.

The use of thrombolytic agents such as urokinase and streptokinase, although limited, has been associated with success in patients with renal-artery thrombosis [91,92] and with limited success in renal-vein thrombosis [93]. The benefits of prolonged therapy with anticoagulants, once a thrombotic episode has been documented, is highly recommended, since recurrence of pulmonary embolism has been reported in patients who have received therapy for prolonged periods after discontinuation of anticoagulation [94].

Acute renal failure

Bleeding disorders are still important factors in the morbidity and mortality of patients with acute renal failure. Regardless of the aetiology of the acute renal failure, the mortality rate associated with a haemorrhagic diathesis ranges from 3 to 15% in different reports [95]. The main sources of bleeding are intracranial, gastrointestinal and disseminated intravascular coagulopathy (DIC).

As in chronic renal failure, different coagulation abnormalities have been reported in acute renal failure. Abnormalities in platelet adhesivity and aggregability *in vivo* and *in vitro* in response to potent stimuli are common. In conditions such as the haemolytic uraemic syndrome (HUS) [96], perhaps mediated by *Escherichia coli* verocytotoxin [97], and thrombotic thrombocytopenic purpura (TTP) [98], particular abnormalities associated with the primary condition can be found, such as circulating high-molecular-weight polymers of vWF and Factor VIII:C along with increased plasma concentrations of β-thromboglobulin, suggesting increased activity of the clotting mechanisms and platelet disruption [99,100]. In some other conditions such as acute renal failure associated with snake bite [101], sepsis, and major obstetric catastrophes [102], DIC may be the main bleeding disorder. In a review of coagulation disorders in acute renal failure, up to 30% of patients presented with overt DIC, mostly associated with obstetric conditions; DIC could still be present in up to 50% of those without clinical manifestations [103]. Correction of DIC often depends upon correction of the primary condition.

Treatment of the bleeding tendency in acute renal failure is orientated to correction of the primary condition. The dramatic improvement in coagulation disturbances seen in chronic renal patients after dialysis may not be seen in acute renal failure, since the primary mechanism responsible for it may be the primary promoter of the bleeding abnormality. Thrombocytopenia can be due to underlying sepsis, trauma and

DIC. Infusion of cryoprecipitate, use of DDAVP [104], and plasmapheresis have been reported to improve the bleeding tendency in special conditions, such as TTP and HUS. These measures are likely to be ineffective in other conditions associated with acute renal failure, such as sepsis and surgical and obstetric complications, where DIC should be corrected with the appropriate selection of antibiotics, dialysis and, if necessary, transfusion of fresh frozen plasma. If liver failure is present, such as in the hepatorenal syndrome, none of these measures is likely to be effective.

Hypercoagulability may also complicate acute renal failure, with extrarenal thrombosis occurring in up to 10% of cases [105,106]. There is also hyperfibrinogenaemia, decreased fibrinolysis [107], and increased 'slow' antiplasmin activity [108].

Urogenital neoplasms

An association between malignant neoplasms and coagulation abnormalities was made by Trousseau in 1865 when he first described the clinical association between venous thrombosis and a solid tumour [109].

Among the most common urological neoplasms, carcinoma of the prostate [110] and renal-cell carcinoma [111] have frequently been cited as likely to present with coagulation abnormalities.

Different components of neoplastic tissues may contribute to the abnormal bleeding tendency, in that some components of malignant tissue may promote bleeding; it is well known that the high fibrinolytic activity of some tissues in the urogenital tract (e.g. bladder, prostate and renal capsule) [109] may produce bleeding, while the release of coagulant-like substances from these tissues may contribute to thromboembolism. Other major causes for abnormal bleeding are decreased bone-marrow platelet production, increased platelet consumption, and a low-grade DIC often seen in some of these patients. Along with platelet abnormalities, production of fibrinolytic and coagulant-like substances from some of these tumours may well account for the increased frequency of thromboembolic disorders observed [112].

Many investigators have described the abnormal haemorrhagic tendency of patients with prostate carcinoma during resective surgery [113]. One logical explanation could relate to the local (normal) action of urinary urokinase, since patients who develop abnormal bleeding due to increased fibrinolytic activity respond to antifibrinolytic therapy or heparin. However, in a recent retrospective study at the M.D. Anderson

Hospital, Houston, Texas [114], no significant abnormal bleeding or thrombotic complications were found in untreated patients with prostate carcinoma compared with other neoplasms.

Some other substances have been isolated from prostatic tissue, which were first identified as the causes of the bleeding tendency, such as a plasmin-like enzyme or plasminogen activator [115] and a tissue thromboplastin [116].

The reported increased tendency to develop thrombotic episodes is on the other hand difficult to relate exclusively to the malignant process, since some patients had received oestrogen therapy (that will induce a reduction in AT-III). In another report [117], six of 20 patients with prostatic carcinoma who exhibited circulating platelet aggregates, abnormally high concentrations of Factor VII, plasminogen and prekallikrein, along with already decreased concentrations of AT-III prior to treatment, developed venous thrombosis or ischaemic vascular disease when they received oestrogen or estramustine phosphate therapy. Other abnormalities noticed in this group of patients with thromboembolic complications were higher concentrations of vWF antigen, fibrinopeptide A, plasminogen activator inhibitor and C_1-inhibitor, decreased urokinase inhibitors as well as decreased tissue plasminogen activator. All these findings are uncommon, and the mechanism of production of thrombohaemorrhagic diatheses not well understood, but identification of coagulation disturbances in this group of patients may make clinical management and prevention of thromboembolic complications in prostatic cancer patients on anticoagulant or oestrogen therapy somewhat simpler.

Another urologic neoplasm frequently associated with bleeding abnormalities is renal-cell carcinoma. Classically described in these patients is the tendency of these tumours to spread to the renal vein and inferior cava, through formed thrombi [118]. The identification of fibrin in the tumour is evidence of coagulation pathway activation by the tumour, and has led to the rationale for the use of anticoagulant and antiplatelet drugs in such patients [119]. Along with evidence for the thromboembolic phenomena described in these patients, DIC has also been reported [120], and it is not unusual for a covert renal-cell cancer to present with a thromboembolic episode [121]. Some of the coagulation abnormalities described in patients with renal-cell cancer are elevated fibrinogen concentrations, an abnormal increased serum content of sialic acid [122] that decreases after nephrectomy [123], increased concentrations of FDPs, which may be particularly high in patients with metastatic carcinoma [124], a plasminogen activator produced by the cancer tissue [125], while others have demonstrated production of a possible diffusible inhibitor of fibrinolysis [126]. An abnormal coagulant substance that does not require coagulation Factor VII (different from tissue thromboplastin) has also been isolated [127], and its presence associated with *in vitro* tumour spreading. Some of the coagulant factors could be related to coagulation Factors IX and VII. A urokinase-like substance has also been isolated that may account for increased fibrinolytic activity in more aggressive renal-cell cancer. A potent inducer of platelet aggregation that also may induce adenocarcinoma cell growth, and is presumably a heparin-binding growth factor, has been isolated in renal adenocarcinoma. This substance also exhibits angiogenic properties and could be responsible for the hypervascularity observed in renal-cell carcinoma [128].

In Wilms' tumour, an acquired form of von Willebrand's disease has been reported, probably due to the adsorption of the coagulation Factor VIII molecular complex by nephroblastic tissue since no immunoglobulin-mediated inhibitor has been yet identified [129]. Another abnormality associated with nephroblastoma is hyperviscosity secondary to the elevated plasma concentrations of hyaluronic acid [130]. Platelet abnormalities are common findings in hyperviscosity states and have been described in patients with paraproteinaemia-related hyperviscosity. These abnormalities seem to be secondary to the interaction of hyaluronic acid and platelets since assays for coagulation Factor VIII Ag and vWF are normal once the hyaluronic acid is removed from the abnormal serum [131].

Prolonged thrombin time and reptilase time and mild elevations in fibrinogen, with increased bleeding have been described in patients with metastatic bladder carcinoma; in a patient with transitional-cell carcinoma of the bladder, the isolation of a heparin-like anticoagulant seemed to be the cause of the abnormality [132].

The transient thrombocytopenia seen in some patients with testicular cancer is a major complication of cisplatin–vinblastine and bleomycin therapy, probably due to the synergistic effect of these drugs and not to the neoplasm itself, since severe thrombocytopenia may follow initial therapy with vinblastine [133].

In summary, it is reasonable to conclude that locally produced procoagulant and fibrinolytic substances are expected causes of coagulation abnormalities in some urological cancer patients. However, the influence of sepsis and antineoplastic agents should be considered, since this may make a susceptible patient develop severe bleeding or thrombosis and their attendant complications.

Renal transplantation

Relative procoagulant activity is noticed during the early period after renal transplantation, expressed by increasing levels of vWF, Factor VIII:c, and decreased levels of prostacyclin and plasminogen [134]. Although within the normal range, concentrations of the components of the fibrinolytic pathway are in the lower limit of normal. Unless other pathological conditions are present, such as sepsis or rejection, no active consumption of coagulation factors is observed.

In hyperacute rejection, very extensive intravascular activation of the coagulation system is present, with severe consumption of platelets and Factors II, V, VIII and fibrinogen. All these blood components can be demonstrated in the rejected allograft [60]. This condition may lead to a severe consumption coagulopathy such as seen in DIC. Along with the activation of the coagulation system, the fibrinolytic pathway is activated as expressed by the activation of Factor XII (Hageman) [60].

In acute rejection, activation of the local fibrinolytic pathway has been demonstrated. FDPs along with Factor VIII are found in urine [60]. Urinary thromboxane B_2 is increased early in transplant rejection [135]. There is also accumulation of platelets in the graft, active circulating platelets and circulating platelet aggregates; platelet lifespan is shortened and platelet Factor 4 (PF_4) can be detected in plasma, and accompanied by increased urinary thromboxane B_2 consistent with platelet activation. Activation of the fibrinolytic pathway, as assessed by the presence of kallikrein inhibition, β-XIIa inhibition, increased plasminogen and AT-III, have been found prior to clinical signs of rejection, which may indicate an acute response to the thrombotic tendency observed in rejection [136]. Most importantly, all of these abnormalities disappear with remission of the rejection episode.

Along with the transplant-induced changes in the coagulation system, immunosuppressive drugs such as prednisone and cyclosporin have been linked to the thrombotic tendency [137,138]. Increased production of thromboxane B_2, platelet activation and release of platelet-activating factor (PAF) [139] that could enhance the postsurgical thromboplastin effect, have been reported in patients receiving cyclosporin. In the long term, increased platelet aggregability, plasma concentrations of Factor

VIII : c, fibrinogen and AT-III, as well as increased thromboembolic complications compared to those patients only receiving azathioprine and antilymphocytic globulin, have been observed [60]. Studies on the use of cyclosporin–platelet aggregation inhibitors, and the possible role of ω_3-polyunsaturated fatty acids [140], in reducing the high incidence of thromboembolic complications are now in progress, with initially encouraging results.

References

1 Bright, R. *Reports of Medical Cases*. Guy's Hospital of London. Longman, Rees, Orme and Brown, London (1827).

2 Gafter, U., Bessler, H., Malachi, T. *et al.* (1987) Platelet count and thrombopoietic activity in patients with chronic renal failure. *Nephron*, **45**, 207–210.

3 Babcock, R.B., Dumper, C.W. and Scharfman, W.B. (1976) Heparin induced immune thrombocytopenia. *New Engl. J. Med.*, **295**, 237–241.

4 George, J.N. and Shattil, S.J. (1991) The clinical importance of acquired abnormalities of platelet function. *New Engl. J. Med.*, **324**, 27–39.

5 Di Minno, G., Martinez, J., McKean, M.L. *et al.* (1985) Platelet dysfunction in uremia. Multifaceted defect corrected by dialysis. *Am. J. Med.*, **79**, 552–559.

6 Winchester, J.F., Forbes, C.D., Lang, S. *et al.* Platelet function regulating agents—Experimental data relevant to renal disease. In: *Thromboembolism: A New Approach to Therapy* (Eds Mitchell, J.R.A. & Domenet, J.G.), pp. 84–103. Academic Press, London (1977).

7 Lindsay, R.M., Friesen, M., Koens, F. *et al.* (1976) Platelet function in patients on long term peritoneal dialysis. *Clin. Nephrol.*, **6**, 335–339.

8 Rabiner, S.F. and Molinas, F. (1970) The role of phenol and phenolic acids on the thrombocytopathy and defective platelet aggregation of patients with renal failure. *Am. J. Med.*, **49**, 346–351.

9 Weiss, H.J. (1972) Acquired qualitative platelet disorders. In: *Hematology* (Eds Williams, W.J., Beutler E., Erslev, A.J. *et al.*), pp. 1171–1175. McGraw-Hill, New York (1972).

10 Eknoyan, G., Wacksman, S.J., Gluek, H.I. *et al.* (1969) Platelet function in renal failure. *New Engl. J. Med.*, **280**, 677–681.

11 Bazilinski, N., Shaykh, M., Dunea, G. *et al.* (1985) Inhibition of platelet function by uremic middle molecules. *Nephron*, **40**, 423–428.

12 Remuzzi, G., Benigni, A., Dodesini, P. *et al.* (1983) Reduced platelet thromboxane formation in uremia. Evidence for a functional cyclooxygenase defect. *J. Clin. Invest.*, **71**, 762–768.

13 Remuzzi, G. (1989) Bleeding disorders in uremia: pathophysiology and treatment. *Adv. Nephrol.*, **18**, 171–186.

14 Gawaz, M.P. and Ward, R.A. (1990) Effects of hemodialysis on platelet-derived thrombospondin (TSP). *Abstr. Am. Soc. Nephrol.*, 398.

15 Knudsen, F. and Dyerberg, J. (1985) Platelets and antithrombin III in uraemia: the acute effect of haemodialysis. *Scand. J. Clin. Lab. Invest.*, **45**, 341–347.

16 Ware, J.A., Clark, B.A., Smith, M. *et al.* (1989) Abnormalities in cytoplasmic Ca^{2+} in platelets from patients with uremia. *Blood*, **73**, 172–176.
17 Steiner, R.W., Coggins, C. and Carvalho, A. (1979) Bleeding time in uremia: a useful test to assess clinical bleeding. *Am. J. Hematol.*, **7**, 107–117.
18 Livio, M., Gotti, E. and Marchesi, D. (1982) Uremic bleeding. Role of anemia and beneficial effect of red cell transfusion. *Lancet*, **ii**, 1013–1015.
19 Di Paolo, N., Capotondo, L., Rossi, P. *et al.* (1989) Bleeding tendency of chronic uremia improved by vascular factor. *Nephron*, **52**, 268–272.
20 Remuzzi, G., Cavenaghi, A.E., Mecca, G. *et al.* (1977) Prostacyclin-like activity and bleeding in renal failure. *Lancet*, **ii**, 1195–1197.
21 Sakariassen, K.S., Bolhuis, P.A. and Sixma, J.J. (1979) Human blood platelet adhesion to artery subendothelium is mediated by Factor VIII–von Willebrand factor bound to the subendothelium. *Nature (London)*, **279**, 636–638.
22 Kazatchkine, N., Sultan, V., Caen, J.P. *et al.* (1976) Bleeding in uremia: A possible cause. *Br. Med. J.*, **2**, 612–615.
23 Howard, M.A., Whitworth, J.A., Hendrix, L. *et al.* (1979) Abnormal Factor VIII in chronic renal failure. *Med. J. Austral.*, **1**, 148–151.
24 Janson, P.A., Jubelirer, S.J. and Weinstein, M.J. (1980) Treatment of the bleeding tendency in uremia with cryoprecipitate. *New Engl. J. Med.*, **303**, 1318–1322.
25 Mannuci, P.M., Remuzzi, G., Pusineri, F. *et al.* (1983) Deamino 8-D-arginine vasopressin shortens the bleeding time in uremia. *New Engl. J. Med.*, **308**, 8–12.
26 Sorensen, P.J., Knudsen, F., Nielsen, A. *et al.* (1989) Protein C assays in uremia. *Thromb. Res.*, **54**, 301–310.
27 Knudsen, F., Sorensen, P.J., Hoj, A. *et al.* (1988) Inhibitors of coagulation in terminal renal failure and hemodialysis. *Nephron*, **49**, 335–336.
28 Quereda, C., Pardo, A., Lamas, S. *et al.* (1988) Lupus-like *in vitro* anticoagulant activity in end-stage renal disease. *Nephron*, **49**, 39–44.
29 D'Agati, V., Kunis, Ch. and Williams, G. (1990) Anticardiolipin antibody and renal disease: A report of three cases. *J. Am. Soc. Nephrol.*, **1**, 777–784.
30 Brand, T.P., Jesperson, J. and Sorensen, L.H. (1981) Antithrombin III and platelets in hemodialysis patients. *Nephron*, **28**, 1–3.
31 Allon, M., Soffer, O., Evatt, B. *et al.* (1989) Protein S and C antigen levels in proteinuric patients. *Am. J. Hematol.*, **31**, 96–101.
32 Bronner, M., Pati, M., Cunningham, C. *et al.* (1986) Estrogen–progesterone therapy for bleeding gastrointestinal telangiectasis in chronic renal failure. An uncontrolled trial. *Ann. Intern. Med.*, **105**, 371–374.
33 Suki, W.N. (1988) Pericarditis. *Kidney Int.*, **33** (Suppl. 24), S10–S12.
34 Maher, J.F. and Schreiner, G.E. (1966) Hazards and complications of dialysis. *New Engl. J. Med.*, **272**, 370–393.
35 Bechar, M., Lakke, J.P. *et al.* (1972) Subdural hematoma during long term hemodialysis. *Arch. Neurol.*, **26**, 513–516.
36 Tietjen, D.P., Moore, J. Jr and Gouge, S.F. (1987) Hemodialysis associated acute subdural hematoma. Interim management with peritoneal dialysis. *Am. J. Nephrol.*, **7**, 478–481.
37 Ingelberg, R. (1989) Non-surgical treatment of subdural hematoma in hemodialysis patients. *Clin. Neurol. Neurosurg.*, **91**, 85–89.
38 Fernandez, F., Goudable, C., Su, P. *et al.* (1985) Low hematocrit and prolonged

bleeding time in uremic patients: Effect of red cell transfusions. *Br. J. Haematol.*, **59**, 139–148.

39 Moia, M., Mannucci, P.M., Vizzotto, I. *et al.* (1987) Improvement in the haemostatic defect of uraemia after treatment with recombinant human erythropoietin. *Lancet*, **ii**, 1227–1229.

40 Rabiner, S.F. and Drake, R.F. (1975) Platelet function as an indicator of adequate dialysis. *Kidney Int.* (Suppl. 2), S144–S146.

41 Liu, Y., Kosfeld, R. and Marcum, S. (1984) Treatment of uraemic bleeding with conjugated oestrogens. *Lancet*, **ii**, 887–890.

42 Zoja, C., Vigano, G., Corna, D. *et al.* (1990) Oral zeranol shortens the prolonged bleeding time of uremic rats. *Kidney Int.*, **38**, 96–100.

43 Cameron, J.S. Coagulation and thromboembolic complications in the nephrotic syndrome. In: *Advances in Nephrology* (Eds Bach, J-F., Crosnier, J., Funck-Brentano, J-L., Grunfeld, J-P. & Maxwell, M.H.), Vol. 14, pp. 75–114. Year Book Medical Publishers, New York (1984).

44 Addis, T. *Glomerular Nephritis, Diagnosis and Treatment.* Macmillan, New York (1948).

45 Llach, F., Papper, S. and Massry, S.G. (1980) The clinical spectrum of renal vein thrombosis: acute and chronic. *Am. J. Med.*, **69**, 819–827.

46 Llach, F., Koffler, A. and Massry, S.G. (1977) Renal vein thrombosis and the nephrotic syndrome. *Nephron*, **19**, 65–68.

47 Harrington, J.T. and Kassirer, J.P. (1982) Renal vein thrombosis. *Ann. Rev. Med.*, **33**, 255–262.

48 Llach, F. (1985) Hypercoagulability and thrombotic complications of nephrotic syndrome. *Kidney Int.*, **28**, 429–439.

49 Velasquez, F. and Garcia, N. (1984) Evaluation of asymptomatic renal vein thrombosis in patients with idiopathic nephrotic syndrome. *Abstr. Am. Soc. Nephrol.*, 254.

50 Levy, P.R. and Jao, W. (1974) Nephrotic syndrome in association with renal vein thrombosis in infancy. *J. Pediatr.*, **85**, 359–361.

51 Cameron, J.S. (1977) Platelets and glomerulonephritis. *Nephron*, **18**, 253–258.

52 Taira, K., Matsunaga, T., Kawahara, S. *et al.* (1989) Fragments of urinary fibrin/fibrinogen degradation products and cross linked fibrin degradation products in various renal diseases. *Thomb. Res.*, **53**, 367–377.

53 Sakakibara, K., Nagase, M., Takada, Y. *et al.* (1987) Relationship between urinary fibrinogen degradation products and various types of chronic nephritis. *Thromb. Res.*, **45**, 403–411.

54 Canavese, C., Strata, P., Salomone, M. *et al.* (1982) Platelet activation in the nephrotic syndrome. *Clin. Nephrol.*, **17**, 268–269.

55 Tomura, S., Ida, T., Kuriyama, P. *et al.* (1982) Activation of platelets in patients with chronic proliferative glomerulonephritis and the nephrotic syndrome. *Clin. Nephrol.*, **17**, 24–30.

56 Adler, A.J., Lundin, A.P., Feinroth, M.V. *et al.* (1980) Beta thromboglobulin levels in the nephrotic syndrome. *Am. J. Med.*, **69**, 551–554.

57 Kuhlman, U., Steurer, J., Bollinger, A. *et al.* (1981) Platelet aggregation and beta thromboglobulin levels in nephrotic patients with and without thrombosis. *Clin. Nephrol.*, **15**, 229–235.

58 Parbtani, A., Frampton, G. and Cameron, J.S. (1980) Measurements of platelet release substances in glomerulonephritis. A comparison of beta thromboglobulin (beta-TG), platelet factor 4 (PF4) and serotonin assays. *Thromb. Res.*, **19**, 177–189.

59 Schiepatti, A., Dodesini, P., Benigni, A. *et al.* (1982) Increased malondialdehyde (MDA) and circulating platelet aggregates in nephrotic syndrome are related to plasma albumin levels. *Kidney Int.*, **21**, 265 (Abstract).

60 Kanfer, A., Kleinknecht, D., Broyer, M. *et al.* (1970) Coagulation studies in 45 cases of nephrotic syndrome without uremia. *Thromb. Diathes. Haemorrh.*, **24**, 562–571.

61 Andrassy, K., Ritz, E. and Bommer, J. (1980) Hypercoagulability in the nephrotic syndrome. *Klin. Wochenschr.*, **58**, 1029–1036.

62 Pareti, F.I., Capitanio, A., Mannucci, L. *et al.* (1980) Acquired dysfunction due to the circulation of 'exhausted' platelets. *Am. J. Med.*, **69**, 235–240.

63 Bang, N., Heidenreich, R.O. and Trygstad, C.W. (1972) Plasma protein requirements for human platelet aggregation. *Ann. NY Acad. Sci.*, **201**, 280–299.

64 Bang, N., Trygstad, C.W., Schroider, J. *et al.* (1973) Enhanced platelet function in glomerular renal diseases. *J. Lab. Clin. Med.*, **81**, 651–660.

65 Remuzzi, G., Mecca, G., Marchesi, D. *et al.* (1979) Platelet hyperaggregability and the nephrotic syndrome. *Thromb. Res.*, **16**, 345–354.

66 Yoshida, N. and Aoki, N. (1978) Release of arachidonic acid from human platelets. A key role for the potentiation of platelet hyperaggregability in normal subjects as well as those with nephrotic syndrome. *Blood*, **52**, 969–977.

67 Benigni, A., Rizzoni, G., Antolino, A. *et al.* (1990) Preliminary report: renal thromboxane A_2 synthesis in children with frequent relapsing nephrotic syndrome. *Lancet*, **ii**, 533–534.

68 Green, D., Arruda, J., Honic, G. *et al.* (1976) Urinary loss of clotting factors due to hereditary membranous nephropathy. *Am. J. Clin. Pathol.*, **65**, 346–351.

69 Vaziri, N., Toohey, J., Paule, P. *et al.* (1984) Urinary excretion and deficiency of prothrombin in nephrotic syndrome. *Am. J. Med.*, **77**, 433–436.

70 Saito, K., Goodnough, L.T., Makker, S.P. *et al.* (1981) Urinary excretion of Hageman factor (Factor XII) and presence of non functional Hageman factor in the nephrotic syndrome. *Am. J. Med.*, **70**, 531–537.

71 Natelson, E.A., Lynch, E.C. and Hettig, R.A. (1970) Acquired Factor IX deficiency in the nephrotic syndrome. *Ann. Intern. Med.*, **73**, 373–378.

72 Kendall, A.G., Lohmann, R.E. and Dossetor, J.B. (1971) Nephrotic syndrome: a hypercoagulable state. *Arch. Intern. Med.*, **127**, 1021–1027.

73 Thompson, C., Forbes, C.D., Prentice, C.R. *et al.* (1974) Changes in blood coagulation and fibrinolysis in the nephrotic syndrome. *Q. J. Med.*, **43**, 399–407.

74 Bonell, B., Boissou, F., Abbal, M. *et al.* (1981) Comparison of progressive antithrombin activity and concentration of three thrombin inhibitors in nephrotic syndrome. *Thromb. Haemost.*, **46**, 623–629.

75 Thaler, E., Balzar, E., Kopsa, H. *et al.* (1978) Acquired antithrombin III deficiency in patients with glomerular proteinuria. *Haemostasis*, **7**, 257–272.

76 Lange, L.G., Carvalho, A., Bagdasarian, D. *et al.* (1974) Activation of Hageman factor in the nephrotic syndrome. *Am. J. Med.*, **56**, 565–569.

77 Scheinman, K.I. and Stiehm, E.R. (1971) Fibrinolytic studies in the nephrotic

syndrome. *Pediatr. Res.*, **5**, 206–211.

78 Marder, V.J., Shulman, N.R. and Carrol, W.R. (1969) High molecular weight derivatives of human fibrinogen produced by plasmin I. Physicochemical and immunological characterization. *J. Biol. Chem.*, **244**, 2117–2119.

79 Collen, D. (1976) Identification of some properties of a new reacting plasmin inhibitor in human plasma. *Eur. J. Biochem.*, **69**, 209–216.

80 Clouse, L. and Comp, P. (1986) The regulation of hemostasis: The protein C system. *New Engl. J. Med.*, **314**, 1298–1304.

81 Allon, M., Soffer, O., Evatt, B. *et al.* (1989) Protein S and C antigen levels in proteinuric patients. Dependence on type of glomerular pathology. *Am. J. Hematol.*, **31**, 96–101.

82 Gandrille, S., Jouvin, M.H., Toulon, P. *et al.* (1988) A study of fibrinogen and fibrinolysis in 10 adults with nephrotic syndrome. *Thromb. Haemost.*, **59**, 445–450.

83 Aoki, N., Moroi, M., Sakata, Y. *et al.* (1978) Abnormal plasminogen. A hereditary molecular abnormality found in patients with recurrent thrombosis. *J. Clin. Invest.*, **61**, 1186–1195.

84 Du, X., Glass-Greenwalt, P., Kant, K.S. *et al.* (1985) Nephrotic syndrome with renal vein thrombosis: Pathogenetic importance of a plasmin inhibitor. *Clin. Nephrol.*, **24**, 186–191.

85 Alkjaersig, N., Fletcher, A.P., Narayanan, M. *et al.* (1987) Course and resolution of the coagulopathy in nephrotic children. *Kidney Int.*, **31**, 772–780.

86 Yamauchi, H. and Hopper, T. (1964) Hypovolemia, shock and hypotension as a complication in the nephrotic syndrome. Report of ten cases. *Ann. Intern. Med.*, **60**, 242–254.

87 Calcagno, P.L. and Rubin, M.I. (1961) Physiological consideration concerning corticosteroids therapy and complications in the nephrotic syndrome. *J. Pediatr.*, **58**, 685–701.

88 Haynes, R.C. and Murad, F. Adrenocorticotropic hormone: adrenocortical steroids and their synthetic analogs; inhibitors of adrenocortical steroid biosynthesis. In: *Goodman and Gilman's The Pharmacological Basis of Therapeutics* (Eds Goodman, A., Gilman, A., Goodman, L., Rale, T. & Murad, F.), 6th edn, pp. 1459–1489. Macmillan, New York (1985).

89 O'Reilly, R. Anticoagulant, antithrombotic and thrombolytic drugs. In: *Goodman and Gilman's The Pharmacological Basis of Therapeutics* (Eds Goodman, A., Gilman, A., Goodman, L., Rale, T. & Murad, F.), 6th edn, pp. 1339–1359. Macmillan, New York (1985).

90 Vermylen, C., Levin, M., Lanham, J. *et al.* (1987) Decreased sensitivity to heparin *in vitro* in steroid responsive nephrotic syndrome. *Kidney Int.*, **31**, 1396–1401.

91 Cameron, J.S., Ogg, C.S., Ellis, F.G. *et al.* (1971) Femoral artery thrombosis in nephrotic syndrome. *Arch. Dis. Child.*, **46**, 215–216.

92 Crowley, J.P., Matarese, R.A., Quevedo, S.F. *et al.* (1984) Fibrinolytic therapy for bilateral renal vein thrombosis. *Arch. Intern. Med.*, **144**, 159–161.

93 Bromberg, W.D. and Firlit, C. (1990) Fibrinolytic therapy for renal vein thrombosis in the child. *J. Urol.*, **143**, 86–88.

94 O'Brien, A.A., O'Donnell, J.P. and Keogh, J.A.B. (1986) Renal vein thrombosis with recurrent pulmonary embolism in the nephrotic syndrome: use of Greenfield

filter. *Postgrad. Med.*, **62**, 223–225.
95 Steinman, T. and Lazarus, J.M. Organ system involvement in acute renal failure. In: *Acute Renal Failure* (Eds Brenner, B.M. & Lazarus, J.M.), pp. 586–617. W.B. Saunders, Philadelphia (1983).
96 White, D.J., Young, F. and McKendrick, M.W. (1988) Haemolytic uraemic syndrome in adults. *Br. Med. J.*, **296**, 899.
97 Kavi, J. and Wise, R. (1989) Causes of the haemolytic uraemic syndrome. It might be verocytoxin produced by *Escherichia coli. Br. Med. J.*, **298**, 65–66.
98 Kelton, J.G., Moore, J.C. and Murphy, W.G. (1987) Studies investigating platelet aggregation and releases initiated by sera from patients with thrombotic thrombocytopenic purpura. *Blood*, **69**, 924–928.
99 Walters, M., Levin, M., Smith, C. *et al.* (1988) Intravascular platelet activation in the hemolytic uremic syndrome. *Kidney Int.*, **33**, 107–115.
100 Monteagudo, J., Pereira, A., Roig, S. *et al.* (1990) Investigation of plasma von Willebrand factor and circulating platelet aggregating activity in mitomycin C-related hemolytic uremic syndrome. *Am. J. Hematol.*, **33**, 46–49.
101 Chugh, K.S., Pal, Y., Chakravarty, R.N. *et al.* (1984) Acute renal failure following poisonous snakebite. *Am. J. Kidney Dis.*, **4**, 30–38.
102 Stratta, P., Canavese, C., Goia, L. *et al.* (1986) Clinical therapeutic correlations in consumption coagulopathy of obstetric acute renal failure. *Clin. Exp. Obstet. Gynecol.*, **13**, 43–49.
103 Kanfer, A. (1982) Coagulation and renal diseases. *Proc. Eur. Dial. Transplant. Assoc.*, **19**, 703–713.
104 Gotti, E., Mecca, G., Valentino, C. *et al.* (1984) Renal biopsy in patients with acute renal failure and prolonged bleeding time. *Lancet*, **ii**, 978–979.
105 McMurray, S.D., Luft, F.C., Maxwell, D.R. *et al.* (1978) Prevailing patterns and predictor variables in patients with acute tubular necrosis. *Arch. Intern. Med.*, **138**, 950–955.
106 Kleinknecht, D., Jungers, P., Chanard, J. *et al.* (1972) Uremic and non-uremic complications in acute renal failure: Evaluation of early and frequent dialysis on prognosis. *Kidney Int.*, **1**, 190–197.
107 Larsson, S.O., Hedner, U., Nilsson, I.M. (1971) On coagulation and fibrinolysis in acute renal insufficiency. *Acta Med. Scand.*, **189**, 443–451.
108 Kanfer, A., Vandewalle, A., Beaufils, M. *et al.* (1975) Enhanced antiplasmin activity in acute renal failure. *Br. Med. J.*, **4**, 195–197.
109 Dvorak, H.F. Abnormalities of hemostasis in malignancy. In: *Hemostasis and Thrombosis: Basic principles and clinical practice* (Eds Coleman, R., Hirsh, J., Marder, V. & Salzman, E.), 2nd edn, pp. 1143–1157. J.B. Lippincott, Philadelphia (1987).
110 Rader, E.S. (1975) Hematologic problems in urology. *Urology*, **5**, 589–593.
111 Naito, S., Kanamori, T., Hisano, S. *et al.* (1982) Human renal cell carcinoma: Establishment and characterization of two new cell lines. *J. Urol.*, **128**, 1117–1120.
112 Kursh, E., Ratnoff, O. and Persky, L. (1976) Current clotting concepts in urology. *J. Urol.*, **116**, 214–217.
113 Pergament, M.L., Swaim, W.R. and Blackard, C.E. (1976) Disseminated intravascular coagulation in the urologic patient. *J. Urol.*, **116**, 1–7.

114 Drewinko, B., Cobb, P., Guinee, V. *et al.* (1987) Untreated prostatic carcinoma is not associated with frequent thrombohemorrhagic disorders. *Urology*, **30**, 11–17.

115 Tagnon, H.J., Whitmore, W.F., Schulman, P. *et al.* (1953) The significance of fibrinolysis occurring in patients with metastatic cancer of the prostate. *Cancer*, **6**, 63–67.

116 Rapaport, S.I., Chapman, C.G. and Ames, S.B. (1959) Coexistent hypercoagulability and acute hypofibrinogenemia in a patient with prostatic carcinoma. *Am. J. Med.*, **27**, 144–149.

117 Blomback, M., Hedlund, P.O. and Sawe, U. (1988) Changes in blood coagulation and fibrinolysis in patients on different treatment regimens for prostatic cancer. Predictors for cardiovascular complications. *Thromb. Res.*, **49**, 111–121.

118 Sogani, P.C., Herr, H.W. and Whitmore, W.F. (1983) Renal cell carcinoma extending into inferior vena cava. *J. Urol.*, **130**, 660–663.

119 Marshall, E.M., Mendelsohn, L., Butler, K. *et al.* (1987) Treatment of metastatic renal cell carcinoma with coumarin (1,2-benzopyrone) and cimetidine: A pilot study. *J. Clin. Oncol.*, **5**, 862–867.

120 Sun, N.C.J., McAfee, W.M., Hum, G.J. *et al.* (1979) Hemostatic abnormalities in malignancy: A prospective study of 108 patients, Part I. Coagulation studies. *Am. J. Clin. Pathol.*, **71**, 10–17.

121 Gore, J.M., Appelbaum, J.S., Greene, H.L. *et al.* (1982) Occult cancer in patients with acute pulmonary embolism. *Ann. Intern. Med.*, **96**, 556–560.

122 Dawson, N.A., Barr, C.F. and Alving, B.M. (1985) Acquired dysfibrinogenemia: Paraneoplastic syndrome in renal cell carcinoma. *Am. J. Med.*, **78**, 682–686.

123 Sufrin, G., Mink, I., Fitzpatrick, J. *et al.* (1978) Coagulation factors in renal adenocarcinoma. *J. Urol.*, **119**, 727–730.

124 Riedmiller, H., Thuroff, J.W. and Jacobi, G.H. (1984) Fibrinogen degradation products in urological malignant tumors. *Urol. Int.*, **39**, 13–17.

125 Cliffton, E.E. and Grossi, C.E. (1955) Fibrinolytic activity of human tumor tissues as measured by the fibrin-plate method. *Cancer*, **8**, 1146–1154.

126 Yuen, P. and Kwaan, H.C. (1983) Fibrinolytic activity in human tumor tissues. *Cancer Invest.*, **1**, 369–375.

127 Gördon, S.G., Franks, J.J. and Lewis, B.J. (1979) Comparison of procoagulant activities in extracts of normal and malignant human tissue. *J. Natl. Cancer Inst.*, **62**, 773–776.

128 Mydlo, J.H., Heston, W.D. and Fair, W.R. (1987) Characterization of a heparin-binding growth factor from adenocarcinoma of the kidney. *J. Urol.*, **140**, 1575–1579.

129 Joist, J.H., Cowan, J.F. and Zimmerman, T.S. (1978) Acquired von Willebrand's disease. Evidence for a quantitative and qualitative Factor VIII disorder. *New Engl. J. Med.*, **298**, 988–991.

130 Morse, B. and Nussbaum, M. (1967) The detection of hyaluronic acid in the serum and urine of a patient with nephroblastoma. *Am. J. Med.*, **42**, 996–1002.

131 Bracey, A., Wu, A., Aceves, J. *et al.* (1987) Platelet dysfunction associated with Wilms' tumor and hyaluronic acid. *Am. J. Hematol.*, **24**, 247–257.

132 Tefferi, A., Owen, B., Nichols, W. *et al.* (1989) Isolation of a heparin-like anti-

coagulant from the plasma of a patient with metastatic bladder carcinoma. *Blood*, **74**, 252–254.

133 Steurer, G., Kusmitz, R., Pavelka, M. *et al.* (1989) Early onset thrombocytopenia during combination chemotherapy in testicular cancer is induced by vinblastine. *Cancer*, **63**, 51–58.

134 Fellstrom, B., Siegbahn, A., Liljenberg, G. *et al.* (1990) Primary haemostasis, plasmatic coagulation and fibrinolysis in renal transplantation. *Thromb. Res.*, **59**, 97–104.

135 Foegh, M.L., Winchester, J.F., Zmudka, M. *et al.* (1981) Urine i-TXB_2 in renal allograft rejection. *Lancet*, **ii**, 431–434.

136 Schrader, J., Gallimore, M., Eisenhauer, T. *et al.* (1988) Parameters of the kallikrein–kinin, coagulation and fibrinolytic systems as early indicators of kidney transplant rejection. *Nephron*, **48**, 183–189.

137 Vanrenterghem, Y., Roels, L., Lerut, T. *et al.* (1985) Thromboembolic complications and haemostatic changes in cyclosporin treated cadaveric kidney allografts recipients. *Lancet*, **i**, 999–1002.

138 Carlsen, E. and Prydz, H. (1985) Effect of cyclosporin A (CyA) on procoagulant activity in mononuclear cells (MNC) and monocytes (M) *in vitro*. *Thromb. Haemost.*, **54**, 202 (Abstract).

139 Pirotzky, E., Egido, J., Colliez, P. *et al.* (1989) Involvement of platelet-activating factor in renal processes. *Adv. Lipid Res.*, **23**, 277–293 (Abstract).

140 Urakaze, M., Hamazaki, T., Kashiwabara, H. *et al.* (1989) Favorable effects of fish oil concentrate on risk factors for thrombosis in renal allograft recipients. *Nephron*, **53**, 102–109.

Chapter 9
Anticoagulated patients

MARK N. LEVINE

The major complication of anticoagulant therapy is haemorrhage. In this chapter, the incidence of haemorrhage in patients receiving anticoagulant therapy (either heparin or oral anticoagulants), the mechanism of anticoagulant-induced haemorrhage, the clinical and the laboratory risk factors that predispose the bleeding, and practical issues related to the bleeding surgical patient are discussed. The information presented was drawn from results of randomized control trials whenever possible. Haemorrhage was classified as major if it was intracranial or retroperitoneal, if it led directly to death, or if it resulted in hospital admission or transfusion. All other bleeding episodes were considered as minor.

Heparin

Heparin is used for both the prevention and treatment of venous thromboembolism, for the treatment of ischaemic coronary syndromes, and as adjuvant treatment following coronary thrombolysis. Heparin is usually given in low doses by subcutaneous injection to prevent venous thrombosis (prophylactic heparin) and higher doses to treat patients with acute venous thromboembolism or with acute coronary syndromes (therapeutic heparin).

Mechanism of heparin-induced bleeding

The major anticoagulant action of heparin when administered at therapeutic concentrations is through its ability to augment the inhibition of a number of activated coagulation factors by antithrombin III [1–3]. Heparin binds to antithrombin III and produces a conformational change in the antithrombin III molecule. This exposes an arginine residue which neutralizes the serine active site on the activated coagulation Factors IIa, IXa and Xa [1–3]. At higher concentrations, heparin has an additional effect by catalysing the inhibition of thrombin by heparin cofactor II [4]. Additional mechanisms for heparin-induced bleeding are inhibition of platelet function [5] and increased capillary permeability [6]. Heparin can also produce thrombocytopenia, but this is rarely an important cause of bleeding.

Risk of bleeding associated with therapeutic heparin administration

The incidence of bleeding during heparin therapy in patients with venous thromboembolism has been reported from randomized trials which have compared continuous intravenous heparin with intermittent intravenous heparin and from trials which have compared intravenous heparin with subcutaneous heparin [7–16]. In these studies, the reported risk of major haemorrhage has varied from 1 to 33% (Table 9.1). Results from clinical trials in patients with acute coronary syndromes indicate that there is no evidence that heparin administered alone increases the risk of bleeding [17–19]. However, when heparin is used as an adjunct to thrombolytic therapy in patients with myocardial infarction, there is an increased risk of minor bleeding, often at the site of angiography-catheter insertion [20–23].

Relationship between risk of bleeding and heparin dose–response

Patients who are on therapeutic heparin are monitored by a test of coagulation, i.e. the activated partial thromboplastin time (APTT). It is customary to try to maintain the APTT within a defined therapeutic range, which is usually 1.5–2-fold normal control plasma.

There have been no randomized trials in patients with established venous thrombosis which directly compare different doses of heparin, but if haemorrhagic rates from individual trials are correlated with the 24 doses of heparin (from the studies in Table 9.1), a significant relationship is observed between heparin dose and bleeding (the correlation coefficient is 0.56) [24].

It is not possible from reported studies to separate the effects of heparin response as measured by the APTT and heparin dose. However, subgroup analysis of randomized trials and prospective cohort studies provides only suggestive evidence for an association between the incidence at bleeding and the anticoagulant response as manifested by an excessively prolonged APTT [24].

Table 9.1 Risk of bleeding associated with therapeutic heparin

Study	Method of administration	Patient no.	Major† haemorrhage no. (%)	24 hour heparin dose (iu)
Salzman *et al.* (1975) [7]	Continuous	69	1 (1.0)	24 480
	vs.		*	
	Intermittent	72	6 (8.3)	31 740
Glazier and Corwell	Continuous	20	0	25 488
(1976) [8]	vs.		*	
	Intermittent	21	7 (33.0)	32 808
Mant *et al.* (1977) [9]	Continuous	40	6 (15.0)	33 074
	vs.			
	Intermittent	36	4 (11.0)	29 861
Wilson and Lampman	Continuous	40	2 (5.0)	27 695
(1979) [10]	vs.			
	Intermittent	40	4 (10.0)	37 015
Fagher and Lundh (1981)	Continuous	15	3 (20.0)	37 371
[11]	vs.			
	Intermittent	13	4 (30.8)	41 380
Wilson *et al.* (1981) [12]	Continuous	36	3 (8.0)	28 440
	vs.			
	Intermittent	29	5 (17.0)	43 570
Bentley *et al.* (1980) [13]	Subcutaneous	50	2 (4.0)	36 998
	vs.			
	Continuous	50	4 (8.0)	36 814
Andersson *et al.*	Subcutaneous	72	2 (2.7)	35 000
(1982) [14]	vs.			
	Continuous	69	2 (2.8)	31 500
Hull *et al.* (1986) [15]	Subcutaneous	57	2 (3.5)	32 317
	vs.			
	Continuous	58	2 (3.4)	29 674
Doyle *et al.* (1987) [16]	Subcutaneous	51	4 (7.8)	29 180
	vs.			
	Continuous	52	2 (3.8)	29 260

* $p<0.05$.
† Three fatal bleeds in all studies combined.

Relationship between risk of bleeding and patient risk factors

There is good evidence that co-morbid conditions, particularly recent surgery or trauma, are important risk factors for heparin-induced bleeding [24–27]. This association was demonstrated in a recent study by

Hull and associates (1990) in patients with proximal vein thrombosis [26]. Patients without clinical risk factors for bleeding were treated with a starting dose of 40 000 iu of heparin by continuous infusion, while those with well-recognized risk factors for bleeding (e.g. recent surgery, trauma) received a starting dose of only 30 000 iu. Bleeding occurred in 1 : 88 patients (1%) who received the higher dose and in 12 : 111 patients (11%) who received the lower dose. There is also evidence that the concurrent use of aspirin, and older age increase the risk of bleeding [25–27].

Risk of bleeding associated with prophylactic low-dose subcutaneous heparin

Low-dose heparin is an effective form of prophylaxis for venous thrombosis in surgical and medical patients. Collins *et al.* (1988) have conducted an overview analysis of randomized trials of prophylactic subcutaneous heparin in general surgical and orthopaedic patients [28]. There was evidence from this analysis that heparin administration was associated with an increased risk of minor bleeding, albeit small, with an absolute increase of 2%. There was no evidence of increased fatal bleeding with heparin prophylaxis.

Clagget and Reisch (1988) have conducted an overview analysis of randomized trials of heparin prophylaxis in general surgical patients [29]. The overall incidence of major haemorrhage was identical (0.33%) among heparin and control patients. However, there was a statistically significant difference in wound haematomas between groups; 6.3% for heparin patients compared to 4.1% in control patients.

Results from randomized trials of heparin prophylaxis in patients undergoing hip surgery suggest that there is an increased risk of minor bleeding, particularly at the operative site, but not an increased risk of major or fatal bleeding [24,28,29].

Oral anticoagulant therapy

Vitamin K antagonists are widely used to prevent recurrent thrombosis in patients with established thromboembolism and to prevent thrombosis in high-risk individuals.

Mechanisms of oral anticoagulant-induced bleeding

Vitamin K catalyses the post-translational carboxylation of glutamic acid residues on several proteins synthesized in the liver. The resulting γ-carboxyglutamic residues may bind calcium ions in the presence of membrane phospholipids, an important requirement for the appropriate function of these proteins. The vitamin K-dependent coagulation proteins are Factors II, VII, IX and X. The non-carboxylated forms are inactive because they can no longer form appropriate complexes with calcium and phospholipid and thus, if the carboxylated forms are excessively depleted, haemorrhage can result.

Monitoring oral anticoagulant therapy

The prothrombin time (PT) test, is the most common method used in monitoring oral anticoagulant therapy. This test is responsive to reductions in three of the vitamin K clotting factors, Factors II, VII and X. This test is performed by adding a phospholipid extract of mammalian tissue (known as thromboplastin) to citrated plasma and clotting the mixture by adding calcium. Thromboplastins are prepared from brain, lung or placental tissues and vary notably in their responsiveness to the anticoagulant effects of warfarin [30–33]. As a consequence of the variability and responsiveness of different thromboplastins, PT results obtained from patients on oral anticoagulant therapy may not be interchangeable between laboratories and as a consequence, could produce potential problems for anticoagulant control.

Over the years a number of attempts have been made to standardize the reporting system for the PT [30–33]. Using a reference thromboplastin prepared by the WHO, an international committee recommended the adoption of a uniform calibration system in which the PT ratio (patient's PT : control PT) is expressed in terms of the International Normalized Ratio (INR) [33,34]. The INR is calculated as follows:

$$\text{INR} = [\text{observed ratio}]^{c}$$

where c is the constant which represents the International Sensitivity Index (ISI). The majority of commercial rabbit brain thromboplastins have an ISI between 2.0 and 2.5, while human brain thromboplastins have an ISI close to 1.0.

Relationship between intensity of anticoagulant therapy and haemorrhage

The recommended therapeutic range for oral anticoagulant therapy for most indications is an INR of 2–3 [31] (Table 9.2). A relationship

Table 9.2 Recommended therapeutic range for oral anticoagulant therapy

Indication	INR
Prophylaxis of venous thromboembolism	2.0–3.0
Treatment of deep vein thrombosis/pulmonary embolism	2.0–3.0
Prevention of arterial thromboembolism	2.0–3.0

Atrial fibrillation, valvular heart disease, tissue heart valves, myocardial infarction all INR 2.0–3.0, except mechanical prosthetic heart valves (INR 3.0–4.5).

between the intensity of anticoagulant therapy and the risk of bleeding has been noted in patients with deep vein thrombosis, tissue heart valves and mechanical heart valves [34–36]. In patients with venous thrombosis, Hull and colleagues (1982) reported a strong relationship between the intensity of warfarin treatment and the risk of bleeding [34]. The patients randomized to receive less intense warfarin (targeted INR = 2.0) had significantly less bleeding (4% vs. 22%) than those patients receiving more intense therapy (targeted to INR = 2.5–4.5).

Turpie *et al.* (1988) randomized patients with tissue heart valves to standard-intensity warfarin (INR 2.5–4.0) or less intense warfarin (INR 2.0–2.5) [35]. The rate of clinically important bleeding was reduced from 14% in the standard-intensity group to 6% in the low-intensity groups without loss of antithrombotic efficacy.

In a recently reported trial, patients with prosthetic heart valves were randomized to either moderate-intensity warfarin (targeted INR = 2.65) or high-intensity warfarin (targeted INR = 9.0) [36]. Bleeding was more common in the higher intensity group.

Relationship between risk of bleeding and patient risk factors

Major bleeding is especially likely in patients with ischaemic cerebral vascular disease and venous thromboembolism, possibly owing to the higher prevalence of associated risk factors in these conditions [37]. In venous thromboembolism, these co-morbid conditions (cancer, recent surgery and paraplegia) predispose the patient to thrombosis. In cerebral vascular disease, major bleeding is usually intracerebral, possibly because of associated hypertension or the vascular disease *per se*.

There have been two recent retrospective studies which have examined the risk factors of bleeding. Gurwitz *et al.* (1988) reported no relationship between age and risk of bleeding in 321 patients on long-term oral anticoagulant therapy [38]. Landefeld *et al.* (1989) however, reported five factors which predicted independently for bleeding in a cohort of patients on long-term anticoagulant therapy [39,40]. These were ≥65 years of age, with a history of stroke, history of gastrointestinal bleeding, atrial fibrillation, and a serious co-morbid condition (recent myocardial infarction, renal insufficiency or severe anaemia). In addition, in this study there was evidence that those patients who experienced a bleeding episode with the PT within the therapeutic range, had an underlying pathological cause for the bleed.

Interaction of oral anticoagulants with other drugs

Certain drugs can influence the absorption, metabolism and excretion of warfarin, and thus can have a clinically important impact on oral anticoagulant control. Certain drugs, such as cholestyramine, liquid paraffin laxatives and some antacids impair warfarin absorption from the gut and consequently, decrease the anticoagulant effect [41,42]. Drugs that displace warfarin from albumin, such as phenylbutazone, phenytoin and oral hypoglycaemic agents, increase the anticoagulant effect [41,42]. Some drugs induce hepatic microsomal drug metabolizing enzymes, thus increasing the metabolism of warfarin and decreasing the anticoagulant effect. Such drugs include barbiturates, rifampin and griseofulvin [41,42]. The use of broad-spectrum antibiotics which sterilize the bacterial gut flora can influence the anticoagulant effect of warfarin [41,42]. Thus, it is very important that when a patient on long-term oral anticoagulant therapy is started on a new medication, the PT be followed more closely for a while.

Risk of haemorrhage and clinical disorder

A previous review of published randomized trials of long-term oral anticoagulant therapy revealed that bleeding rates (pooled rates) during long-term anticoagulant therapy can be substantial (Table 9.3) [37]. Depending on the indication, major bleeding ranged from 1 to 8%. The highest rates occurred in patients with cerebral vascular disease and venous thromboembolism.

Table 9.3 Haemorrhage during warfarin therapy

Indication	Patient no.	Major bleed (%)	Fatal bleed (%)
Ischaemic cerebrovascular	588	41 (7.0)	28 (4.8)
Prosthetic mechanical heart valves	405	10 (2.4)	7 (1.7)
Atrial fibrillation	536	24 (4.5)	1 (0.2)
Ischaemic heart	1890	88 (4.7)	19 (1.0)
Venous thromboembolism	159	13 (8.1)	0

Management of the bleeding patient

Heparin

Bleeding due to heparin therapy can be life threatening. When bleeding is serious, the anticoagulant effect of heparin should be reversed with protamine sulphate, a strongly basic drug that combines with and neutralizes heparin. The appropriate neutralizing dose depends on both the dose of heparin and the time of its administration. If protamine sulphate is given within minutes of intravenous heparin injection, then a full neutralizing dose (1 mg protamine/100 iu heparin) should be given. Rapid infusion of protamine sulphate can cause hypotension and therefore it should be infused slowly over a 10 min period. Since the plasma half-life of heparin is approximately 60 min, >50 mg of protamine sulphate is seldom required, since this dose reverses the anticoagulant effect of 10 000 iu of heparin administered 30 min previously. Only 50% of the calculated dose of protamine sulphate should be given if heparin neutralization is required 60 min after heparin injection and only 25% of the calculated dose is required if heparin was administered 2 h previously. Treatment with protamine sulphate may have to be repeated because the drug is cleared from the blood more rapidly than heparin.

Oral anticoagulant therapy

The approach to treatment is influenced by whether the PT is in the targeted therapeutic range at the time of bleeding, or whether it is excessively prolonged. If haemorrhage occurs when the PT is within the therapeutic range, an underlying cause of bleeding should be sought [40]. Bleeding associated with oral anticoagulants is usually managed by one or more of the following approaches:

1 Cessation of anticoagulant.

2 Administration of vitamin K.

3 Administration of plasma derivatives containing vitamin K-dependent clotting factors.

4 Volume replacement if indicated.

If the PT is only slightly outside the therapeutic range, and bleeding is not life threatening, the patient can be treated by omitting the next two or three doses of warfarin and by carefully monitoring the patient's progress. If the PT is markedly prolonged, but the bleeding is not life threatening, the PT can be reduced within 8 h by the intravenous or subcutaneous administration of vitamin K. A dose of >25 mg causes the patient to become refractory to further anticoagulant therapy for days. The dose of 5–10 mg allows anticoagulant therapy to be continued if indicated. If bleeding is potentially life threatening and the PT is prolonged, the coagulation defect may be reversed immediately by infusion of fresh frozen plasma or Factors II, VII, IX and X concentrate. The administration of plasma may be problematic in a patient with poor cardiac reserve because of fluid overload. If plasma cannot be given, then factor concentrate may be used; however, factor concentrate should not be used in the presence of liver failure.

The bleeding patient with established venous thrombosis

Results of randomized trials have firmly established the need for adequate heparin therapy in the treatment of acute venous thrombosis and the need for long-term oral anticoagulant therapy to prevent recurrent thrombosis in patients with venous thrombosis, atrial fibrillation or prosthetic heart valves. Thus, the bleeding patient who requires continuing anticoagulant therapy obviously poses a difficult clinical dilemma. In such cases, the first step is to stabilize the patient and control the bleeding. Anticoagulant therapy should not be resumed during this critical period. However, once the patient has been stabilized and the bleeding stopped, then a decision concerning further anticoagulant therapy should be made. If a patient with acute proximal deep vein thrombosis and/or pulmonary embolism has had an anticoagulant-associated bleed and the bleeding has stopped, then two approaches can be considered. If bleeding was associated with an excessively prolonged APTT (in the case of heparin) or PT (in the case of oral anticoagulants), then antithrombotic therapy can be resumed, with closer monitoring and maintaining the test within the targeted therapeutic range (perhaps towards the lower end of the therapeutic range). A second approach for such a patient would be to interrupt the vena cava by a Greenfield filter.

Management of the anticoagulated patient who requires elective surgery

Patients with acute venous thrombosis are traditionally treated with heparin for a period of 7–10 days, with oral anticoagulants being started on day 5 and overlapping with heparin for 4–5 days. Oral anticoagulants are then continued for 3 months, providing there is no continuing risk factors such as antithrombin III or protein C deficiency.

Patients who require surgery soon after an initial acute venous thromboembolic event are likely to be at increased risk of postoperative venous thrombosis. Hence, our approach to such patients is to recommend delaying the elective surgery until 3 months of oral anticoagulants are completed. Then, when such a patient undergoes surgery, prophylactic measures are used. If the patient is undergoing general surgery, subcutaneous heparin (5000 iu twice daily) commencing 2 h preoperatively is used. In addition, because of the recent history of venous thrombosis, we would also use graduated compression stockings postoperatively. In the orthopaedic patient, prophylaxis with either low-dose oral anticoagulant therapy (targeted INR = 2.0–3.0), subcutaneous heparin or low-molecular-weight heparin if available would be recommended.

The situation arises however, where a patient is on oral anticoagulant therapy for either venous thrombosis, atrial fibrillation or prosthetic heart valves and requires the continuation of such treatment postoperatively. There are several approaches to such patients. One approach has been to stop oral anticoagulants approximately 1 week before the elective surgery and let the prothrombin time drift down to the normal range. However, such an approach would not be considered optimal because the patient would be at increased risk for thrombosis during the period when the coagulation test is subtherapeutic. Our approach has been to admit such patients electively to hospital and administer subcutaneous vitamin K, 10 mg daily for 2 days. Intravenous heparin is started on the 2nd day with a bolus of 5000 iu intravenously, followed by a continuous infusion of approximately 1000 iu/h adjusted to maintain the APTT at 1.5–2 times normal; 4–6 h preoperatively, the heparin infusion is discontinued; postoperatively, once primary haemostasis is achieved, the heparin infusion can be restarted. Generally, we wait at least 24 h before resuming the heparin infusion. Once the patient is making a satisfactory postoperative recovery and capable of taking adequate oral intake, oral anticoagulants can be restarted. When the PT is within the therapeutic range, the heparin can be discontinued.

References

1 Rosenberg, R.D. and Lam, L. (1979) Correlation between structure and function of heparin. *Proc. Natl. Acad. Sci. USA*, **76**(2), 1218–1222.

2 Rosenberg, R.D. The heparin–antithrombin system: a natural anticoagulant mechanism. In: *Hemostasis and Thrombosis; Basic Principles and Clinical Practice* (Eds Colman, R.W., Hirsh, J., Marder V.J. & Salzman, E.W.), 2nd edn, pp. 1373–1392. J.B. Lippincott, Philadelphia (1987).

3 Lindahl, U., Backstrom, G., Hook, M. *et al.* (1979) Structure of the antithrombin-binding site of heparin. *Proc. Natl. Acad. Sci. USA*, **76**(4), 3198–3202.

4 Ofosu, F.A., Modi, G.J., Hirsh, J. (1986) Mechanisms for inhibition of the generation of thrombin activity by sulfated polysaccharides. *Ann. NY Acad. Sci.*, **485**, 41–55.

5 Fernandez, F., Nguyen, P., van Ryn, J. *et al.* (1986) Haemorrhagic doses of heparin and other glycosaminoglycans induce a platelet defect. *Thromb. Res.*, **43**, 491–495.

6 Blajchman, M.A., Young, E. and Ofosu, F.A. (1989) Effects of unfractionated heparin, dermatan sulfate and low molecular weight heparin on vessel wall permeability in rabbits. *Ann. NY Acad. Sci.*, **556**, 245–253.

7 Salzman, E.W., Deykin, D., Shapiro, R.M. and Rosenberg R. (1975) Management of heparin therapy. *New Engl. J. Med.*, **292**, 1046–1050.

8 Glazier, R.L. and Corwell, E.B. (1976) Randomized prospective trial of continuous vs. intermittent heparin therapy. *JAMA*, **236**, 1365–1367.

9 Mant, M.J., O'Brien, B.D., Thong, K.L. *et al.* (1977) Haemorrhagic complications of heparin therapy. *Lancet*, **i**, 1133.

10 Wilson, J.R. and Lampman, J. (1979) Heparin therapy: a randomized prospective study. *Am. Heart J.*, **97**, 155–158.

11 Fagher, B. and Lundh, B. (1981) Heparin treatment of deep vein thrombosis. *Acta Med. Scand.*, **210**, 357–361.

12 Wilson, J.E., Bynum, L.J. and Parkey, R.W. (1981) Heparin therapy in venous thromboembolism. *Am. J. Med.*, **70**, 808–816.

13 Bentley, P.G., Kakkar, V.V., Scully, M.F. *et al.* (1980) An objective study of alternative methods of heparin administration. *Thromb. Res.*, **18**(1–2), 177–187.

14 Andersson, G., Fagrell, B., Holmgren, K. *et al.* (1982) Subcutaneous administration of heparin: A randomized comparison with intravenous administration of heparin to patients with deep vein thrombosis. *Thromb. Res.*, **27**, 631–639.

15 Hull, R.D., Raskob, G.E., Hirsh, J. *et al.* (1986) Continuous intravenous heparin

compared with intermittent subcutaneous heparin in the initial treatment of proximal-vein thrombosis. *New Engl. J. Med.*, **315**, 1109–1214.

16 Doyle, D.J., Turpie, A.G.G., Hirsh, J. *et al.* (1987) Adjusted subcutaneous heparin or continuous intravenous heparin in patients with acute deep vein thrombosis. A randomized trial. *Ann. Intern. Med.*, **107**(4), 441–445.

17 Theroux, P. Ouimet, H., McCans, J. *et al.* (1988) Aspirin, heparin or both to treat acute unstable angina? *New Engl. J. Med.*, **319**, 1105–1111.

18 Seneri, G.G.N., Roveli, F., Gensini, G.F. *et al.* (1987) Effectiveness of low-dose heparin in prevention of myocardial reinfarction. *Lancet*, **i**, 937–942.

19 Turpie, A.G.G., Robinson, J.G., Doyle, D.J. *et al.* (1989) Comparison of high-dose with low-dose subcutaneous heparin to prevent left ventricular mural thrombosis in patients with acute transmural anterior myocardial infarction. *New Engl. J. Med.*, **320**, 352–394.

20 The SCATI Group (1989) Randomized controlled trial of subcutaneous calcium–heparin in acute myocardial infarction. *Lancet*, **ii**, 182–185.

21 Seneri, G.G.N., Gensini, G.R., Poggesi, L. *et al.* (1990) Effect of heparin, aspirin, or alteplase in reduction of myocardial ischaemia in refractory unstable angina. *Lancet*, **i**, 615–618.

22 Topol, E.J., George, B.S., Kereiakes, D.J. *et al.* (1989) A randomized controlled trial of intravenous tissue plasminogen activator and early intravenous heparin in acute myocardial infarction. *Circulation*, **79**, 281–286.

23 Gruppo Italiano per lo Studio della Sopravvivenza nell'Infarto Miocardio. (1990) GISSI-2: A factorial randomized trial of alteplase versus streptokinase and heparin versus no heparin among 12 490 patients with acute myocardial infarction. *Lancet*, **ii**(336), 65–70.

24 Levine, M.N., Hirsh, J. and Kelton, J.G. Heparin-induced bleeding. In: *Heparin: Chemical and Biological Properties Clinical Applications* (Eds Lane, D.A. & Lindahl, U.) pp. 517–532. Edward Arnold, London (1989).

25 Jick, H., Slone, D., Borda, I.T. and Chapiro, S. (1968) Efficacy and toxicity of heparin in relation to age and sex. *New Engl. J. Med.*, **279**, 284–286

26 Hull, R.D., Raskob, G.E., Rosenbloom, D. *et al.* (1990) Heparin for 5 days versus for 10 days in the initial treatment of proximal venous thrombosis. *New Engl. J. Med*, **322**, 1260–1264.

27 Yett, H.S., Skillman, J.J. and Salzman, E.W. (1978) The hazards of heparin plus aspirin. *New Engl. J. Med.*, **298**, 1092.

28 Collins, R., Scrimgeour, A., Yusuf, S. *et al.* (1988) Reduction in fatal pulmonary embolism and venous thrombosis by perioperative administration of subcutaneous heparin. *New Engl. J. Med.*, **318**, 1162–1173.

29 Clagett, G.P. and Reisch, J.S. (1988) Prevention of venous thromboembolism in general surgical patients. *Ann. Surg.*, **208**, 227–240.

30 Hirsh, J., Poller, L., Deykin, D. *et al.* (1989) Optimal therapeutic range for oral anticoagulants. *Chest* (Suppl.), **95**(2), 5S–11S.

31 Hirsh, J. (1987) Is the dose of warfarin prescribed by American Physicians unnecessarily high? *Arch. Intern. Med.*, **147**, 769–777.

32 Poller, L. (1987) Progress in standardisation in anticoagulant control. *Haematol. Rev.*, **1**, 225–241.

33 Hirsh, J. and Levine, M. (1988) Confusion over the therapeutic range for monitoring

oral anticoagulant therapy in North America. *Thromb. Haemost.*, **59**(2), 129–132.

34 Hull, R., Hirsh, J., Jay, R. *et al.* (1982) Different intensities of oral anticoagulant therapy in the treatment of proximal-vein thrombosis. *New Engl. J. Med.*, **307**, 1676–1681.

35 Turpie, A.G.G., Gunstensen, J., Hirsh, J. *et al.* (1988) Randomized comparison of two intensities of oral anticoagulant therapy after tissue heart valve replacement. *Lancet*, **i**, 1242–1245.

36 Saour, J.N., Sieck, J.O., Mamo, L.A.R. and Gallus, A.S. (1990) Trial of different intensities of anticoagulation in patients with prosthetic heart valves. *New Engl. J. Med.*, **322**(7), 428–432.

37 Levine, M.N., Raskob, G. and Hirsh, J. (1989) Hemorrhagic complications of long-term anticoagulant therapy. *Chest* (Suppl.), **95**(2), 26S–36S.

38 Gurwitz, J.H., Goldberg, R.J., Holden, A. *et al.* (1988) Age-related risks of long term oral anticoagulant therapy. *Arch. Intern. Med.*, **148**, 1733–1736.

39 Landefeld, C.S. and Rosenblatt, M.W. (1989) Bleeding in outpatients treated with warfarin: relation to the prothombin time and important remediable lesions. *Am. J. Med.*, **87**, 153–159.

40 Landefeld, C.S. and Goldman, L. (1989) Major bleeding in outpatients treated with warfarin: incidence and prediction by factors known at the start of outpatient therapy. *Am. J. Med.*, **87**, 144–152.

41 Koch-Weser, J. and Sellers, D.M. (1971) Drug interactions with oral anticoagulants. *New Engl. J. Med.*, **285**, 487–498.

42 Sellers, D.M. and Koch-Weser, J. (1971) Drug interactions with coumarin anti-coagulants. *New Engl. J. Med.*, **285**, 547–548.

Chapter 10
Bleeding and thrombolytic therapy

GORDON D.O. LOWE

There is increasing evidence for a balance between haemostasis and thrombosis (Fig. 10.1). Excessive bleeding after surgery may arise from vascular defects (including technical failures and vessel wall disorders such as vitamin C deficiency), platelet defects (including platelet functional defects such as aspirin ingestion), coagulation defects (including anticoagulant treatment or prophylaxis), and excessive fibrinolysis (including that due to recent thrombolytic therapy—the subject of this chapter). On the other hand, there is increasing evidence that postoperative thrombosis is associated with vessel wall lesions, hyperactivity of platelets and coagulation as a response to surgical trauma, and underactive fibrinolysis [1]. Perioperative antiplatelet or anticoagulant therapy significantly lowers the risk of postoperative thromboembolism, and this benefit outweighs the increased risk of bleeding [2,3]. Surgeons and physicians must therefore try to balance the risks of bleeding and thromboembolism, and this is particularly important when using thrombolytic therapy, which has powerful effects on both processes.

Thrombolytic therapy is an increasingly important part of the management of cardiovascular disease [4,5]. Its importance to surgeons is twofold

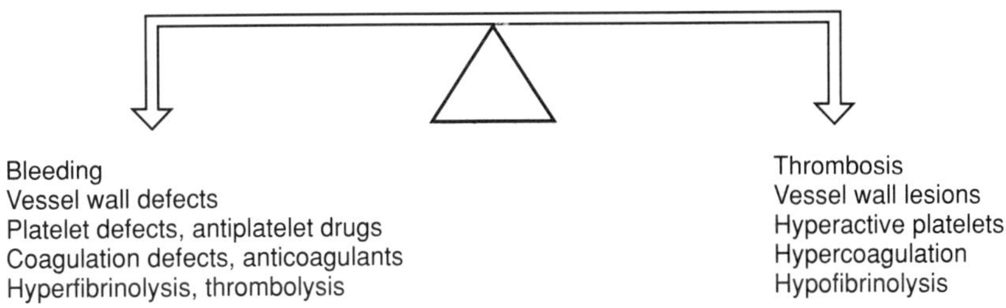

Fig. 10.1 The physiological balance between haemostasis and thrombosis. Thrombolytic therapy lyses thrombi, but also increases the risk of bleeding by lysing recently formed haemostatic plugs in vessel wall defects, and also by its systemic effects on platelets and coagulation. (From [6] with permission.)

1 Surgeons may use thrombolytic therapy on their patients, e.g. in arterial thromboembolism of the limbs, or in extensive venous thromboembolism.

2 Surgeons may be faced with the need for urgent surgery in these or other patients who have recently received thrombolytic therapy (e.g. for recent myocardial infarction) and who are therefore at increased risk of bleeding, as well as of further thromboembolism.

This chapter briefly outlines the drugs used for thrombolytic therapy, their antithrombotic and haemorrhagic effects, their indications and contraindications, laboratory monitoring, and the prevention and management of bleeding during or after treatment. For more detailed reviews, the reader is referred to recent publications [4–7].

Drugs used in thrombolytic therapy

Four thrombolytic agents are currently licensed for use in the UK: streptokinase, anistreplase, urokinase and alteplase. All are plasminogen activators, which activate plasminogen to plasmin (Fig. 10.2). Streptokinase and anistreplase are exogenous activators from streptococci. Alteplase is one form of the endogenous, extrinsic, tissue-type plasminogen activator (tPA) which is produced by recombinant gene technology. Urokinase is one form of the endogenous, intrinsic, urinary-type plasminogen activator (uPA), which is produced by tissue culture of kidney cells. Saruplase is a recombinant form of single-chain uPA, not yet licensed for clinical use.

When these activators are infused into veins or arteries in doses which exceed the neutralizing capacity of their inhibitors (antistreptococcal antibodies in the case of streptokinase or anistreplase; or the endogenous plasminogen activator inhibitors (PAIs) such as PAI-1 and PAI-2 in the case of urokinase, alteplase or saruplase), plasmin is formed. When plasmin generation exceeds the neutralizing capacity of its inhibitors (α_2-antiplasmin, α_2-macroglobulin), free plasmin can digest crosslinked fibrin, fibrinogen and coagulation Factors V and VIII, resulting in prolongation of clotting times (thrombin time, prothrombin time and activated partial thromboplastin time) (Figs 10.2 and 10.3).

High plasma concentrations of fibrinogen/fibrin degradation products (FDPs) are present during and for several hours after thrombolytic therapy. Together with fibrinogen depletion, they prolong the thrombin time (by inhibiting thrombin) and inhibit platelet aggregation (prolonging the skin bleeding time). Plasmin splits off the 1–42 fragment of the Bβ

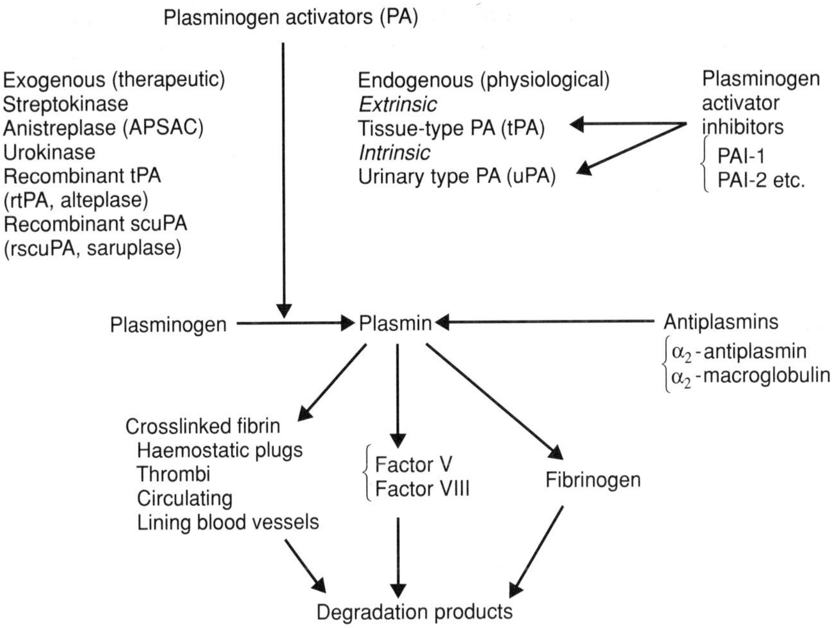

Fig. 10.2 The fibrinolytic system. (From [6] with permission.)

chain of fibrinogen, then digests it to high- and low-molecular-weight FDPs. With crosslinked fibrin, plasmin splits off the 15–42 fragment of the Bβ chain, then digests it to high- and low molecular-weight crosslinked FDP (XL-FDP), which can be detected immunologically by monoclonal antibodies against crosslinked fragments [6,7]. While digestion of crosslinked fibrin was thought by some to be a potential marker of lysis of thrombi, plasma XL-FDP levels show poor correlations with angiographic thrombolysis [6], and it is now appreciated that thrombolytic therapy also digests crosslinked fibrin in haemostatic plugs (causing bleeding), in the circulation, and lining blood vessels (Figs 10.2 and 10.3).

Streptokinase

This is currently the 'gold standard' thrombolytic agent because there is most experience in its use, because it is the cheapest, and because no other thrombolytic agents have been proven in randomized controlled trials to achieve superior clinical results, or to reduce overall adverse

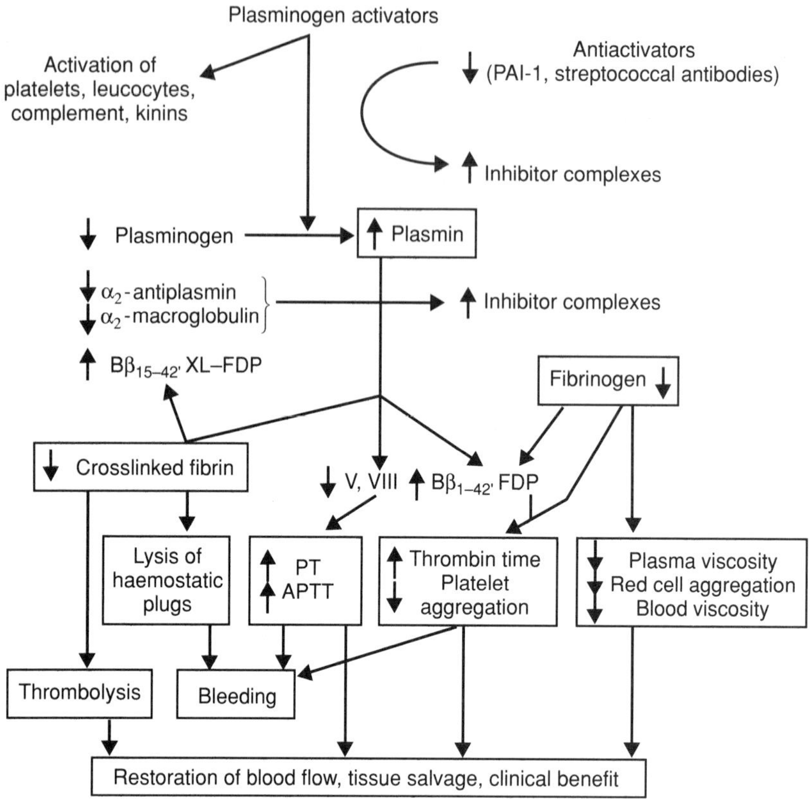

Fig. 10.3 Systemic effects of thrombolytic therapy. (From [5] with permission.)

reactions, which would justify their higher costs in routine use [5,8]. As a foreign protein, its disadvantages are a higher risk of hypotension and allergic reactions [9,10], and antibody formation which may render standard doses ineffective in patients treated within the previous year [11]. Urokinase or alteplase may therefore be considered in patients with hypotension, allergy to streptokinase (or multiple allergies), or recent (5 days to 12 months) streptokinase therapy or streptococcal infections. Streptokinase has a half-life of about 25 min.

Anistreplase

Anistreplase or anisoylated streptokinase–plasminogen activator complex (APSAC) is a proenzyme, whose catalytic serine active site is temporarily masked by an anisoyl group. Following intravenous infusion, it is slowly activated by sustained deacylation, and has a half-life of about 90 min. Unlike streptokinase, it can be given as a bolus infusion over 5 min. Its systemic effects, adverse effects, and clinical efficacy appear comparable to streptokinase: however, it may have a higher risk of haemorrhagic stroke [8]. It is currently licensed in the UK for use in acute myocardial infarction.

Urokinase

This is less antigenic than streptokinase, but has similar systemic effects on the blood. It is not currently licensed for use in acute myocardial infarction in the UK, but is licensed for use in venous thromboembolism, peripheral arterial thromboembolism and clotted arteriovenous shunts.

Alteplase

This is less antigenic than streptokinase, has fewer systemic effects on the blood (fibrinogen depletion and prolongation of clotting times), and shows a higher degree of binding to fibrin. Its 'clot-selectivity' was initially hypothesized to result in greater clinical efficacy and less haemorrhagic risk; however, these potential advantages have not been demonstrated in large randomized trials of alteplase (or the similar preparation, duteplase) against streptokinase in acute myocardial infarction [8–10]. In the GISSI-2 and ISIS-3 studies, mortality with alteplase or duteplase was similar to that with streptokinase, although previous studies had shown higher early coronary patency rates [5,8–10]. Explanations include the similar *later* patency rates, and the beneficial effects of marked streptokinase-induced fibrinogen depletion and FDP formation on plasma and blood viscosity, restoration of blood flow, and prevention of rethrombosis [5] (Fig. 10.3). Streptokinase also has a lower risk of bleeding, especially cerebral bleeding, than alteplase or duteplase [8–10]. Along with other evidence [5,6,12], this finding suggests that the most important cause of bleeding after thrombolytic therapy is digestion of recently-formed haemostatic fibrin plugs, which is probably higher with 'clot-selective' agents because no plasminogen activator can differentiate between haemostatic fibrin and thrombotic fibrin [5,12]. The antiplatelet and anticoagulant effects of plasma FDPs (Figs 10.1 and 10.3) appear to play lesser roles in bleeding, and this limits the value of laboratory monitoring [5,6,12].

Indications for thrombolytic therapy

Acute myocardial infarction

This is now the prime indication for thrombolytic therapy, which has been shown in large, randomized controlled trials to reduce infarct size and consequently to reduce total mortality [4,5,13]. Streptokinase is effective when given up to 24 h after the onset of symptoms [13], showing that coronary thrombosis and myocardial infarction are evolving, dynamic processes rather than short-lived, all-or-none events; however, it is most effective when given early. Streptokinase is usually combined with aspirin, with which there is a synergistic reduction in mortality [13], showing the equal importance of platelet and fibrin components of coronary thrombi. The need for anticoagulant therapy as well as aspirin after thrombolysis in myocardial infarction remains to be established; it increases the risk of bleeding more than aspirin [8,9,13].

Three randomized controlled trials have now shown that immediate percutaneous transluminal coronary angioplasty (PTCA) is not advantageous after thrombolytic therapy, and may be associated with increased risks of reinfarction and mortality [5]. Likewise, studies of immediate versus delayed coronary grafting have shown high risks of bleeding and mortality in patients undergoing surgery within 12–24 h of thrombolytic therapy [14]. As with other invasive procedures, surgery should therefore be delayed if possible for 24 h after thrombolytic therapy for myocardial infarction. Some have advocated the use of clot-selective agents such as alteplase rather than streptokinase in patients with acute infarction who are at high risk of requiring invasive procedures or surgery, because of its shorter half-life and lesser systemic effects on the blood [15]. Others have pointed out that the digestive effects of clot-selective agents on haemostatic plugs may last longer than their effects on the blood [12]; moreover they carry a higher risk of stroke [8–10].

Peripheral arterial thrombolysis

This now has an accepted place in management of acute or subacute limb ischaemia, and is usually given as a local, low-dose infusion into the thrombus which occludes the artery or graft, with repeated angiography to monitor the extent of lysis (which occurs in about 70% of cases). Details of management are given in recent reviews [12,16–19].

Despite local infusion, systemic effects on the blood are often observed in practice, especially after reperfusion which increases systemic circulation of plasminogen activator. Bleeding at the site of catheter insertion is common, but can usually be controlled by local compression. Major bleeding requiring transfusion or surgery occurs in about 5% of cases, and is poorly related to changes in the blood [6,12,16–19]. Angioplasty or surgery may be required to deal with residual stenoses or failed thrombolysis. Angioplasty (and clot aspiration) may usefully and safely be performed before removal of the catheter. Heparin (monitored by the APTT) followed by aspirin is usually given after thrombolysis, to reduce the risk of reocclusion.

Venous thromboembolism

This is a controversial indication for thrombolytic therapy, with wide variations in practice. This reflects doubt as to whether the increased risk of bleeding and higher cost, relative to conventional anticoagulant therapy, are justified by clinical benefit (mortality, prevention of the post-thrombotic leg syndrome) as distinct from angiographic lysis [5]. Future randomized trials may clarify this doubt. Meanwhile, thrombolytic therapy should be considered in massive thromboembolism which threatens life (pulmonary embolism with marked haemodynamic effects) or limb (impending venous gangrene) [5]. Such therapy may have to be sustained for a few days, in contrast to the few hours required for acute myocardial infarction or local arterial infusion in limb ischaemia. Monitoring of laboratory tests is recommended in such patients [5,6,12], to exclude systemic bleeding disorders prior to therapy, to confirm a systemic lytic effect after 2–4 h, and to determine the timing of initiation of heparin after cessation of therapy. Table 10.1 gives some guidelines for management [5].

Unstable angina and thromboembolic stroke

These are theoretical situations in which thrombolytic therapy may be beneficial; however, clinical benefit has not yet been shown in randomized trials [4,5,17]. Thrombolytic therapy in stroke has been associated with intracranial bleeding and reperfusion oedema; it should however be considered in severe vertebrobasilar occlusion, which has a poor prognosis.

Table 10.1 Guidelines for monitoring of sustained thrombolytic therapy with streptokinase or urokinase (e.g. for deep vein thrombosis, pulmonary embolism). (From [5] with permission)

1 *Patient selection*
- Confirm recent, potentially lysable thrombus by objective test
- Carefully evaluate potential benefit of thrombolysis against contraindications (Table 10.2)
- Minimize iatrogenic bleeding (Table 10.3)

2 *Baseline haemostatic screen*
- Haematocrit or haemoglobin, platelet count
- APTT, PT, thrombin time
- Save plasma for fibrinogen, fibrin degradation products, euglobulin clot lysis time (ECLT) and streptokinase resistance test if required
- Save serum for blood group and crossmatch

3 *Initiate thrombolytic treatment with standard dose*

4 *Establish systemic fibrinolytic state (2–4 h)*
Repeat thrombin time (most sensitive) and/or APTT. If no lytic state (<1.5 times baseline), measure fibrinogen, FDP, ECLT (pre- and post-treatment) ± streptokinase resistance test. Consider:
- Repetition of tests after short interval
- Increasing dose
- Changing thrombolytic agent
- Stopping thrombolytic therapy

5 *After cessation of thrombolytic therapy*
- Monitor thrombin time and/or APTT
- Do not start heparin until less than twice control value

Contraindications and precautions

Table 10.2 lists some traditional contraindications to thrombolytic therapy: many are relative rather than absolute, and the risks of bleeding must be balanced against the benefits of thrombolysis, especially when thromboembolism threatens life or limb. In myocardial infarction, increasing clinical trial experience may suggest that the balance of benefit over risk does in fact favour thrombolytic therapy in some groups of patients in Table 10.2 traditionally considered to have contraindications, e.g. those with previous ulcer or stroke, or aged >75 years [8]. Much bleeding after thrombolysis is iatrogenic, following invasive procedures, which should therefore be minimized [20] (Table 10.3).

Table 10.2 Some contraindications to thrombolytic therapy*

- Current or recent (6 months) internal bleeding or stroke
- Known bleeding disorder (e.g. thrombocytopenia, haemophilias, severe liver or kidney disease)
- Possible aortic dissection } *Note*: may mimic acute myocardial infarction
- Acute pericarditis, oesophagitis } or pulmonary embolism
- Oesophageal varices
- Active peptic ulcer, ulcerative colitis or gastrointestinal neoplasm; acute pancreatitis
- Previous intracranial haemorrhage (at any time)
- Severe arterial hypertension (risk of intracranial haemorrhage): systolic >200 mmHg or diastolic >120 mmHg
- Haemorrhagic retinopathy (e.g. diabetic)
- Bacterial endocarditis
- Left heart thrombus (e.g. in mitral valve disease and atrial fibrillation: risk of thromboembolism)
- Active genitourinary lesion
- Active lung cavitation (e.g. tuberculous)
- Active intracranial disease (e.g. neoplasm)
- Recent (2–4 weeks):
  Surgery or trauma (especially cranial or ocular)
  Organ biopsy
  Puncture of non-compressible vessels (e.g. subclavian)
  Prolonged cardiopulmonary resuscitation
  Abortion or obstetric delivery
- Pregnancy (risk of retroplacental haemorrhage)
- Aged >75 years

Contraindications to streptokinase or anistreplase (consider alteplase or urokinase)
- Known hypersensitivity
- Recent streptococcal infection
- Recent (5 days to 12 months) treatment with either drug (unless clinical situation can await measurement of streptokinase resistance)

* See also manufacturers' data sheets. *Note*: many contraindications are relative rather than absolute (e.g. life-threatening pulmonary thromboembolism in a pregnant (or elderly) patient may well justify thrombolytic therapy despite the increased risk of placental (or intracranial) bleeds). (From [5] with permission.)

Management of bleeding during or after thrombolytic therapy

During and for several days after thrombolytic therapy, patients must be carefully observed for bleeding in specialist units which have adequate

Table 10.3 Minimizing iatrogenic bleeding complications in thrombolytic therapy. (With acknowledgements to [20])

1 *Intramuscular injection sites*
Avoid intramuscular injections: use intravenous or subcutaneous routes

2 *Peripheral venepuncture sites*
Avoid multiple venepunctures. Use a large cannula in each arm, flushed with heparin–saline (one for blood sampling, and one for intravenous medication including thrombolytic drug, heparin, etc.)

3 *Central venous access sites* (e.g. for central venous pressure measurements or temporary electrical pacing)
Avoid subclavian vein, if possible, which cannot be compressed. Use basilic vein in antecubital fossa; or jugular or femoral vein (if expert)

4 *Arterial puncture sites*
Avoid if possible. If essential, seal during thrombolytic therapy by indwelling cannula, sheath or suture

staff and facilities for observation, haemostatic investigations and replacement therapy, diagnostic imaging, and surgical evacuation of life-threatening haematomas. Pulse, blood pressure and haemoglobin level should be monitored, and patients assessed at least daily, especially for intracranial, retroperitoneal or gastrointestinal bleeding, which are potentially fatal.

Significant bleeding is managed as follows:

1 *Stop the infusion of plasminogen activator* (and heparin if this is also being given). The normal liver rapidly clears the activator from the circulation, and corrects depletion of clotting factors by synthesis of fibrinogen, Factor V and Factor VIII. However, activators with high fibrin affinity (e.g. alteplase) may continue to exert local lytic effects on fibrin haemostatic plugs for some hours, while high plasma FDP levels also persist for several hours and may interfere with fibrin polymerization, reducing the tensile strength of haemostatic plugs [12].

2 *If bleeding is severe,* plasmin activity on haemostatic plugs can be inhibited by intravenous infusions of protease inhibitors (Chapter 15), e.g. aprotinin (500 000 kallikrein inactivator units (KIU) over 10 min, then 200 000 iu 4-hourly until the bleeding stops), or the more specific plasmin inhibitor tranexamic acid (10 mg/kg body weight over 10 min, repeated if necessary after 6–8 h until the bleeding stops). Administration of the latter drug carries an increased risk of arterial thrombosis [7], as shown, for example, in controlled trials of subarachnoid haemorrhage [21,22]. On the other hand, a meta-analysis of controlled trials

has shown its value in acute gastrointestinal bleeding [23], presumably by inhibiting local gastrointestinal fibrinolysis of haemostatic plugs. Aprotinin has been shown to reduce blood loss after cardiopulmonary bypass, presumably by inhibiting contact-activated fibrinolysis (Chapter 12).

3 *A coagulation screen* (platelet count, thrombin time, PT, APTT, fibrinogen level) should be performed, the haematocrit checked, and red blood cells or whole blood crossmatched and infused to replace blood loss as required. In patients in whom bleeding is not controlled by the above measures, marked prolongation of clotting times (or marked fibrinogen depletion) should lead to consideration of correcting depletion of fibrinogen, Factor V and Factor VIII by fresh frozen plasma or cryoprecipitate. However, the risks of transfusion reactions and viral transmission (hepatitis B, hepatitis C, HIV) with blood products must also be considered (Chapter 16). Because plasma or cryoprecipitate also replenish plasminogen, concurrent aprotinin or tranexamic acid therapy has been recommended [20]. Platelet transfusion may be indicated for continued bleeding associated with thrombocytopenia (platelet count $<100 \times 10^9/l$) or platelet dysfunction (skin bleeding time >10 min with platelet count $>100 \times 10^9/l$): the latter has been associated with clinical bleeding in one study [24]. Other laboratory tests have not been shown to be of clinical value in the management of bleeding [6].

4 *Intracranial haemorrhage* must be suspected in all patients with headache, vomiting, drowsiness or focal signs: it is commoner with anistreplase, alteplase or duteplase than with streptokinase [8]. Lumbar puncture should be avoided as it wastes time and carries a bleeding risk. Thrombolytic therapy and/or anticoagulants should be reversed urgently, and immediate neurological consultation obtained regarding computed tomography brain scanning and evacuation of intracranial haematomas.

5 *Retroperitoneal haemorrhage* may follow the Seldinger technique of arterial puncture, cardiac resuscitation, or twisting movements of the trunk. It should be suspected in patients with unexplained falls in blood pressure or haemoglobin level, and in those with pain in the abdomen, loin or shoulder-tip. Abdominal ultrasound or CT scanning, laparoscopy or paracentesis may reveal the bleeding, and urgent surgical consultation and reversal of thrombolytic therapy and/or anticoagulants are required.

6 *Gastrointestinal bleeding* may reflect previous peptic ulcer, acute stress ulceration, or other lesions. Tranexamic acid may be appropriate [23]. Past history of ulcer or dyspepsia need not contraindicate thrombolysis, but prophylactic H_2-antagonist drugs may be wise [20].

7 *Haematuria* is common, and if heavy or persistent merits intravenous urography and cystoscopy to exclude an underlying lesion.
8 *Aortic or pericardial bleeding* can be lethal when aortic dissection or pericarditis are misdiagnosed as acute myocardial infarction [25] or possibly as pulmonary embolism.

Prevention of bleeding when surgery is required after thrombolytic therapy

As previously noted, surgery—along with other invasive procedures—should be delayed if possible for at least 24 h after recent thrombolytic therapy, because of the increased risk of bleeding associated with impaired formation and/or premature lysis of haemostatic plugs, as well as the increased risk of postoperative thrombosis in patients with current thrombosis. Nevertheless, early surgery may be required (e.g. for life-threatening bleeding, for life- or limb-threatening thrombosis despite thrombolytic therapy, or for other surgical emergencies). In such cases the surgeon may deem it prudent to advise the patient and/or relatives of the increased risks of bleeding and of thrombosis; haematological advice should also be sought.

Management to minimize bleeding prior to surgery is similar to the management of bleeding outlined above. The infusion of plasminogen activator (and heparin) should be stopped, and if possible surgery delayed for an hour or so to allow clearance. If this is not possible, or if there is active bleeding, plasmin activity may be reversed by aprotinin or tranexamic acid, if the risk of unlysable fibrin is accepted; the on-call haematologist should be consulted; a coagulation screen, platelet count, haematocrit and crossmatch performed; and fresh frozen plasma, cryoprecipitate or platelets considered as indicated by test results, balancing the risks of bleeding against the risks of transfusion reactions and viral infections (Chapter 16). Meticulous haemostatic technique is important, including the tying of vessels rather than cautery, to minimize dependence on haemostatic plugs. Finally, the balance between haemostasis and thrombosis should be remembered (Fig. 10.1): patients are at risk of postoperative thrombosis, especially in the presence of current thrombosis, plasmin inhibitor therapy, and transfusion of clotting factors or platelets. The minimum prophylaxis is graduated elastic compression stockings or intermittent calf compression; aspirin or anticoagulants should also be considered according to the relative risks of thrombosis and bleeding in the individual patient.

References

1 Lowe, G.D.O. (1991) Aetiology of deep vein thrombosis. *Curr. Pract. Surg.*, **3**, 131–136.

2 Salzman, E.W. and Davies, G.C. (1980) Prophylaxis of venous thromboembolism. Analysis of cost-effectiveness. *Ann. Surg.*, **191**, 207–218.

3 Clagett, G.P. and Reisch, J.S. (1988) Prevention of venous thromboembolism in general surgical patients. Results of meta-analysis. *Ann. Surg.*, **208**, 227–240.

4 Julian, D., Kubler, W., Norris, R.M., *et al.* (Eds) *Thrombolysis in Cardiovascular Disease.* Marcel Dekker, Basel (1989).

5 Lowe, G.D.O. Clinical and laboratory aspects of thrombolytic therapy. In: *Recent Advances in Blood Coagulation 5* (Ed. Poller, L.), pp. 265–291. Churchill Livingstone, Edinburgh (1991).

6 Lowe, G.D.O. and Rumley, A. Laboratory aspects of thrombolytic therapy. In: *Blood Coagulation and Haemostasis—A Practical Guide* (Ed. Thomson, J.M.), 4th edn, pp. 177–208. Churchill Livingstone, Edinburgh (1991).

7 Bennett, B. and Ogston, D. Fibrinolytic bleeding syndromes. In: *Disorders of Hemostasis* (Eds Ratnoff, O.D. & Forbes, C.D.), 2nd edn, pp. 327–351. W.B. Saunders, Philadelphia (1991).

8 ISIS-3 Collaborative Group (1992) ISIS-3: a randomised trial of streptokinase vs. tissue plasminogen activator vs. anistreplase and of aspirin plus heparin vs. aspirin alone among 41 299 cases of suspected acute myocardial infarction. *Lancet*, **339**, 753–770.

9 GISSI (1990) GISSI-2: a factorial randomised trial of alteplase versus streptokinase and heparin versus no heparin among 12 490 patients with acute myocardial infarction. *Lancet*, **336**, 65–71.

10 International Study Group (1990) In-hospital mortality and clinical course of 20 981 patients with suspected acute myocardial infarction randomised between alteplase and streptokinase with or without heparin. *Lancet*, **336**, 71–75.

11 Jalihal, S. and Morris, G.K. (1990) Antistreptokinase titres after intravenous streptokinase. *Lancet*, **335**, 184–185.

12 Marder, V.J. and Sherry, S. (1988) Thrombolytic therapy; current status. *New Engl. J. Med.*, **318**, 1512–1520 and 1585–1595.

13 ISIS-2 Collaborative Study Group (1988) Randomised trial of intravenous streptokinase, oral aspirin, both, or neither, among 17 987 cases of suspected acute myocardial infarction: ISIS-2. *Lancet*, **ii**, 349–360.

14 Lee, K.F., Mandell, J., Rankin, J.S. *et al.* (1988) Immediate versus delayed coronary grafting after streptokinase treatment: postoperative blood loss and clinical results. *J. Thorac. Cardiovasc. Surg.*, **95**, 216–222.

15 Tiefenbrunn, A. and Sobel, B.S. (1989) The impact of coronary thrombolysis on myocardial infarction. *Fibrinolysis*, **3**, 1–15.

16 Graor, R.A. and Olin, J.W. Regional thrombolysis in peripheral arterial occlusions. In: *Thrombolysis in Cardiovascular Disease* (Eds Julian, D., Kubler, W., Norris, R.M., Swan, H.J.C., Collen, D. & Verstraete, M.) pp. 381–395. Marcel Dekker, Basel (1989).

17 Editorial (1990) Non-coronary thrombolysis. *Lancet*, **335**, 691–693.

18 Earnshaw, J.J. (Ed.) *The Current Status of Peripheral Arterial Thrombolysis.* Inte-

grated Medical Communications, Fleet, Hampshire (1991).
19 Gaines, P.A. and Beard, J.D. (1991) Radiological management of acute lower limb ischaemia. *Br. J. Hosp. Med.*, **45**, 343–353.
20 De Bono, D. Problems in thrombolysis. In: *Thrombolysis in Cardiovascular Disease* (Eds Julian, D., Kubler, W., Norris, R.M., Swan, H.J.C., Collen, D. & Verstraete, M.), pp. 279–292. Marcel Dekker, Basel (1989).
21 Kassell, N.F., Torner, T.C. and Adams, H.P. Jr. (1984) Antifibrinolytic therapy in the acute period following aneurysmal subarachnoid hemorrhage. Preliminary observations from the Cooperative Aneurysm Study. *J. Neurosurg.*, **61**, 225–231.
22 Vermeulen, M., Lindsay, K.W., Murray, G.D. *et al.* (1984) Antifibrinolytic treatment in subarachnoid hemorrhage. *New Engl. J. Med.*, **311**, 342–347.
23 Henry, D.A. and O'Connell, D.L. (1989) Effects of fibrinolytic inhibitors on mortality from upper gastrointestinal haemorrhage. *Br. Med. J.*, **298**, 1142–1146.
24 Gimple, L.W., Gold, H.K., Leinbach, R.C. *et al.* (1989) Correlation between template bleeding time and spontaneous bleeding during treatment of acute myocardial infarction with recombinant tissue-type plasminogen activator. *Circulation*, **80**, 581–588.
25 Petch, M.C. (1990) Dangers of thrombolysis. *Br. Med. J.*, **300**, 483–484.

Chapter 11
Infection, trauma, shock and burns

JENNIFER L. HANSLIP

This chapter outlines the particular bleeding problems associated with conditions which may be seen in surgical patients, namely, infection, trauma, shock and burns.

Infections

Infection in surgical patients may be seen in three main situations:

1 Preoperatively, in elective admissions found to have infection unrelated to their surgical problem (e.g. HIV infection).

2 As a presenting problem (e.g. rupture of a diverticular abscess causing peritonitis and Gram-negative septicaemia or a breast abscess due to *Staphylococcus aureus*).

3 Postoperatively as an early or late complication of surgery (e.g. septicaemia or wound infection, aspiration pneumonia).

In these different situations, the organism(s) responsible for the infection will vary. Bleeding problems arise from a variety of infections and can be due to:

1 Disseminated intravascular coagulation (DIC).

2 Thrombocytopenia.

3 Thrombocytosis: primary (thrombocythaemia) and secondary (reactive).

4 Vascular abnormalities, including vasculitis.

Each of these bleeding problems will be considered in relation to infection.

Disseminated intravascular coagulation (defibrination syndrome; consumption coagulopathy; intravascular coagulation with fibrinolysis)

DIC, an acquired disorder of haemostasis, is a disruption of haemostasis in response to various 'trigger' mechanisms which can paradoxically produce simultaneous thrombosis and haemorrhage by concurrent activation of both the coagulation and the fibrinolytic systems. Normal haemostasis relies on a delicate balance between the coagulation and fibrinolytic systems; however, this balance is disrupted in DIC. As a result, there can be excessive bleeding, ischaemic lesions or even tissue necrosis due to thrombosis in small and large vessels by fibrin and platelet deposition. All organs can be affected, with the most commonly affected being the kidneys, brain, heart and adrenals. As a result, multiple organ failure can occur. Thrombosis can be both arterial and venous (Fig. 11.1).

DIC is not a disease in itself but an acquired disorder of haemostasis in response to certain clinical conditions and a wide spectrum of diseases. Both the nature of the haemostatic 'trigger' and the general status of the patient prior to illness are important determinants of whether the presentation and subsequent course of DIC is acute, subacute or chronic, and whether the effects of DIC will be mild or severe.

Pathogenesis

DIC is initiated by the activation of the coagulation system in response to various 'triggered' mechanisms. Activation of the coagulation system leads to thrombin production and consumption of coagulation factors and platelets. Perpetuation of the DIC process is thought to be largely due to thrombin generated intravascularly at the start of DIC. Our understanding of the pathogenesis of DIC is based on experimental observations. Many authors have presented DIC models in animals caused by intravenous injection of thrombin [1–4]. Animal models have also been used to demonstrate that intravenous injection of homogenized thromboplastin-rich tissue resulted in a DIC state [4–6]. Thrombin is involved in many haemostatic processes and the effects of thrombin production are seen in DIC and are now outlined.

Role of thrombin

1 In the presence of thrombin, fibrinogen loses fibrinopeptides A and B, resulting in soluble fibrin monomers. Definite increases in levels of fibrinopeptide A (FPA) have been shown in DIC [7]. Soluble fibrin is either cleared by the reticuloendothelial system (RES) or becomes precipitated and polymerized to an insoluble gel which can occlude blood vessels. This polymerization reaction also involves thrombin and Factor XIII (transamidase).

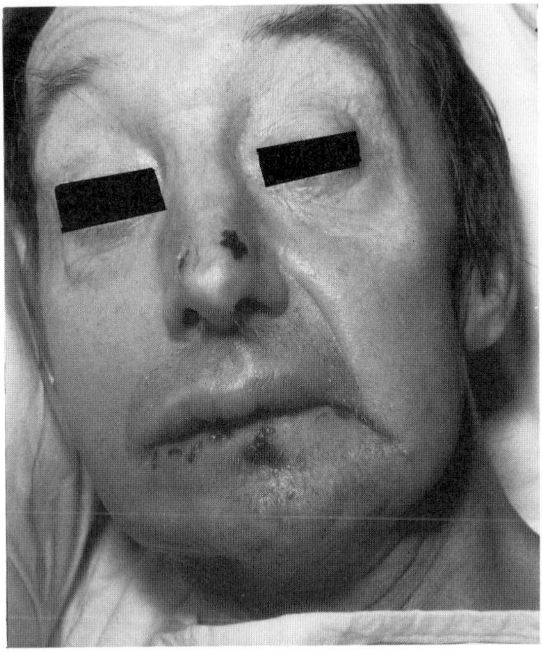

(a)

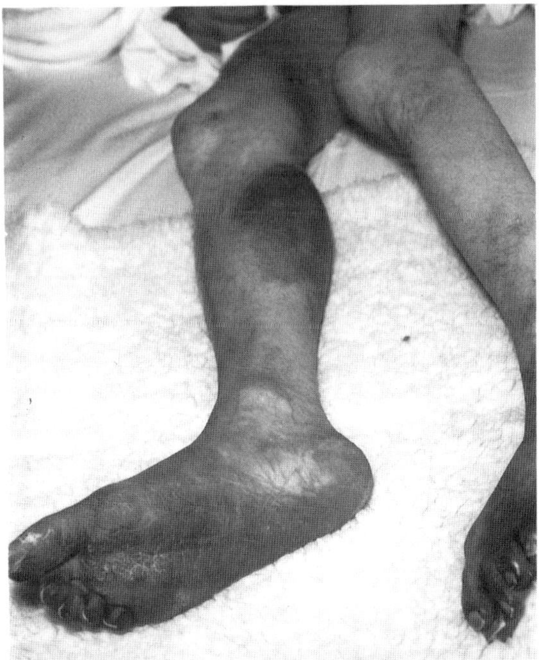

(b)

Fig. 11.1 This patient presented following an episode of urinary-tract infection with Gram-negative septicaemia. He was anuric, hypotensive and had areas of skin necrosis on nose and lips (a) and ischaemia of the feet. He also had areas of skin haemorrhage and purpura (b) and bled excessively from venepuncture sites.

2 Thrombin-mediated peptide release from Factors VIII:C and V leads to decreased concentrations of these factors [8].
3 Thrombin binds to platelets leading to platelet aggregation. These platelet aggregates can be cleared by the RES or are deposited in the microcirculation.

Role of fibrinolysis

During DIC, fibrin is formed inappropriately within the circulation. Fibrinolysis (usually secondary rather than primary) is an important compensatory mechanism which prevents widespread organ damage due to vascular occlusion by fibrin. Antifibrinolytic agents have been shown to enhance DIC in man [9].

Plasmin, the main enzyme involved in fibrin degradation, cleaves fibrin into fibrin degradation products (FDPs) which, in turn, form a complex with unstable fibrin monomers to produce stable fibrin monomers which cannot polymerize [10–12]. Fibrinolysis clearly has beneficial antithrombotic effects. However, adverse anticoagulant effects can occur from the following mechanisms:
1 Platelet dysfunction due to coating of the surface of platelets by FDPs.
2 Degradation of clotting Factors V, VIII, IX and XI (which are already reduced in amount due to coagulation activation) by excessive plasmin (hyperplasminaemia) [13–15].
3 Dissolution of haemostatic thrombi as well as fibrin by hyperplasminaemia.
4 Presence of circulating fibrin and FDPs.

Thrombosis and bleeding

Normal haemostasis relies on a fine balance between coagulation activation and compensatory fibrinolysis. Disruption of this balance, as in DIC, produces different degrees of thrombosis and/or bleeding depending upon the haemostatic 'trigger'.

Many conditions can cause mild DIC which may go unnoticed, causing few clinical problems. In such situations, small thrombi form which, due to their size, cause no haemodynamic upset. The fibrinolytic system, triggered at the onset of DIC, removes these thrombi as they form. No major vascular occlusion occurs and the haemostatic balance is restored. In severe DIC, haemostasis can be activated to such a degree that fibrinolysis may be inadequate and there is an imbalance favouring thrombus formation. Fibrin and platelets are deposited in the microcirculation, leading to organ ischaemia and microangiopathic haemolytic anaemia. This overwhelming activation of coagulation in severe DIC can lead to both thrombotic and bleeding problems. Bleeding occurs because the coagulation factors and platelets are consumed and when fibrinolysis is excessive.

Whether the process of DIC is acute, chronic, mild or severe is determined by the degree of disruption of the balance between coagulation and fibrinolysis, the general state of the patient pre-DIC, the underlying 'trigger' to haemostasis and other non-haemostatic factors (e.g. an intact RES [16,17]), catecholamines [18], lipids [19], pregnancy and liver disease. DIC tends to occur more readily in those whose ability to replace haemostatic molecules is already compromised (e.g. patients with liver failure or neonates). The 'triggers' to DIC give rise to DIC by three main initiating mechanisms, which are now described.

Initiation

DIC can be initiated by the following three main mechanisms which occur in response to the underlying 'trigger' or cause of DIC.

1 *Tissue damage→release of tissue factor and activation of extrinsic pathway.* Any tissue damage (e.g. septicaemia, surgical and obstetric trauma, burns and head injuries [20]) can lead to tissue thromboplastin release into the circulation via breached vessels, causing direct activation of the extrinsic coagulation pathway.

2 *Cell damage→release of procoagulant molecules.* Damage to red blood cells (RBCs), e.g. due to haemolysis, gives rise to the release of procoagulant material from RBCs causing DIC in situations such as malaria, sickle-cell disease or mismatched transfusion. Granulocytes may release procoagulant molecules from their granules, especially when the granule content is increased (e.g. in septicaemia [21–24]).

3 *Endothelial damage→activation of Factor XII and the intrinsic pathway.* Intact endothelium has an anticoagulant effect. Its cells contain thrombomodulin, which enhances the activation of protein C, heparins which combine with and activate antithrombin III [25] and prostaglandin PGI_2 (prostacyclin), a potent inhibitor of platelet aggregation. Platelet aggregation and adherence to the endothelium rarely occurs in 'normal' situations (i.e. free-flowing blood and normal endothelium due to the balance between production of thromboxane A_2—a potent platelet aggregating agent—by circulating platelets and prostacyclin from endothelial cells).

Bacterial endotoxins (especially those from Gram-negative organisms), extensive burns, acidosis, anoxia, viraemia, antigen–antibody complexes, vasculitis and hypotension are examples of some of the factors which can give rise to endothelial damage. The lipid A portion of the bacterial endotoxin molecule is known to penetrate and damage vascular membranes and to generate procoagulant activity by stimulating human mononuclear cells [26,27]. When subendothelial collagen becomes exposed, as in the conditions described above, there is direct activation of Factor XII which, in turn, directly or indirectly activates the intrinsic coagulation system, complement cascade, kinin formation and fibrinolysis.

In septicaemia, bacterial endotoxin (usually produced by Gram-negative organisms) can cause not only endothelial damage but platelet aggregation. Experimental evidence suggests that platelets may have a role in the initiation of DIC. Bacterial isolates, particularly *Staphylococcus aureus* and *Pseudomonas aeruginosa*, have been shown, *in vitro*, to induce irreversible platelet aggregation. Both these types of bacteria were associated with a high incidence of DIC in the infected individuals from whom they were isolated [28].

The three mechanisms described above are the main ways in which DIC is initiated. Occasionally, massive amounts of procoagulant molecules or tissue factor can be released into the circulation directly, i.e. with no evidence of tissue or vascular damage.

Severe snake venom poisonings (e.g. the venom of the snake *Echis carinatus*) cause rapid DIC *in vivo* due to direct activation of prothrombin and subsequent thrombin release. Such snake bites releasing venom are an important example of DIC occurring in the absence of widespread vascular injury [8,29]. Direct proteolytic cleavage of serine proteases of the coagulation cascade can lead to DIC in acute pancreatitis when pancreatic enzymes enter the circulation.

In practice, more than one of the initiating mechanisms of DIC is usually involved (e.g. in septicaemia there is both endothelial damage and white-cell procoagulant release). However, during septicaemia, associated complications (e.g. hypoxia and acidosis) can cause more cell damage, procoagulant release and acceleration of the coagulation process.

In a single case of DIC, one or all of the initiating mechanisms may be involved depending upon the cause or 'trigger' of the DIC process. These will now be discussed.

Causes or 'triggers'

DIC can be caused or 'triggered' by many different disorders (see Chapter 3). The next section specifically deals with the role of infection as a cause or 'trigger' of DIC. As many as two-thirds of all cases of DIC are believed to be precipitated by infection [30].

Table 11.1 lists the various bacterial, viral, rickettsial, fungal and protozoan infections that have been associated with DIC. While DIC has been shown to be associated with these infections, it should be noted that DIC is not invariable and that other studies have failed to detect it in patients with these infections [39–45]. In some reported cases of DIC, the only evidence has been from laboratory abnormalities as there was absence of any associated clinically significant bleeding.

Meningococcal septicaemia was the first infection in which DIC was described. A fulminant, potentially fatal, haemorrhagic picture is seen with profound shock, cutaneous ecchymoses and petechiae (Fig. 11.2). At autopsy, visceral petechiae, especially in the adrenal cortex, are seen — the classic Waterhouse–Friderichsen syndrome [46]. Thrombi can also be demonstrated, at autopsy, in the small blood vessels of the adrenal cortex, renal cortex and other organs. Such patients may demonstrate all the typical laboratory features of DIC. Not all patients with meningo-

Table 11.1 Infections which cause or 'trigger' DIC

Bacterial	*Viral [31–34]*
Escherichia coli	Hepatitis A and B
Pseudomonas aeruginosa	Non-A, non-B hepatitis
Klebsiella	Cytomegalovirus
Neisseria meningococcus	Varicella
Haemophilus influenzae	Influenza
Streptococcus pneumoniae	Haemorrhagic fevers (e.g. dengue)
Staphylococcus aureus	Herpes simplex and zoster
Clostridium perfringens	*Protozoan [36–38]*
Chlamydia psittaci	Malaria
Mycoplasma pneumoniae	Trypanosomiasis
Mycobacterium tuberculosis	Schistosomiasis
Rickettsial [35]	*Fungal*
Rocky mountain spotted fever	*Aspergillus*
Scrub typhus	*Candida albicans*

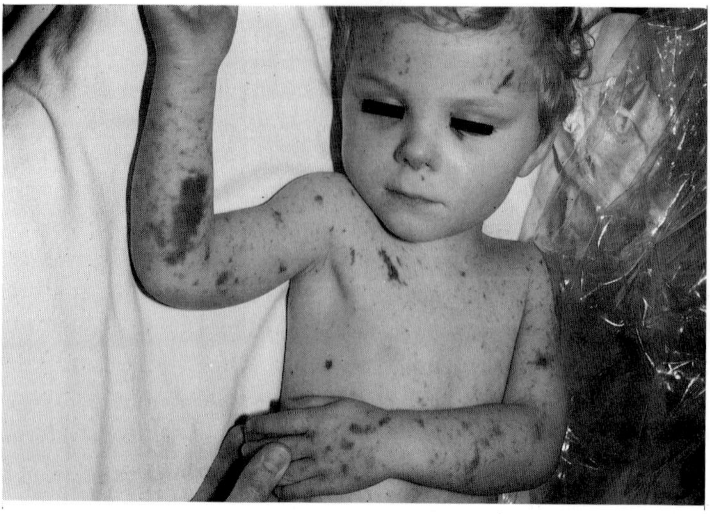

Fig. 11.2 This child was diagnosed as suffering from meningococcal septicaemia but died before treatment was effective. Typical purpuric lesions are present in the skin. These are probably vasculitic. Acute DIC changes were present in the blood. Death resulted from adrenal haemorrhage.

coccal septicaemia develop these severe problems. However, should they arise, the prognosis is poor.

The fulminant haemorrhagic picture described above is not only seen with meningococcal septicaemia. Other Gram-negative organisms (e.g. *Escherichia coli*, *Pseudomonas* and *Klebsiella* and infection with streptococci, staphylococci and *Clostridium*) can also cause a similar picture. Patients who have undergone splenectomy, or who are immunosuppressed, are particularly vulnerable to infection from *Streptococcus pneumoniae* and can develop septicaemia and a Waterhouse–Friderichsen-like syndrome. Routine prophylaxis with pneumococcal vaccine in asplenic patients does not uniformly prevent this complication [47,48].

Revaccination and antibiotic prophylaxis may be needed in such patients [49]. Gram-negative infections can be responsible for a subacute form of DIC where haemorrhage is less severe.

The initiation of DIC in infections is complex, ultimately producing activation of polymorphonuclear leucocytes, mononuclear phagocytes, platelets, vascular endothelium and blood coagulation by the mechanisms outlined earlier.

Thrombocytopenia

If disordered haemostasis is due to an abnormality of platelets, this can be quickly established by measuring the bleeding time and peripheral platelet count. If both these tests are in the 'normal' range, it is unlikely that the bleeding problem is caused by platelet dysfunction. Platelet defects can be qualitative or quantitative. Thrombocytopenia (i.e. a reduction in the number of circulating platelets) is a quantitative platelet defect. The normal range for the peripheral platelet count is $150-400 \times 10^9/l$. While spontaneous bleeding can occur once the platelet count is $<50 \times 10^9/l$, it does not usually occur until the count has fallen to $\leq 20 \times 10^9/l$ (Fig. 11.3a–c). Any peripheral platelet count which is low should be confirmed by checking the count on a freshly stained blood film. Platelet agglutinins can sometimes cause spurious thrombocytopenia. A prolonged bleeding time occurs when the platelet count falls below approximately $100 \times 10^9/l$ and there is a progressive increase in the bleeding time as the platelet count falls below this level [50].

Infection

Severe infections, particularly those involving bacteraemia, commonly cause thrombocytopenia [30]. An analysis of 11 studies (which included 1074 patients), in which data were available, indicates that approximately 62% of patients with severe bacterial infections (most of whom had documented septicaemia) were thrombocytopenic [51]. Thrombocytopenia is the commonest haemostatic disorder seen with infection and the mechanisms by which it occurs will now be considered.

Mechanisms

There are several different mechanisms (outlined below) by which infection can cause thrombocytopenia. Often, more than one of these mechanisms is responsible for the development of thrombocytopenia in infected patients.

Inadequate production of platelets

Infection has been shown to suppress erythropoiesis and it is likely that platelet production from the bone marrow (thrombopoiesis) is suppressed as a result of infection. However, more clinical evidence is needed to

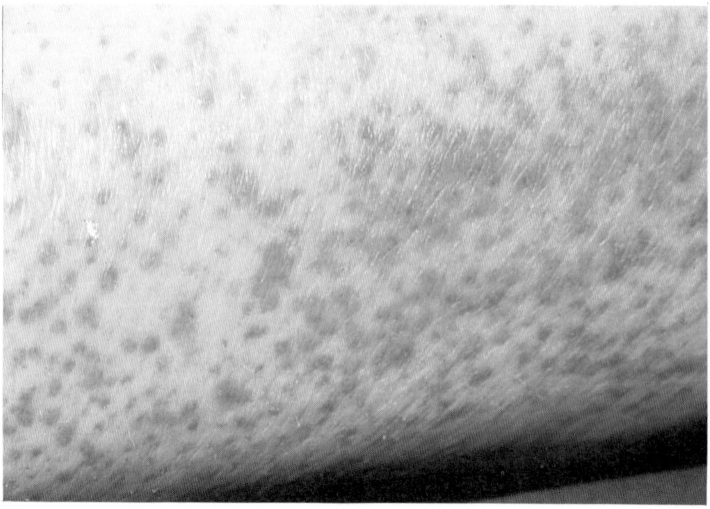

(a)

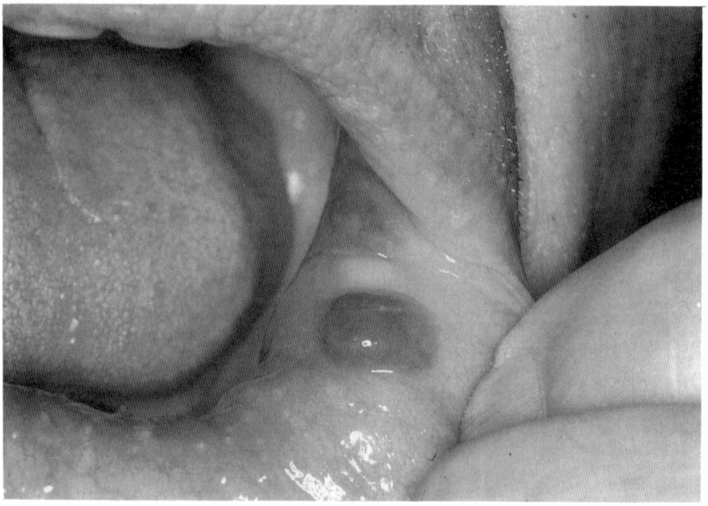

(b)

Fig. 11.3 (a) Extensive skin purpura—the lesions do not blanch with pressure. The cause was septicaemia associated with gallstone disease and ascending cholangitis. There was associated acute hepatic failure with disturbance of blood coagulation. (b) Blood blisters on gums and cheek associated with a virus infection and thrombocytopenia. (c) Ecchymosis associated with acute DIC, with platelet, coagulation and fibrinolytic disturbances.

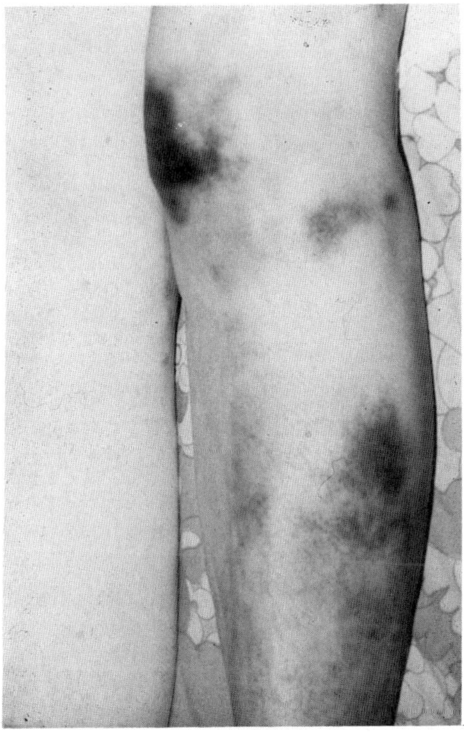

(c)

confirm this. Platelet suppression has been shown to occur with live measles vaccine [52], murine cytomegalovirus [53] and B19 parvovirus [54]. Some viral infections seem to be associated with platelet suppression. However, the role of platelet suppression in causing thrombocytopenia in bacterial infections is not yet established.

Increased destruction of platelets

1 Increased platelet destruction in patients with infection can occur due to associated DIC which consumes platelets. When thrombocytopenia is seen in infected patients, there is often laboratory evidence of DIC. Increased turnover of platelets and fibrinogen in bacteraemic patients who were thrombocytopenic but not hypofibrinogenaemic has been shown [55].

2 Infection can alter the reticuloendothelial system in such a way that platelets are rapidly cleared from the circulation.

3 Some infections cause splenomegaly and, as a result, there is sequestration of platelets in the spleen and decreased numbers of circulating platelets.

4 In some infections, immunological mechanisms cause platelet destruction and thrombocytopenia. Antibodies, produced in response to bacterial and viral infections, may destroy circulating platelets if bacteria or virus particles are adherent to platelets.

Immune complexes

Circulating immune complexes play an important role in the production of thrombocytopenia in infection. Human platelets have been shown to possess an Fc receptor that can bind the Fc portion of circulating immune complexes [56] in a reaction that does not require complement. Human platelets have been shown, *in vitro*, to bind either DNA or DNA–anti-DNA complexes [57]. This mechanism has been shown to play a part in the thrombocytopenia caused by rubella [58], malaria [39], Gram-negative and Gram-positive sepsis [59]. Immunological thrombocytopenic purpura (ITP) often seems to follow both clinical and subclinical viral infections. Several studies have demonstrated that patients with ITP have circulating immune complexes in the blood [60,61]. It is thought that many cases of ITP may arise as a consequence of a viral infection, rather than being due to autoimmune disease.

Direct bacterial (or viral) damage

Platelets can be damaged by the direct action of bacteria or viruses on them and this results in decreased numbers of circulating platelets. Staphylococci have been shown to stimulate human platelets to undergo the release reaction [62]. Platelet interactions with bacteria, viruses or parasites can cause platelet aggregation, release of platelet contents, binding of platelet aggregates by polymorphonuclear leucocytes and phagocytosis by these leucocytes of the infectious agent and occasionally platelets [63]—the end result being decreased numbers of circulating platelets. In some situations, platelets may be altered by an infectious agent but not destroyed, and this leads to a qualitative rather than a quantitative platelet defect, i.e. the circulating platelets are not reduced in number (as in thrombocytopenia), but their function may be abnormal resulting in bleeding or platelet thrombus formation.

Endothelial injury

In bacterial and viral infections, infectious particles may damage the endothelium. Circulating platelets become adherent to this damaged endothelium resulting in a decrease in their numbers.

These mechanisms are the main ways in which thrombocytopenia is initiated in patients with infection. Animal studies have shown that bacterial lipopolysaccharide (LPS), a bacterial endotoxin contained in the cell walls of Gram-negative bacteria, aggregates and binds to platelets, altering surface proteins [64,65]. Although animal studies show that LPS can produce thrombocytopenia, the role of bacterial LPS in causing thrombocytopenia in humans is not yet fully established.

Causes

A wide variety of infections can cause thrombocytopenia and the types of infection are similar to those causing DIC. Table 11.2 lists some infections and infectious diseases that are associated with thrombocytopenia. The degree of thrombocytopenia, in the majority of cases, is not severe.

Bacterial infection with both Gram-positive and Gram-negative organisms can cause thrombocytopenia [66–68] and in the majority of cases,

Table 11.2 Infections and infectious diseases associated with thrombocytopenia

Bacterial	*Fungal*
Sepsis due to Gram-negative or Gram-positive organisms	Toxoplasmosis
Brucellosis	Histoplasmosis
Typhoid fever	*Spirochaetal*
Diphtheria	Congenital syphilis
Tuberculosis	*Viral*
Subacute bacterial endocarditis (SBE)	Rubella/mumps/rubeola/varicella/vaccinia
Psittacosis	Epstein–Barr
Rickettsial	Cytomegalovirus
Rocky mountain spotted fever	Haemorrhagic fevers (e.g. dengue)
Scrub typhus	Hepatitis
Protozoan	Herpes simplex infection
Malaria	Influenza
Trypanosomiasis	HIV
Visceral leishmaniasis	(Measles vaccine)

it is of a mild degree. Studies have shown that approximately 60–65% of patients with thrombocytopenia secondary to infection have platelet counts $>50 \times 10^9/l$ [69,70]. Several studies demonstrate the fact that haemorrhage occurs only rarely in patients who have thrombocytopenia arising from infection [67,71–73]. A circulating platelet count of $>50 \times 10^9/l$ is usually sufficient for adequate haemostasis to occur in the absence of any other haemostatic defect.

Acquired immunodeficiency syndrome

The acquired immunodeficiency syndrome (AIDS), caused by human immunodeficiency virus (HIV) infection, can cause anaemia and leucopenia in association with a normocellular or hypercellular bone marrow [74–82]. Thrombocytopenia is found less frequently [75,77–80,83] than either anaemia or leucopenia. The exact mechanism(s) by which peripheral cytopenia occurs in AIDS is unknown. Marked immunological abnormalities are seen in AIDS [84]. Thrombocytopenia in patients with AIDS is thought to be due to a combination of mechanisms, one of which is likely to be inadequate platelet production due to marrow suppression by HIV. Another likely cause is excessive peripheral destruction of circulating platelets by immune mechanisms. Intercurrent infections in patients with AIDS may contribute to bone-marrow suppression and may enhance peripheral destruction of platelets, thus worsening thrombocytopenia. The degree of thrombocytopenia in patients with AIDS can be severe enough to cause clinically significant bleeding.

Platelet levels tend to improve when specific therapy given with the aim of treating AIDS and any associated infections is successful. Bone-marrow suppression is one of the many side-effects associated with the use of azidothymidine (AZT) in the treatment of patients with AIDS or AIDS-related complex (ARC) [85].

Thrombocytosis

Bleeding problems due to platelet disorders can occur when there is a decrease in platelets (thrombocytopenia, as already discussed), or when there is an increase in the number of circulating platelets (thrombocytosis). Both thrombocytopenia and thrombocytosis are quantitative platelet defects. A different form of platelet dysfunction is a qualitative platelet defect where platelets can be reduced, normal or increased in number but their function is abnormal, causing either excessive bleeding or thrombosis. Thrombocytosis, a cause of qualitative platelet defects, will now be discussed.

Thrombocytosis is a common clinical finding and can be either primary ('thrombocythaemia', due to disease of the bone marrow, e.g. myeloproliferative disease) or secondary ('reactive thrombocytosis', due to a variety of conditions including infections). The commonest causes of the reactive thrombocytosis are haemorrhage, postsurgery states, malignancy, inflammatory conditions (e.g. rheumatoid arthritis, Crohn's disease, chronic and (less commonly) acute infections) and splenectomy.

Thrombocytosis is defined as a rise in the blood platelet count to over 400×10^9/l. In a study of 372 patients with thrombocytosis where platelet counts were $>500 \times 10^9$/l, 24% were related to infection, 19% to surgery, 17% to iron deficiency and bleeding, 9% to malignancy, 9% to splenectomy, and 21% to miscellaneous causes [86]. Particular infections which cause reactive thrombocytosis are bacterial pulmonary infections (e.g. tuberculosis) and osteomyelitis. Thrombocytosis due to infections usually resolves when the infection has been appropriately treated.

Qualitative platelet defects

A prolonged bleeding time usually suggests thrombocytopenia. However, a prolonged bleeding time in the presence of a normal or high platelet count can be caused by a qualitative platelet defect. These defects can be inherited (e.g. Bernard–Soulier syndrome) or acquired (due to myeloproliferative diseases, reactive thrombocytosis, uraemia, paraproteinaemia or drugs such as aspirin and other non-steroidal anti-inflammatory agents). They may also arise indirectly from infection, i.e. when infections cause a reactive thrombocytosis, or in DIC, when fibrin degradation products coat platelets altering their function. Qualitative platelet defects usually cause an increased bleeding tendency. However, thrombosis can also occur.

Vascular abnormalities

Vascular abnormalities can cause bleeding problems but infection is rarely a cause. The main types of vascular abnormalities which cause bleeding are listed below.

1 *Congenital vascular disorders*. An example is hereditary haemorrhagic telangiectasia (Rendu–Weber–Osler disease) [87–89].

Table 11.3 Causes of vasculitis

Infections	*Malignancy*
Streptococcal	Gastrointestinal
Subacute bacterial endocarditis	Haemopoietic
Viral haemorrhagic fevers (e.g. dengue)	*'Collagen diseases'*
Drugs	Systemic lupus erythematosus
Antibiotics	Systemic sclerosis
Non-steroidal anti-inflammatory agents	Dermatomyositis
Hypnotics	
Anticoagulants	

2 *Hereditary connective tissue disorders.* Examples include Ehlers–Danlos syndrome [90], pseudoxanthoma elasticum [91], Marfan's syndrome [92] and osteogenesis imperfecta [93].
3 *Mechanical purpura,* for example increased venous pressure after coughing or vomiting and skin trauma.
4 *Metabolic purpura,* for example scurvy, diabetes mellitus, amyloid and dysproteinaemias [94–101].
5 *Drug-related purpura,* for example long-term steroid therapy and warfarin and protein C deficiency [102,103].
6 *Vasculitis (allergic purpura/non-thrombocytopenic purpura).* Inflammation and infiltration of the walls of blood vessels (vasculitis) may occur in response to a variety of agents. This form of vascular damage can also be described as non-thrombocytopenic purpura and be regarded as an 'aseptic vasculitis' [104]. Chemicals (including drugs), toxins, infections, and physical stimuli are some agents known to cause vasculitis (see Table 11.3).

Vasculitis

Infection-induced vasculitis appears to be mediated by deposition of immune complexes in the walls of the affected blood vessels. Histological examination of affected skin shows a lymphocytic infiltrate. Antigen–antibody complex deposition and activation of the complement system results in endothelial damage, platelet adhesion and aggregation and fibrin formation [105].

Leakage of red cells from the damaged vessel produces purpura which is palpable to the finger, itchy, and uncomfortable. Skin necrosis and ulceration can occur. Non-thrombocytopenic purpura can be readily distinguished from thrombocytopenic purpura by the characteristic skin lesions and the absence of low levels of circulating platelets in the former.

Henoch–Schönlein purpura

Special mention should be made of Henoch–Schönlein purpura which, although rare, is probably the commonest form of vasculitic purpura. Skin, joints, alimentary tract, kidneys, heart and the central nervous system can be involved. The condition is more common in children than adults and can occur acutely in epidemics with a seasonal increase in the spring [106]. Often, there will be a history of a preceding upper respiratory tract infection. Although β-haemolytic *Streptococcus* has often been implicated by either culture or rising antistreptolysin-O (ASO) titres, a causal relation between the Henoch–Schönlein syndrome and streptococcal infection has not been established.

Clinically, a fever occurs, followed by a purpuric, often palpable, skin rash which affects the pretibial region, thighs and buttocks. The rash, which can continue to form in crops over several weeks, is characteristically symmetrical in its distribution and (unlike thrombocytopenic purpura) is often uncomfortable and urticarial rather than purpuric. Involvement of other systems leads to acute arthritis, intestinal pain and bleeding, nephritis and proteinuria, pleurisy, pericarditis, iritis, CNS bleeding, acute intussusception or renal failure.

The condition is often self-limiting in children. Corticosteroids and occasionally cytotoxic drugs can be used and symptoms usually rapidly respond to such treatment

The only demonstrable abnormality of haemostatic tests in some patients with Henoch–Schönlein purpura has been a lack of prostacyclin-stimulating factor in their blood. Close relatives have also shown this abnormality [107]. Renal and skin biopsies may reveal deposits of IgA surrounding blood vessels in the affected site. In addition, some patients have been shown to have an elevated serum IgA.

Clinical features of bleeding problems related to infections

Infection can lead to inadequate haemostasis by the different mechanisms previously described. Often, more than one of these mechanisms is responsible for altered haemostasis occurring in relation to a single infection (e.g. a single infection in a patient could give rise to bleeding problems caused by the occurrence of disordered coagulation, platelet abnormalities and vessel-wall abnormalities). Alternatively, another infection may produce only platelet abnormalities. Whether clinically significant bleeding occurs in the presence of such altered haemostasis depends on several other factors (e.g. the general state of the patient, underlying diseases and drug therapy).

Thrombocytopenia

Thrombocytopenia associated with infection is usually not severe. Corrigan [69] and Riedler *et al.* [70] reported that approximately 60–65% of patients who had thrombocytopenia secondary to infection had platelet counts of $>50 \times 10^9/l$.

Haemorrhage due to thrombocytopenia caused by infection is rare if a low platelet count is the only haemostatic abnormality, as a circulating platelet count of $50 \times 10^9/l$ provides adequate haemostasis. Pure 'platelet bleeding' (i.e. when there is intact whole blood coagulation), causes a recognized clinical syndrome. Superficial capillaries leak blood causing pinpoint petechiae or larger purpuric lesions and mucosal bleeding. Epistaxis, haematuria, melaena and menorrhagia can all occur. A minor superficial cut may bleed excessively and dental extractions can be complicated by protracted blood loss.

Excessive bleeding due to thrombocytopenia or defective platelet function (for example in thrombocythaemia) can usually be controlled by prolonged local pressure. Platelet bleeding starts immediately after the initial trauma but does not recur once it has been stopped.

Disseminated intravascular coagulation

DIC is not always clinically apparent. Mild cases may only be diagnosed from minor abnormalities in clotting studies. Severe DIC can have florid clinical features. DIC can be regarded as acute, subacute or chronic. The underlying 'trigger' or cause of DIC determines the acuteness or chronicity of DIC. Acute DIC is often associated with severe clinical consequences. There is gross activation of coagulation, uncompensated consumption of coagulation factors and platelets and secondary fibrinolysis — all of which result in simultaneous haemorrhage and thrombosis. The fine balance between coagulation activation and adequate compensatory fibrinolysis is upset. Clinically, patients in such situations are often extremely ill with signs of fever, hypotension, acidosis, hypoxia and proteinuria. The onset of acute DIC can be explosive. Both DIC and the underlying cause or 'trigger' of the DIC process cause similar clinical features, often making it difficult to determine whether the former or the latter is predominantly responsible for the clinical features.

Haemorrhage is the commonest clinical manifestation in severe cases of DIC. Skin bleeding in the form of petechiae, purpura and ecchymoses all occur. Bleeding into muscles can occur. Mucosal bleeding leads to epistaxis, gum bleeding, vaginal haemorrhage, haematemesis and melaena. Particular care needs to be taken of venepuncture sites which may bleed excessively. Postoperative wounds, drain and catheter sites are all prone to haemorrhage. There may be cerebral or pulmonary haemorrhage. Haemorrhage can increase the dysfunction of major organs which are often already damaged by thrombosis and ischaemia.

In mild, usually subacute and chronic cases of DIC, there is a greater balance between haemorrhage and thrombosis. As a result, DIC may not be clinically evident (i.e. there is neither thrombosis nor bleeding). If other factors (e.g. stasis or atheroma) are present, these may encourage thrombosis. The diagnosis in mild cases of DIC is often suggested by laboratory abnormalities of clotting studies (see later).

Only 7% of patients have clinical signs of thrombosis at presentation and thrombosis is apparent during the course of DIC in approximately 25% of cases [108]. Micro- and macrovascular thrombosis can lead to a wide range of ischaemic organ damage, which, in turn, causes renal impairment, coma, confusion and cardiorespiratory failure. Thrombotic complications also include acral cyanosis, thrombophlebitis, digital and skin gangrene.

The kidneys are particularly vulnerable in DIC and impairment of renal function occurs due to (i) ischaemic cortical necrosis secondary to thrombosis in glomerular capillaries and arterioles (from DIC) and (ii) acute tubular necrosis resulting from hypovolaemia or hypotension (for example in septic shock). Haematuria, anuria or oliguria can all occur. Microangiopathic haemolytic anaemia is sometimes seen because of fragmentation of red cells which are trapped by fibrin within the microvasculature. Figure 11.4 outlines the clinical features of DIC.

An analysis of studies with available data indicates that even in patients with DIC who have thrombocytopenia in association with sepsis, clinically significant bleeding (i.e. generalized bleeding in addition to cutaneous purpura) is rare [109]. Only 7–10% of patients with sepsis and thrombocytopenia (with or without DIC) were described as having generalized haemorrhage [66,67,72,73].

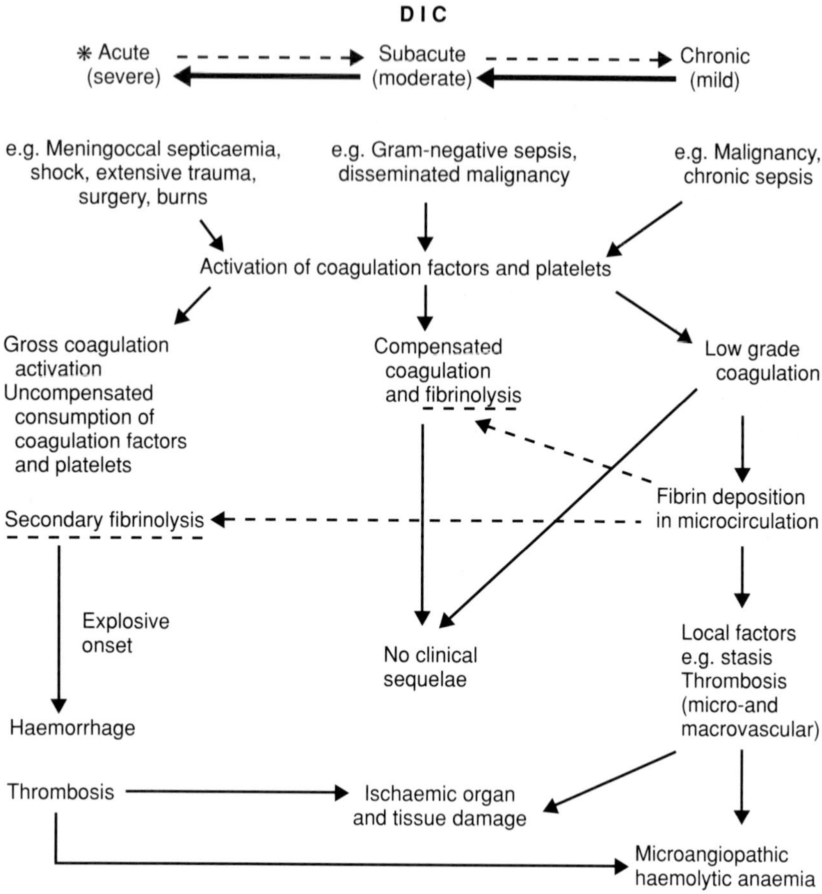

Fig. 11.4 Clinical features of DIC. * Acute DIC can progress (←) from chronic DIC. Less commonly, acute DIC can become (---→) chronic DIC.

It is important to remember that the major organ dysfunction which can affect patients with DIC may be due to a combination of the underlying cause of DIC, associated circulatory failure, acidosis and disordered coagulation. Circulatory failure and acidosis are frequent complications of septic shock. Finally, other determinants as to whether DIC, platelet disorders and vasculitis will cause clinically significant haemorrhage include the general status of the patient, the presence and nature of underlying diseases and drug therapy.

Laboratory diagnosis of bleeding problems

When a bleeding problem in an infected patient is suggested clinically (e.g. by the presence of petechiae, purpura or gum bleeding), laboratory investigations are carried out to determine the exact nature of this bleeding problem. Vasculitis (non-thrombocytopenic purpura) is easily distinguished from thrombocytopenic purpura by the nature of the cutaneous lesions and the presence of normal levels of circulating platelets. Thrombocytosis and thrombocytopenia are diagnosed by a platelet count and blood film. Laboratory tests which detect evidence of platelet and coagulation activation and fibrinolysis are used to diagnose DIC. However, no single laboratory test or particular combination of tests can be used to make a definite diagnosis of DIC [110]. Abnormalities of coagulation tests can help to confirm a suspected diagnosis of DIC if a patient has a condition predisposing to DIC and/or has clinical evidence of DIC.

Before considering the laboratory tests required, it is important to remember that samples must be obtained from a fresh venepuncture (not from an indwelling intravenous cannula). Samples should be sent to the laboratory without delay.

Tests

1 *Blood count, blood film and platelet count* give an indication of the numbers of platelets. A low haemoglobin may be due to haemolysis or bleeding. The blood film may show thrombocytopenia or fragmentation of red blood cells caused by red cell damage (e.g. in intravascular haemolysis or renal disease). An elevated white cell count indicates underlying infection.

2 *Prothrombin time (PT)* measures extrinsic coagulation pathway activity. The PT is prolonged in moderate and severe DIC due to factor consumption and the presence of fibrin degradation products (FDPs). The PT can be normal in mild cases of DIC.

3 *Activated partial thromboplastin time (APTT) with kaolin* measures intrinsic coagulation pathway activity. In severe DIC, the APTT is prolonged due to factor consumption and the presence of FDPs. Like the PT, the APTT can be normal in mild DIC. Note, however, that septic patients may have conditions other than DIC that are responsible for prolongation of both the PT and APTT [67].

4 *Thrombin time (TT)* measures the conversion of fibrinogen to fibrin. The TT is usually prolonged in DIC. Prolongation of the TT occurs when there is a lack of clottable fibrinogen or interference with the reaction (e.g. by heparin or FDPs). In the presence of heparin, the reptilase time (see later) is normal while the TT is prolonged.

5 *Fibrinogen concentration* is usually reduced in severe DIC. Clot formation can be observed in a glass tube at the bedside. With severe fibrinogen depletion, a small clot forms which is difficult to see.

6 *FDP concentration* reflects fibrinolytic activity and is usually very high in moderate and severe DIC. FDP concentration is also higher after surgery or blood transfusion.

7 *Ethanol gelation test/protamine sulphate precipitation test.* Both of these tests are positive in the presence of fibrin monomer complexes in the blood and are usually positive in DIC. However, they are non-specific tests as fibrin monomer complexes can be found in trauma and infection (without DIC).

8 *Bleeding time (BT)* is measured using a standard spring-loaded template device. The BT is prolonged by thrombocytopenia and platelet dysfunction.

9 *Platelet aggregation studies* can assess potential platelet dysfunction (e.g. in thrombocythaemia and DIC).

10 *Coagulation factor assays* will accurately diagnose factor deficiencies. There are usually decreased levels of multiple factors in DIC. However, assay of individual factors is seldom helpful if the deficiencies are due to DIC.

11 *Euglobulin lysis time* is a measure of fibrinolytic activity. In early DIC, the lysis time is shortened and in late DIC it is prolonged.

12 *Reptilase time* is prolonged in DIC. As mentioned earlier, this test is unaffected by heparin. Thus, a reptilase time can distinguish between coagulation abnormalities due to heparin or DIC if the patient is on heparin. The test can be unreliable in the presence of high levels of circulating FDPs.

13 *$B\beta_{15-42}$ peptide levels* reflect the digestion of fibrin monomers by plasmin. Increased levels are found in DIC.

14 *FPA and FPB* are sensitive indicators of thrombin generation. Increased levels are found in DIC, tissue inflammation and injury.

15 *β-Thromboglobulin (BTG) and platelet factors 3 and 4* are indicators of platelet activation and release of granules. Levels of these substances are increased in the initial stages of DIC due to intravascular damage to platelets.

16 *Antithrombin III levels (AT-III)* are decreased in DIC, liver disease and congenital AT-III deficiency.
17 *Plasminogen concentration* reflects fibrinolytic activity. In DIC, plasminogen concentration is reduced.
18 α_2*-Antiplasmin* also reflects fibrinolysis and decreased levels are found in DIC.
19 *Plasminogen activator (tPA)* There may be increased levels of this in DIC due to fibrinolysis.
20 *Plasmin–antiplasmin complexes* are present in DIC.

Of the tests described above, 1–8 are the most useful initial screening investigations that should be used to diagnose the nature of a bleeding problem. In acute DIC, speedy confirmation of the diagnosis is important to enable the institution of prompt treatment. The initial screening tests used to diagnose DIC (1–6) are sensitive but lack specificity. As a result, these tests can be affected by the underlying condition which has 'triggered' the DIC process. Similarly, thrombocytopenia is frequently seen in DIC but it too may be due to the underlying 'trigger' of DIC (e.g. infection). In DIC, FDP assay is probably the most useful test as many authorities require an elevation in its level before a diagnosis of DIC is entertained [110,111]. During DIC, coagulation test results are continually changing due to the dynamic nature of the DIC process. Sequential testing of coagulation is more useful than a single set of test results considered in isolation, as the former gives more information about the progress of DIC, i.e. indicates any improvement or deterioration with time. Initial screening tests used to diagnose DIC may indicate whether the process is acute or chronic. Acute DIC is associated with gross abnormalities of coagulation tests, whereas chronic DIC may produce only minor coagulation abnormalities.

Tests 9–20 are additional laboratory investigations that can be used to diagnose a bleeding problem. These tests are sometimes impractical and are not usually immediately necessary. Often, they are only available in specialist centres.

Management of bleeding problems

The principles of management of a patient with bleeding problems are similar whether the bleeding has been caused by infection or any other cause. In general, the first step is to establish the nature and severity of the haemostatic defect both clinically and in the laboratory in order that the most appropriate treatment is given. Secondly, repeat testing of haemostatic function following treatment is necessary, particularly if surgery is contemplated, and if the treatment has been given specifically to prevent bleeding during this surgical procedure. Thirdly, a local cause for bleeding should be sought if, despite adequate replacement treatment, the bleeding has not improved.

More specifically, the management of bleeding problems arising from infection involves effective replacement therapy (if clinically indicated) and control of the underlying infection.

Thrombocytopenia

The management of thrombocytopenia caused by infection is usually conservative as the platelet count generally recovers as the infection is adequately treated. Spontaneous bleeding generally occurs when the platelet count is $<20 \times 10^9$/l unless there is platelet dysfunction or severe infection, in which cases bleeding can arise at higher platelet counts. Platelet transfusions are given when clinically indicated by the condition of the patient. Platelet transfusions often need to be repeated every 24–48 h depending on the nature and extent of the bleeding. Regular platelet counts should be carried out. Severe thrombocytopenia without evidence of bleeding is not usually an indication for platelet transfusion. However, thrombocytopenic patients must be regularly examined to check for any fresh purpuric or petechial lesions appearing on the skin, mucous membranes or optic fundi. Sudden intracranial haemorrhage, the major cause of death in thrombocytopenic patients, does not usually occur until after petechial lesions on the skin and mucous membranes have developed. Frequently, infection-induced purpura is caused by peripheral destruction of platelets and, in these cases, the effect of platelet transfusions is very short-lived. A platelet count checked 1 h after transfusion should show an increment. No increment suggests that the transfused platelets are being rapidly consumed (e.g. due to DIC) and that further platelet transfusions will be of little benefit.

Disseminated intravascular coagulation

General management

An essential first step in the management of a patient with DIC is the removal or treatment of the precipitating cause or 'trigger' of the DIC process [112]. Correction of the underlying cause or 'trigger' is usually followed by normalization of coagulation. In septicaemia, appropriate intravenous antibiotics in high doses should be started. In acute DIC, patients can be critically ill because of both the underlying cause of DIC and the disordered coagulation. Such patients need acute management in an intensive care unit. If the patient has septic shock or is bleeding profusely, it is vital to restore the circulating blood volume to normal. While this needs to be done fairly rapidly, caution should be taken to ensure that cardiac function is not compromised by transfusion of large volumes of fluid. The heart may already be affected by ischaemia caused by thrombosis. Close monitoring of renal function is necessary to detect evidence of renal failure. If generalized bleeding is present, it may cause local problems when inserting arterial or venous catheters, which are usually required for monitoring the progress of the patient. In contrast to thrombocytopenia, intracranial bleeding occurs rarely in DIC.

Patients with shock may develop the adult respiratory distress syndrome (ARDS) which impairs oxygenation, making it difficult to achieve adequate arterial oxygenation. DIC and ARDS are closely associated [113,114] but the cause–effect relationship between them is unclear. Tissue oxygenation is adversely affected by the micro- and macrovascular thromboses seen in DIC. The resulting acidosis then enhances thrombosis. Thus, it is important to diagnose and promptly treat associated acidosis.

Specific therapy

Replacement therapy

1 It is generally recommended that in DIC, coagulation factor replacement should not be introduced solely on the basis of an abnormal coagulation screen. It should be instituted if there is uncontrolled bleeding or if the precipitating cause cannot be rapidly treated [115]. Fresh frozen plasma (FFP) and cryoprecipitate provide the necessary coagulation factors. FFP is less useful in practice than in theory because large volumes of FFP are necessary to ensure the maintenance of adequate levels of coagulation factors. In DIC, transfusion with concentrates of coagulation factors can 'add fuel to the fire' (i.e. these coagulation factors can be rapidly consumed and may exacerbate the thrombotic process in the microvasculature) [116,117]. Thus, therapy with coagulation factor concentrates is not usually given in cases of DIC with abnormal coagulation tests but no overt bleeding. In such cases, it is anticipated that appropriate and vigorous treatment of the underlying cause of DIC (e.g. infection) will correct the coagulation abnormalities.

2 Severe bleeding in DIC may warrant treatment with blood and platelet transfusions.

3 Prothrombin complex concentrates and fibrinogen concentrates are potentially thrombogenic and their use is inadvisable. They may also transmit hepatitis and HIV infection.

Inhibition of activated coagulation

Specific coagulation inhibitors such as heparin and AT-III are sometimes used in the treatment of DIC in an attempt to stop the activated coagulation process and, in turn, remove the drive to compensatory fibrinolysis.

1 The use of heparin in DIC is *not* standard practice and its use is controversial because of the lack of controlled clinical trials [118], variation of response to heparin and possible potentiation of the risk of bleeding. The main indication for heparin therapy in DIC is when thrombosis is the predominant problem and when thrombosis is either responsible for organ damage or is potentially detrimental (e.g. pulmonary embolism or peripheral gangrene). In the case of DIC secondary to septicaemia, heparin therapy has not been proved to be of value [119].

2 AT-III concentrate has been use with success as a single therapy in treating small groups of patients with DIC. It is not routinely used to treat patients with DIC secondary to septicaemia.

3 Oral anticoagulants have no place in the treatment of DIC.

Inhibition of excessive fibrinolysis

If laboratory tests indicate that fibrinolysis is a major factor in the DIC process, treatment with antifibrinolytic drugs such as ε-aminocaproic acid (EACA) or tranexamic acid (Cyclokapron) may be tried, particularly if haemorrhage is a problem. EACA acts as both a competitive and non-competitive inhibitor of plasminogen, depending on the concentration used. EACA is administered orally at a dose of 3 g 6-hourly. Tranexamic acid can be given orally or intravenously. Antifibrinolytic drugs, when used to treat bleeding in DIC, give rise to the formation of unlysable thrombus which may appear in blood vessels or, in the presence of haematuria, can cause an obstructive uropathy. In an effort to prevent widespread thrombotic complications, simultaneous low-dose heparin is sometimes administered.

Antiplatelet agents

In cases of DIC where platelet aggregation is thought to be an initiating mechanism, antiplatelet drugs (e.g. prostacyclin) have occasionally been successfully used to treat the DIC process. However, their use in DIC secondary to septicaemia has not yet been proved to be of value [119].

Synthetic thrombin inhibitors

An essential pathogenic factor in the initiation of the DIC process is the intravascular generation of thrombin. Using this concept, animal models of DIC have been used to study the effects of synthetic thrombin inhibitors [4,8]. It is postulated that synthetic thrombin inhibitors may have a prophylactic and therapeutic use in the treatment of DIC.

Removal of already formed thrombi

Animal experiments have successfully demonstrated the removal of fibrin from occluded vessels by both streptokinase and urokinase [120] but there is little evidence to support the use of these agents to treat DIC in man.

Prophylaxis

DIC accompanies the fulminant (usually pneumococcal) sepsis that can affect people with asplenia. Routine prophylaxis of splenectomized patients with pneumococcal vaccine is currently performed [47] but it does not uniformly prevent this complication [48].

Summary

Therapy for bleeding problems which are secondary to infection and septicaemia should be directed at the underlying problem, i.e. effective, prompt and vigorous treatment of infections with antibiotics and, if required, resuscitation of the patient from septic shock which may involve using replacement therapy (e.g. coagulation factor, blood and platelet transfusions), if clinically indicated.

Finally, it should be noted that some of the drugs used to treat infections can also produce thrombocytopenia (secondary to peripheral destruction or bone-marrow suppression) and abnormalities of blood coagulation [121,122].

Trauma

Specific bleeding problems associated with trauma will now be discussed. The various stresses associated with trauma (e.g. pain, infection and bacterial toxins, dead tissue, hypotension and hypovolaemia) can cause activation of a wide variety of cell mediators to which cells in various tissues respond. Such responses can be:

1 Haemostatic (to be discussed here).

2 Physiological (e.g. increased cardiac output, provision of adequate oxygen, substrate and metabolic transport, prevention of shock, acidosis, uraemia and jaundice).

3 Metabolic (e.g. increased energy expenditure, increased synthesis of proteins to sufficiently meet needs for immunological defence, maintenance of cellular functions and healing).

4 Immunological (e.g. inflammation limits the spread of infection).

These responses are necessary for patient survival, control and elimination of infection, wound healing and patient recovery. Without them, shock or overwhelming infection may develop, with resulting multisystem organ failure and death. The following discussion will focus on the bleeding problems associated with trauma.

Physical trauma can cause endothelial injury which causes activation of Factor XII (Hageman factor) and of the intrinsic coagulation cascade. This, in turn, activates the complement cascade (which can itself be activated by trauma), kinins and causes generation of fibrin with subsequent activation of fibrinolysis. Tissue damage due to trauma leads to tissue thromboplastin release directly into the circulation, which results in activation of the extrinsic coagulation pathway. The end result of activation of both the coagulation and complement cascades is (i) altered metabolism which produces fever, proteolysis in muscle and gut, lipolysis and acute phase protein synthesis, (ii) inflammation and (iii) activation of fibrinolysis and production of vasoactive fibrinopeptides.

An inadequate haemostatic response in trauma (and shock) may lead to haemorrhage and DIC (see earlier for DIC). For a patient to recover from trauma, cellular injury caused by trauma has to be effectively balanced by adequate defensive responses. In addition, appropriate supportive treatment (e.g. ventilation, administration of intravenous fluids, antibiotics and nutritional support) may all be required to aid recovery. Surgical debridement of wounds may be necessary. In common with DIC caused by infection, DIC due to trauma should respond to treatment of the trauma (e.g. removal of dead tissue, antibiotic therapy for wound infections and supportive treatment if the patient has shock; see also earlier—management of DIC, p. 220).

Three specific clinical situations of trauma will be described: head injury, fat embolism and drowning.

Head injury

Special mention should be made of bleeding problems associated with head injuries. Massive DIC is a well-recognized complication of traumatic brain damage. In head injuries which cause brain trauma, it is likely that brain tissue (which is highly thromboplastic) enters the systemic circulation and initiates intravascular coagulation via the extrinsic pathway [123]. A study of 13 individuals who suffered brain trauma as a result of gunshot wounds or massive blunt trauma found four who had 'striking clinical and laboratory evidence of hemostatic failure due to acute defibrination' [20]. There were less marked abnormalities in five other patients. However, these abnormalities were thought to be severe enough to be a contributory factor in intracranial haemorrhage. Patients sustaining head injuries with loss of consciousness but without evidence of brain destruction have not been shown to have symptoms or laboratory results to suggest defibrination [123,124].

In the management of patients with DIC due to brain trauma, the use of replacement therapy (i.e. cryoprecipitate to replace fibrinogen, platelet transfusions, whole blood transfusion or FFP to replace clotting factors) can be beneficial [20,125].

Fat embolism

Fat embolism is a complication of a variety of conditions (see Table 11.4) [126–128].

In fat embolism, marrow fat droplets enter the circulation. Embolization to the lung, brain and other organs can cause hypoxia and respiratory failure, altered level of consciousness and focal cerebral signs. The patient will often have a high fever. When the cause is bone injury, petechial haemorrhages are frequently seen on the upper half of

Table 11.4 Causes of fat embolism

- Fractures (e.g. tibia, femur)
- Joint-replacement surgery
- Extensive trauma
- Burns
- Severe infection
- Pancreatitis
- Sickle-cell crises
- Cardiopulmonary bypass surgery
- Renal transplant surgery

the body on the skin (usually sparing the face), conjunctivae, optic fundi, palate and buccal mucosa. Physical signs of fat embolism tend to develop late. The earliest change is hypoxaemia and the chest X-ray may show scattered consolidation (snowstorm appearance). In severe cases, there may be fat in the urine. At postmortem, microthrombi may be found in the cerebral microcirculation. Studies have shown that in patients with lower limb fractures who had hypoxaemia suggesting fat embolism, the platelet count was moderately reduced transiently and the level of fibrinogen-related antigens (FRAs) was elevated [129,130]. (FRAs can be likened to FDPs [143].) Although these changes may be taken to mean that fat droplets initiate DIC, it is suggested that such changes are, in part, secondary to thrombin formation in pulmonary vessels as in experimental fat embolism [131]. Another reason for DIC arising in patients with fat embolism is likely to be the severe acidosis and hypoxia which occurs as a result of circulatory failure induced by fat embolism.

Drowning

Near-drowning in fresh water causes intravascular haemolysis. Haemolysed red cells then 'trigger' DIC [132,133]. Hypoxaemia, cardiorespiratory failure and associated acidosis can augment the DIC process. Cryoprecipitates, platelet transfusions and fresh plasma can be used to treat DIC associated with near-drowning.

Shock

Shock results when tissue/organ blood flow is inadequate to maintain normal cellular activity. Whatever the type of shock (i.e. hypovolaemic, septic, cardiogenic, neurogenic or anaphylactic), it may be complicated by DIC. Widespread vascular damage from endotoxins, infection, immune complexes, hypoxia and acidosis is a major aetiological factor which leads to the development of DIC in patients with shock. It is postulated that platelet aggregation and microthrombus formation 'trigger' DIC in patients with shock [134]. At the onset of DIC in a patient with shock, there is often evidence of bleeding and tissue damage from the underlying cause of the shock. The DIC process worsens both the bleeding and tissue damage. Thrombosis can cause ischaemia to vital organs (e.g. brain and kidney). These organs may already be compromised by the underlying cause of the shock. Thrombosis is especially likely to occur when there is low blood flow, as in shock.

In shocked patients, DIC is usually acute with gross clinical evidence of the process (e.g. acral cyanosis and gangrene or patchy cutaneous gangrene on the extremities [135,136]). Shock secondary to sepsis has already been discussed earlier. It should be emphasized that, in cases of DIC secondary to septic shock, specific therapy for DIC is seldom indicated in the management of shock unless there is clinical evidence of haemostatic failure (see earlier). Treatment of patients with shock and DIC in whom haemostatic failure is clinically apparent again involves replacement therapy as described earlier. AT-III preparations have been given to patients with DIC and shock in an effort to increase AT-III levels, which are reduced in patients with shock. No apparent benefit has been shown on survival [137]. As well as treatment for defective haemostasis, patients with shock need vigorous, appropriate, supportive treatment (depending on the type of shock) and may need to be managed in an intensive care unit. Recently, it has been suggested that avoidance or correction of hypothermia may be critical in preventing or correcting coagulopathy in trauma patients receiving massive transfusion [138].

Another complication seen in patients with shock is ARDS, which impairs oxygenation (see also p. 221). It is thought that thrombosis in the pulmonary microcirculation causing respiratory failure may either occur as a result of ARDS or, as a result of DIC which may, in turn, cause ARDS, i.e. DIC and ARDS seem closely associated but the cause–effect relationship between them is not yet firmly established [139]. A recent report indicates that plasminogen activators can lyse pulmonary microthrombi and prevent the onset of ARDS even when given several hours after trauma [140].

Burns

Acute DIC is frquently seen in patients with burns. In severe cases, patients may develop thrombocytopenia, hypofibrinogenaemia and reduced levels of plasminogen and coagulation factors except Factor VIII [141,142] and, as a result, there can be severe bleeding problems. The haemostatic abnormalities seen in patients with burns are likely to be due to a combination of local consumption of coagulation factors and platelets in the burn-damaged area and generalized DIC. Several factors contribute to the development of DIC in burn patients. Endothelial injury (from the burn) may activate Factor XII and the intrinsic pathway to initiate DIC. Endothelial damage is increased by complications caused by burns, i.e. associated septic or hypovolaemic shock, hypoxia and acidosis. In severe burns, DIC may be initiated by activation of the extrinsic coagulation pathway due to thromboplastin release into the circulation from burn-damaged tissue and red cells. Acute haemolysis may also contribute to the development of DIC in burn patients.

General management of a patient with burns involves analgesia, ensuring an adequate airway, correction of fluid depletion, accurate fluid balance, appropriate treatment of infection and nutritional supplements. Local burn management may involve debridement (to remove necrotic material) and skin grafts.

Heparin therapy to treat the haemostatic defects in patients with severe burns has been advocated but there is little evidence to suggest that it is beneficial. Replacement therapy with blood, platelets and coagulation factors should be given if clinically indicated (see earlier—shock and DIC, p. 220).

References

1 Busch, C. and Saleen, T. (1973) Amount of fibrin in different organs after intravenous, intraportal and intraaortal injection of thrombin in rat. *Thrombos. Diathes. Haemorrh.*, **29**, 87–93.

2 Markwardt, F., Nowak, G., Meerbach, W. and Rudiger, K. (1975) Studies in experimental animals on DIC. *Thrombos. Diathes. Haemorrh.*, **34**, 513–521.

3 Markwardt, F., Nowak, G. and Hoffman, J. (1983) Comparative studies on thrombin inhibitors in experimental microthrombosis. *Thromb. Haemost.*, **49**, 235–237.

4 Hara, H., Tamao, Y., Kikunoto, R. and Okamoto, S. (1987) Effect of a synthetic thrombin inhibitor MCI-9038 on experimental models of disseminated intravascular coagulation in rabbits. *Thromb. Haemost.*, **57**, 165–170.

5 Slaastad, R. and Jeremic, M. (1973) The laboratory diagnosis of low-grade disseminated intravascular coagulation. *Scand. J. Haematol.*, **11**, 50–58.

6 Pflug, J., Calnan, J. and Oslen, G.J. (1968) An experimental model for the study of thrombosis. *Br. J. Surg.*, **25**, 63–69.

7 Cronlund, M., Hardin, J., Burton, J. *et al.* (1976) Fibrinopeptide in plasma of normal subjects and patients with disseminated intravascular coagulation and systemic lupus erythematosus. *J. Clin. Invest.*, **58**, 142–151.

8 Schaeffer, R.C., Briston, C., Chilton, S.-M. and Carlson, R.W. (1986) Disseminated intravascular coagulation following *Echis carinatus* venom in dogs: Effects of a synthetic thrombin inhibitor. *J. Lab. Clin. Med.*, **107**, 488–497.

9 McKay, D.G. and Muller-Berghaus, G. (1967) Therapeutic implications of disseminated intravascular coagulation. *Am. J. Cardiol.*, **20**, 392–410.

10 Bang, N.U. and Chang, M. (1974) Soluble fibrin complexes. *Semin. Thromb. Hemost.*, **1**, 91–103.

11 Jakobsen, E., Ly, B. and Kieulf, P. (1974) Incorporation of fibrinogen with soluble fibrin complexes. *Thromb. Res.*, **4**, 499–501.

12 Fletcher, A.P., Alkjaersig, N., Fisher, S. and Sherry, S. (1966) The proteolysis of fibrinogen by plasmin: the identification of thrombin-clottable fibrinogen derivatives which polymerise abnormally. *J. Lab. Clin. Med.*, **68**, 780–802.

13 Sharp, A.A. (1964) Pathological fibrinolysis. *Br. Med. Bull.*, **20**, 240–243.

14 Pechet, L. (1965) Fibrinolysis. *New Engl. J. Med.*, **273**, 966–967.

15 Donaldson, V. (1960) Effect of plasmin *in vitro* on clotting factors in plasma. *J. Lab. Clin. Med.*, **56**, 644–646.

16 Beller, F.K. (1969) The role of endotoxin in disseminated intravascular coagulation. *Thrombos. Diathes. Haemorrh.*, **36** (Suppl.), 125–150.

17 Evensen, S.A. and Hjort, P.F. Pathogenesis of disseminated intravascular clotting. Plenary sessions, scientific contributions. *XIII International Congress of Haematology, Munich*, pp. 109–120 (1970).

18 Muller-Berghaus, G. (1977) Pathophysiology of generalised intravascular coagulation. *Semin. Thromb. Hemost.*, **3**, 209–246.

19 Huth, K., Schoenborn, W. and Knorpp, K. (1967) Experimentelle Verbranchskoagulopathie nach intravenoser Zufuhr von Fett und Endotoxin. *Thrombos. Diathes, Haemorrh.*, **16**, 228–242.

20 Goodnight, S.H., Kenoyer, G., Rappaport, S.I. *et al.* Defibrination after brain-tissue destruction: A serious complication of head injury. *New Engl. J. Med.*, **290**, 1043–1047.

21 Niemetz, J. (1972) Coagulant activity in leukocytes: tissue factor activity. *J. Clin. Invest.*, **51**, 307–313.

22 Thiagarajan, P. and Niemetz, J. (1980) Procoagulant–tissue factor activity of circulating peripheral blood leukocytes: results of *in vivo* studies. *Thromb. Res.*, **17**, 891–896.

23 Edwards, R.L., Rickles, F.R. and Bobrove, A.M. (1979) Mononuclear cell tissue factor: cell of origin and requirements for activation. *Blood*, **54**, 359–370.

24 Muhlfelder, T.W., Kahn, I. and Niemetz, J. (1978) Factors influencing the release of procoagulant–tissue factor activity from leukocytes. *J. Lab. Clin. Med.*, **92**, 65–72.

25 Kay, L.A. Acquired disorders of coagulation. In: *Essentials of Haemostasis and Thrombosis* (Eds Poller, L. & Thomson, J.), p. 84. Churchill Livingstone, Edinburgh (1988).

26 Rickles, F.R., Rick, P.D., Van Why, M. and Kay, L.A. (1977) Structural features of *Salmonella typhimurium* lipopolysaccharide required for activation of tissue factor in human mononuclear cells. *J. Clin. Invest.*, **59**, 1188–1195.

27 Niemetz, J. and Morrison, D.C. (1977) Lipid A as the biologically active moiety in bacterial endotoxin (LPS)-initiated generation of procoagulant activity by peripheral blood leukocytes. *Blood*, **49**, 947–956.

28 Kessler, C.M., Nussbaum, E. and Tuazon, C.U. (1987) *In vitro* correlation of platelet aggregation with occurrence of disseminated intravascular coagulation and subacute bacterial endocarditis. *J. Lab. Clin. Med.*, **109**, 647–652.

29 Kornalik, F. and Blomback, B. (1975) Prothrombin activation induced by ecarin—a prothrombin converting enzyme from *Echis carinatus* venom. *Thromb. Res.*, **6**, 53–63.

30 Wilson, J.J., Neame, P.B. and Kelton, J.G. (1982) Infection-induced thrombocytopaenia. *Semin. Thromb. Hemost.*, **8**, 217–233.

31 McKay, D.G. and Margaretten, W. (1967) Disseminated intravascular coagulation in virus diseases. *Arch. Intern. Med.*, **120**, 129–152.

32 Davison, A.M., Thomson, D. and Robson, J.S. (1973) Intravascular coagulation complicating influenza A virus infection. *Br. Med. J.*, **1**, 654–655.

33 Srichaikul, T., Nimmanitaya, S., Artchararit, N. *et al.* (1977) Fibrinogen metabolism and disseminated intravascular coagulation in dengue hemorrhagic fever. *Am. J. Trop. Med. Hyg.*, **26**, 525–532.

34 Mitrakul, C., Poshyachinda, M., Futrakul, P. *et al.* (1977) Hemostatic and platelet kinetic studies in dengue hemorrhagic fever. *Am. J. Trop. Med. Hyg.*, **26**, 975–984.

35 Ognibene, A.J., O'Leary, D.S., Czarnecki, S.W. *et al.* (1971) Myocarditis and disseminated intravascular coagulation in scrub typhus. *Am. J. Med. Sci.*, **262**, 233–239.

36 Dennis, L.H., Eichelberger, J.W., Inman, M.M. *et al.* (1967) Depletion of coagulation factors in drug-resistant *Plasmodium falciparum* malaria. *Blood*, **29**, 713–721.

37 Punyagupta, S., Srichaikul, T., Nitiyanant, P. *et al.* (1974) Acute pulmonary insufficiency in falciparum malaria: summary of 12 cases with evidence of disseminated intravascular coagulation. *Am. J. Trop. Med. Hyg.*, **23**, 551–559.

38 Barrett-Connor, E., Ugoretz, R.J. and Braude, A.I. (1973) Disseminated intravascular coagulation in trypanosomiasis. *Arch. Intern. Med.*, **131**, 574–577.

39 Kelton, J.G., Keystone, J., Moore, J. *et al.* (1983) Immune-mediated thrombocytopaenia of malaria. *J. Clin. Invest.*, **71**, 832–836.

40 Neva, F.A., Sheagren, J.N., Shulman, N.R. *et al.* (1970) Malaria: host–defense mechanisms and complications. *Ann. Intern. Med.*, **73**, 295–306.

41 Nelson, E.R., Bierman, H.R. and Chulajata, R. (1964) Hematologic findings in the 1960 hemorrhagic fever epidemic (dengue) in Thailand. *Am. J. Trop. Med. Hyg.*, **13**, 642–649.

42 Butler, T., Tong, M.J., Fletcher, J.R. *et al.* (1973) Blood coagulation studies in *Plasmodium falciparum* malaria. *Am. J. Med. Sci.*, **265**, 63–67.

43 Halstead, S.B. (1982) Dengue: hematologic aspects. *Semin. Hematol.*, **19**, 116–131.

44 Perrin, L.H., Mackey, L.J. and Miescher, P.A. (1982) The hematology of malaria in man. *Semin. Hematol.*, **19**, 70–82.

45 Cosgriff, T.M. (1989) Hemorrhagic fever with renal syndrome: four decades of research. *Ann. Intern. Med.*, **110**, 313–316.

46 McGehee, W.G., Rapaport, S.I. and Hjort, P.F. (1967) Intravascular coagulation in fulminant meningococcaemia. *Ann. Intern. Med.*, **67**, 250–260.

47 Ammann, A.J., Addiego, J., Wara, D.W. *et al.* (1977) Polyvalent pneumococcal–polysaccharide immunization of patients with sickle-cell anaemia and patients with splenectomy. *New Engl. J. Med.*, **297**, 897–900.

48 Overturf, G.D., Field, R., Edmonds, R. (1979) Death from type 6 pneumococcal septicaemia in a vaccinated child with sickle-cell disease. *New Engl. J. Med.*, **300**, 143. (Letter.)

49 Lindblad, B.E. and Lindblad, L.N. (1990) Fatal pneumococcal bacteraemia with disseminated intravascular coagulation and Waterhouse–Friderichsen syndrome in a vaccinated splenectomized adult. Case report. *Acta. Chir. Scand.*, **156**, 487–488.

50 Harker, L.A. and Schlichter, S.J. (1972) The bleeding time as a screening test for the evaluation of platelet function. *New Engl. J. Med.*, **287**, 155–159.

51 Levin, J. Bleeding with infectious diseases. In: *Disorders of Hemostasis* (Eds Ratnoff, O. & Forbes, C.D.), p. 369. W.B. Saunders, London (1991).

52 Oski, F.A. and Naiman, J.L. (1966) Effect of live measles vaccine on the platelet count. *New Engl. J. Med.*, **275**, 352–356.

53 Osborn, J.E. and Shahidi, N.T. (1973) Thombocytopaenia in murine cytomegalovirus infection. *J. Lab. Clin. Med.*, **81**, 53–63.

54 Young, N. (1988) Hematologic and hematopoietic consequences of B19 parvovirus infection. *Semin. Hematol.*, **25**, 159–172.

55 Harker, L.A. and Schlichter, S.J. (1972) Platelet and fibrinogen consumption in man. *New Engl. J. Med.*, **287**, 999–1005.

56 Israels, E.D., Nisli, G., Paraskevas, F. *et al.* (1973) Platelet Fc receptor as a mechanism for Ag–Ab complex-induced platelet injury. *Thromb. Diathes. Haemorrh.*, **29**, 434–444.

57 Clejan, L. and Menahem, H. (1977) Binding of deoxyribonucleic acid to the surface of human platelets. *Acta Haematol. (Basel)*, **58**, 84–88.

58 Myllyla, G., Vaheri, A., Vesikari, T. *et al.* (1969) Interaction between human blood platelets, viruses and antibodies. IV. Post-rubella thrombocytopenic purpura and platelet aggregation by rubella antigen–antibody interaction. *Clin. Exp. Immunol.*, **4**, 323–332.

59 Kelton, J.G., Neame, P.B., Gauldie, J. *et al.* (1979) Elevated platelet-associated IgG in the thrombocytopenia of septicemia. *New Engl. J. Med.*, **300**, 760–764.

60 Wautier, J.L., Boizard, B., Wautier, M.P. *et al.* (1980) Platelet-associated IgG and circulating immune complexes in thrombocytopenic purpura. *Nouv. Rev. Fr. Hematol.*, **22**, 29–36.

61 Lurhuma, A.Z., Riccomi, H., Masson, P.L. (1977) The occurrence of circulating immune complexes and viral antigens in idiopathic thrombocytopenic purpura. *Clin. Exp. Immunol.*, **28**, 49–55.

62 Clawson, C.C., Rao, G.H.R. and White, J.G. (1975) Platelet interaction with bacteria. IV. Stimulation of the release reaction. *Am. J. Pathol.*, **81**, 411–419.

63 Smith, S.B. (1972) Platelets in host resistance: *in vitro* interaction of platelets, bacteria and polymorphonuclear leukocytes. *Blut*, **25**, 104–107.

64 MacIntyre, D.E., Allen, A.P., Thorne, K.J.I. *et al.* (1977) Endotoxin-induced platelet aggregation and secretion. I. Morphological changes and pharmacological effects. *J. Cell. Sci.*, **28**, 211–223.

65 Thorne, K.J.I., Oliver, R.C., MacIntyre, D.E. *et al.* (1977) Endotoxin-induced platelet aggregation and secretion. II. Changes in plasma membrane proteins. *J. Cell Sci.*, **28**, 225–236.

66 Emerson, W.A., Zieve, P.D. and Krevans, J.R. (1970) Hematologic changes in septicaemia. *Johns Hopkins Med J.*, **126**, 69–76.

67 Goldenfarb, P.B., Zucker, S., Corrigan, J.J. Jr. *et al.* (1970) The coagulation mechanism in acute bacterial infection. *Br. J. Haematol.*, **18**, 643–652.

68 Pembrey, R.G., Handley, D.A. and Kimber, R.J. (1971) Causes of thrombocytopenia in a hospital population: a six-months survey of 7750 patients. *Med. J. Austral.*, **i**, 583–588.

69 Corrigan, J.J. (1974) Thrombocytopenia: a laboratory sign of septicemia in infants and children. *J. Pediatr.*, **85**, 219–221.

70 Riedler, G.F., Straub, P.W. and Frick, P.G. (1971) Thrombocytopenia in septicemia: a clinical study for the evaluation of its incidence and diagnostic value. *Helv. Med. Acta*, **36**, 23–38.

71 Oppenheimer, L., Hryniuk, W.M. and Bishop, A.J. (1976) Thrombocytopenia in severe bacterial infections. *J. Surg. Res.*, **20**, 211–214.

72 Milligan, G.F., MacDonald, J.A.E., Mellon, A. *et al.* (1974) Pulmonary and hematologic disturbances during septic shock. *Surg. Gynecol. Obstet.*, **138**, 43–49.

73 Kregar, B.E., Craven, D.E. and McCabe, W.R. (1980) Gram-negative bacteria. IV. Reevaluation of clinical features and treatment in 612 patients. *Am. J. Med.*, **68**, 344–355.

74 Geller, S.A., Muller, R., Greenberg, M.L. and Siegal, F.P. (1985) Acquired immunodeficiency syndrome: distinctive features of bone marrow biopsies. *Arch. Pathol. Lab. Med.*, **109**, 138–141.

75 Spivak, J.L., Bender, B.S. and Quinn, T.C. (1984) Hematologic abnormalities in the acquired immune deficiency syndrome. *Am. J. Med.*, **77**, 224–228.

76 Abrams, D.I., Chinn, E.K., Lewis, B.J. *et al.* (1984) Hematologic manifestations in homosexual men with Kaposi's sarcoma. *Am. J. Clin. Pathol.*, **81**, 13–18.

77 Frontiera, M. and Myers, A.M. (1987) Peripheral blood and bone marrow abnormalities in the acquired immunodeficiency syndrome. *West. J. Med.*, **147**, 157–160.

78 Castella, A., Croxson, T.S., Mildvan, D. *et al.* (1985) The bone marrow in AIDS: a histologic, hematologic, and microbiologic study. *Am. J. Clin. Pathol.*, **84**, 425–432.

79 Shenov, D.M. and Lin, J.H. (1986) Bone marrow findings in acquired immunodeficiency syndrome (AIDS). *Am. J. Med. Sci.*, **292**, 372–375.

80 Schneider, D.R. and Picker, L.J. (1985) Myelodysplasia in the acquired immune deficiency syndrome. *Am. J. Clin. Pathol.*, **84**, 144–152.

81 Laulund, S., Visfeldt, J. and Klinken, L. (1986) Patho-anatomical studies in patients dying of AIDS. *Acta Pathol. Microbiol. Immunol. Scand. (A)*, **94**, 201–221.

82 Metroka, C.E., Cunningham-Rundles, S., Pollack, M.S. *et al.* (1983) Generalized lymphadenopathy in homosexual men. *Ann. Intern. Med.*, **99**, 585–591.

83 Zon, L.I. and Groopman, J.E. (1988) Hematologic manifestations of the human immune deficiency virus (HIV). *Semin. Hematol.*, **25**, 208–218.

84 Fauci, A.S. (1984) Immunologic abnormalities in the acquired immunodeficiency syndrome (AIDS). *Clin. Res.*, **32**, 491–499.

85 Richman, D.D., Fischl, M.A., Grieco, M.H. *et al.* (1987) The toxicity of azidothymidine (AZT) in the treatment of patients with AIDS and AIDS-related complex: a double-blind, placebo-controlled trial. *New Engl. J. Med.*, **317**, 192–197.

86 Robbins, G. and Barnard, D.L. (1983) Thrombocytosis and microthrombocytosis: A clinical evaluation of 372 cases. *Acta Haematol.*, **70**, 175–182.

87 Rendu, M. (1896) Epistaxis répétees. Chez un sujet porteur de petits angiomes cutanés et muqueux. *Bull. Mem. Soc. Med. Paris*, **13**, 731–733.

88 Weber, F.P. (1907) Multiple hereditary developmental angiomata (telangiectases) of skin and mucous membranes associated with recurring haemorrhages. *Lancet*, **ii**, 160–168.

89 Osler, W. (1901) On a family form of recurrent epistaxis associated with multiple telangiectases of the skin and mucous membranes. *Bull. Johns Hopkins Hosp.*, **12**, 333.

90 Beighton, P. *The Ehlers–Danlos Syndrome*. Heinemann, London (1970).

91 Goodman, R.M., Smith, E.W. and Paton, D. (1963) Pseudoxanthoma elasticum: A clinical and histopathological study. *Medicine*, **42**, 297–334.

92 Priest, R.E., Moinuddin, J.F. and Priest, J.H. (1973) Collagen of Marfan syndrome is abnormally soluble. *Nature (London)*, **245**, 264–266.

93 Siegel, B.M., Friedman, I.A. and Schwartz, S.O. (1957) Haemorrhagic disease in osteogenesis imperfecta: Studies of platelet function defect. *Am. J. Med.*, **22**, 315–321.

94 Born, G.V.R. and Wright, H.P. (1967) Platelet adhesiveness in experimental scurvy. *Lancet*, **i**, 477–478.

95 Wilson, P.A., McNicol, G.P. and Douglas, A.S. (1967) Platelet abnormality in human scurvy. *Lancet*, **i**, 975–978.

96 Wallerstein, R.O. and Wallerstein, R.O. Jr. (1976) Scurvy. *Semin. Hematol.*, **13**, 211–218.

97 Lowe, G.D.O., Lowe, J.M., Drummond, M.M. *et al.* (1980) Blood viscosity in young male diabetics with and without retinopathy. *Diabetologia*, **18**, 359–363.

98 Somer, T. (1975) Hyperviscosity syndrome in plasma cell dyscrasias. *Adv. Microcirc.*, **6**, 1–55.

99 Preston, E., Cooke, K.B., Foster, M.F. *et al.* (1978) Myelomatosis and the hyperviscosity syndrome. *Br. J. Haematol.*, **38**, 517–530.

100 Lackner, H., Hunt, V., Zucker, M.B. and Pearson, J. (1970) Abnormal fibrin ultrastructure, polymerisation and clot retraction in multiple myeloma. *Br. J. Haematol.*, **18**, 625–636.

101 Pachter, M.R., Johnson, S.A., Neblett, T.R. and Truant, J.P. (1959) Bleeding, platelets and macroglobulinaemia. *Am. J. Clin. Pathol.*, **31**, 467–482.

102 Scarborough, H. and Shuster, S. (1960) Corticosteroid purpura. *Lancet*, **i**, 93–94.

103 Broekmans, A.W., Bertina, R.M. and Loeliger, E.A. (1983) Protein C and the development of skin necrosis during anticoagulant therapy. *Thromb. Haemost.*, **49**, 251–257.

104 Levin, J. Bleeding with infectious diseases. In: *Disorders of Hemostasis* (Eds Ratnoff, O. & Forbes, C.D.), p. 377. W.B. Saunders, London (1991).
105 Fauci, A.S., Haynes, B.F. and Katz, P. (1978) The spectrum of vasculitis: clinical, pathologic, immunologic and therapeutic considerations. *Ann. Intern. Med.*, **89**, 660–676.
106 Meadow, S.R., Glasgow, E.F., White, R.H.R. *et al.* (1972) Schönlein–Henoch nephritis. *Q. J. Med.*, **41**, 241–258.
107 Turi, S., Belch, J.J.F., Beattie, T.J. and Forbes, C.D. (1986) Abnormalities of vascular prostaglandins in Henoch–Schönlein purpura. *Arch. Dis. Child.*, **61**, 173–177.
108 Hewitt, P.E. and Davies, S.C. (1983) The current state of DIC. *Intensive Care Med.*, **9**, 249–252.
109 Levin, J. Bleeding with infectious diseases. In: *Disorders of Hemostasis* (Eds Ratnoff, O. & Forbes, C.D.), p. 376. W.B. Saunders, London (1991).
110 Bick, R. (1981) Disseminated intravascular coagulation: A clinical/laboratory study of 48 patients. *Ann. NY Acad. Sci.*, **370**, 843–850.
111 Spero, J.A., Lewis, J.H. and Hasiba, U. (1980) Disseminated intravascular coagulation: Findings in 346 patients. *Thromb. Haemost.*, **38**, 28–33.
112 Hamilton, P.J., Stalker, A.L. and Douglas, A.S. (1978) Disseminated intravascular coagulation: A review. *J. Clin. Pathol.*, **31**, 609.
113 El-Kassimi, F.A., Al-Mashhadani, S. and Akhtar, J. (1986) Adult respiratory distress syndrome and disseminated intravascular coagulation complicating heat stroke. *Chest*, **90**, 571–574.
114 Bone, R.C., Bailey, F.P. and Pierce, A. (1976) Intravascular coagulation associated with the adult respiratory distress syndrome. *Am. J. Med.*, **61**, 585–589.
115 Bick, R.L., Schmelhost, W.R. and Fekete, L.F. (1976) Disseminated intravascular coagulation and blood component therapy. *Transfusion*, **16**, 361–368.
116 Preston, F.E. (1982) Disseminated intravascular coagulation. *Br. J. Hosp. Med.*, **28**, 129–133.
117 Prentice, C.R.M. (1985) Acquired coagulation disorders. In: *Clinics in Haematology. Coagulation Disorders* (Ed. Ruggeri, Z.M.), pp. 414–420. W.B. Saunders Co., Eastbourne (1985).
118 Prentice, C.R.M. Heparin and disseminated intravascular coagulation. In: *Heparin: Clinical Chemistry and Usage* (Eds Kakkar, W. & Thomas, D.P.), p. 219. Academic Press, London (1976).
119 Ratnoff, O. Disseminated intravascular coagulation. In: *Disorders of Hemostasis* (Eds Ratnoff, O. and Forbes, CD.), p. 308, W.B. Saunders, London (1991).
120 Heene, D.L. (1977) Disseminated intravascular coagulation. Evaluation of therapeutic approaches. *Semin. Thromb. Hemost.*, **3**, 291–317.
121 Levin, J. Chemotherapy and thrombopoiesis. In: *Cancer Chemotherapy III* (Eds Brodsky, I., Kahn, S.B. & Conroy, J.F.), p. 313. Grune & Stratton, London (1978).
122 Beris, P. and Miescher, P.A. (1988) Hematological complications of antiinfectious agents. *Semin. Hematol.*, **25**, 123–139.
123 Clark, J.A., Finelli, R.E. and Netsky, M.G. (1980) Disseminated intravascular coagulation following cranial trauma. *J. Neurosurg.*, **52**, 266–269.
124 Miner, M.E., Graham, S.H. Gildenberg, P.L. (1982) Disseminated intravascular coagulation fibrinolytic syndrome following head injury in children: frequency

and pragmatic implications. *J. Pediatr.*, **100**, 687–691.

125 Editorial. (1982) Disseminated intravascular coagulation and head injury. *Lancet*, **ii**, 531.

126 Thomas, J.E. and Ayyar, D.R. (1972) Systemic fat embolism: a diagnostic profile in 24 patients. *Arch. Neurol.*, **26**, 517–523.

127 Dines, D.E., Burgher, L.W. and Okazaki, H. (1975) The clinical and pathologic correlation of fat embolism syndrome. *Mayo Clin. Proc.*, **50**, 407–411.

128 Horne, R.H. and Horne, J.H. (1974) Fat embolization prophylaxis. *Arch. Intern. Med.*, **133**, 288–291.

129 Riseborough, E.J. and Herndon, J.H. (1976) Alterations in pulmonary function, coagulation and fat metabolism in patients with fractures of the lower limbs. *Clin. Orthop.*, **115**, 248–267.

130 Bradford, D.S., Foster, R.R. and Nossel, H.L. (1970) Coagulation alterations, hypoxemia and fat embolism in fracture patients. *J. Trauma*, **10**, 307–321.

131 Saldeen, T. (1970) The importance of intravascular coagulation and inhibition of the fibrinolytic system in experimental fat embolism. *J. Trauma*, **10**, 287–298.

132 Culpepper, R.M. (1975) Bleeding diathesis in fresh water drowning. *Ann. Intern. Med.*, **83**, 675. (Letter.)

133 Ports, T.A. and Deuel, T.F. (1977) Intravascular coagulation in fresh-water submersion: report of three cases. *Ann. Intern. Med.*, **87**, 60–61.

134 Hardaway, R.M. (1967) Disseminated intravascular coagulation in experimental and clinical shock. *Am. J. Cardiol.*, **20**, 161–165.

135 Minna, J.D., Robboy, S.J. and Colman, R.W. *Disseminated Intravascular Coagulation*. Charles C. Thomas, Springfield, IL (1974).

136 Hardaway, R.M. III *Syndrome of Disseminated Intravascular Coagulation with Special Reference to Shock and Hemorrhage*. Charles C. Thomas, Springfield, IL (1966).

137 Ferrara, A., MacArthur, J.D., Wright, H.K. *et al.* (1990) Hypothermia and acidosis worsen coagulopathy in the patient requiring massive transfusion. *Am. J. Surg.*, **160**, 515–518.

138 Blauhut, B., Kramar, H., Vinazzer, H. *et al.* (1985) Substitution of antithrombin III in shock and DIC: a randomized study. *Thromb. Res.*, **39**, 81–89.

139 Rinaldo, V.F. and Rogers, R.M. (1982) Adult respiratory-distress syndrome: changing concepts of lung injury and repair. *New Engl. J. Med.*, **306**, 900–909.

140 Hardaway, R.M. and Williams, C.H. (1990) A new treatment for traumatic shock and ARDS. *Resuscitation*, **19**, 61–76.

141 Caprini, J.A., Lipp, V., Zuckerman, L. *et al.* (1977) Hematologic changes following burns. *J. Surg. Res.*, **22**, 626–635.

142 Simon, T.L., Curreri, P.W. and Harker, L.A. (1977) Kinetic characterization of hemostasis in thermal injury. *J. Lab. Clin. Med.*, **89**, 702–711.

143 Merskey, C. Defibrination syndrome. In: *Human Blood Coagulation, Haemostasis and Thrombosis* (Ed. Biggs, R.), 2nd edn, p. 442. Blackwell Scientific Publications, Oxford (1976).

Chapter 12
Extracorporeal circulation: biocompatibility of biomaterials

JAMES M. COURTNEY, SUMUK SUNDARAM AND CHARLES D. FORBES

Biomaterials and biocompatibility

Almost every critically ill patient admitted to hospital has a procedure in which his or her blood is exposed to a foreign surface, be it a pacing wire, indwelling intravenous catheter, dialysis membrane, etc. The problems are the risk of local thrombosis on the material and on the other hand the risks of bleeding from antithrombotic agents and consumption of haemostatic factors. The blood response to extracorporeal circulation involves consideration of the choice of biomaterials and the consequences of their clinical use. This highlights the topic of thrombosis and consumption of coagulation factors on artificial surfaces [1,2] and the potential for bleeding during exposure.

The extracorporeal situations to be considered include haemodialysis and related procedures, membrane plasma separation, cardiopulmonary bypass, artificial heart valves, artificial heart and assist devices, and arterial grafts. A biomaterial is defined as a material of synthetic or natural origin, used in contact with tissues, blood or other biological fluids. Knowledge of the applications of biomaterials extends over a period of about 100 years [3], but improvements in technology and clinical procedures since 1980 have resulted in a dramatic increase in the number of biomaterials now available, in the range of applications, and in their properties and clinical performance [4–10]. The need for improvement still exists for procedures which are experimental such as the artificial heart [11,12], and for long-established and proven procedures, such as the artificial kidney [13,14].

The influence of a biomaterial on blood must be investigated and considered along with the functional characteristic necessary for the intended clinical purpose (e.g. permeability for a haemodialysis membrane or flexibility for blood tubing). The fundamental properties of a biomaterial are its functional characteristic, mechanical strength and compatibility.

The importance of understanding the response of blood to biomaterials has led to detailed studies of blood–biomaterial interactions and the events which induce thrombus formation and coagulation factor consumption on artificial surfaces [1,2,15–19].

Monitoring of the blood response

Blood–biomaterial interactions demonstrate that the contact of blood with an artificial surface inevitably leads to blood component alterations and the formation of a thrombus on the surface. Consumption of factors and use of anticoagulants may lead to bleeding. An understanding of these reactions depends on knowledge of haemostasis and thrombosis which is induced by surface contact.

Haemostasis and thrombosis and artificial surfaces

Haemostasis and thrombosis include the complex reactions between the endothelium, platelets and the coagulation, fibrinolytic and complement systems and active chemical sites on artificial surfaces [20].

The reactions of platelets are adhesion, release and aggregation. While platelets do not normally adhere to the luminal surface of endothelial cells [21–25], platelet adhesion occurs following vascular injury [26–28]. Contact with a foreign surface invariably results in platelet adhesion. The adhesion of platelets initiates a series of reactions leading to platelet secretion, with the discharge of the contents of the platelet granules (the platelet release reaction [29]). This results in the synergistic action of released adenosine diphosphate (ADP) and synthesized thromboxane A_2 (TxA_2) in enhancing the formation of platelet thrombi on to the artificial surface. The formation of a mechanically stable thrombus requires activation of the blood coagulation factors with production of fibrin.

The activation of the blood coagulation factors is normally summarized under the headings of intrinsic, extrinsic and common pathways. In the intrinsic pathway, initiation by contact of blood with an artificial surface leads to the activation of Factor XII. This leads to the activation of Factor XI and Factor IX, with the subsequent conversion of Factor X into its activated form Factor Xa. In the extrinsic pathway, the activation of Factor X results from the initiation by contact of blood with an injured vessel. In the common pathway, Factor Xa catalyses the transformation of prothrombin to thrombin. The conversion of fibrinogen by thrombin into soluble fibrin is followed by the formation of a cross-linked, insoluble or stabilized fibrin. Details of these reactions appear in Chapter 1.

The fibrinolytic system, with its ability to dissolve formed fibrin [30], normally balances the activity of the blood coagulation process in promoting the conversion of soluble fibrinogen to insoluble fibrin. The enzyme plasmin is the essential end product of the fibrinolytic system [31] and the key reaction is the conversion of plasminogen to plasmin, which acts within the thrombus, digesting fibrin to give thrombus dissolution.

The complement system [32] comprises a group of proteins interacting sequentially to bring about inflammation. The activation of the complement system takes place through two major pathways, the classical pathway and the alternative pathway. The component C3 is pivotal in both pathways. In the classical pathway, antigen–antibody complexes provide a site for binding component C1, which promotes activation of components C4 and C2. A complex formed by these components is an activator of C3. In the alternative pathway, activation of C3 involves substances which can bind C3 directly and there is no participation of earlier complement components. Although some components, such as C3b, become bound to the activating surface, the molecules C3a, C4a and C5a are released into the liquid phase. These molecules, which are low-molecular-weight products (anaphylatoxins), are responsible for the biological effects resulting from the activation of the complement system.

The blood response in extracorporeal situations involves the interaction of platelet adhesion, release and aggregation, the coagulation system, in particular the intrinsic pathway, the fibrinolytic system and the complement system, in particular the activation of component C3. In addition to these features, there may be effects due to erythrocytes and leucocytes.

Factors which influence blood–surface interactions

The behaviour of an artificial surface in contact with blood is markedly different from that of endothelium. The lack of adhesion of platelets, erythrocytes and leucocytes to endothelial cells shows that the endothelium presents a non-attractive surface to blood cells [24]. The endothelium also limits thrombus formation by the release of platelet antiaggregating substances [33] and the complexing of thrombin with

Table 12.1 Features relevant to a study of blood–biomaterial interactions

• Proteins
• Platelets
• Intrinsic coagulation
• Erythrocytes
• Leucocytes
• Complement
• Fibrinolysis

antithrombin III [34] and initiation of fibrinolysis [35,36]. In general, biomaterials cannot provide a non-attractive surface comparable to that of the endothelium and cannot perform an active role similar to that achieved by the endothelium. Furthermore, while the endothelium does not seem to adsorb proteins under physiological conditions [4], protein adsorption is an important aspect of blood–biomaterial interactions [1].

Table 12.1 summarizes the features of the blood response relevant to extracorporeal circuits and biomaterials. However, the biomaterial is only one of the factors which influence the response to blood in clinical use. The situation is illustrated in Fig. 12.1, with additional factors such as the presence of an antithrombotic agent, the condition of the blood and the physical conditions imposed by the particular application.

Biomaterials and blood interactions

Protein adsorption to artificial surfaces is rapid from protein solutions [37,38], plasma [39] or whole blood [40] and interactions subsequent to

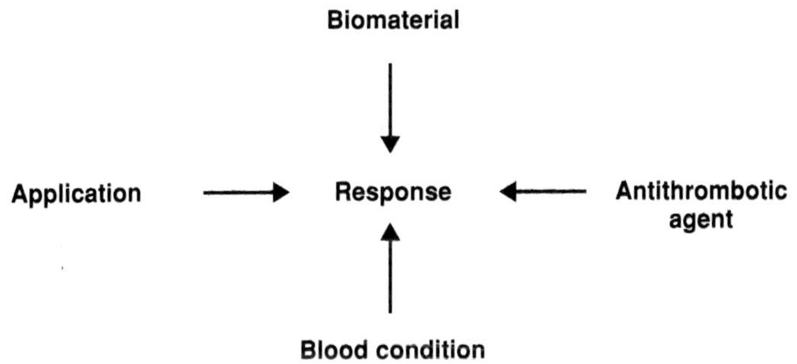

Fig. 12.1 Factors influencing the response of blood in the clinical application of biomaterials.

protein adsorption are strongly influenced by the composition of the adsorbed protein layer [41,42]. In fact, the critical role of the adsorbed protein in blood–biomaterial interactions has led to the term 'conditioning layer' [43–45], although the adsorbed protein should not be regarded as 'passive' [4]. There is evidence of transient adsorption, denaturation, or changes in configuration [46,47]. The relationship between protein adsorption and platelet reactivity has been widely studied, with the general conclusion that platelet adhesion to artificial surfaces is inhibited by prior adsorption of albumin and promoted by prior adsorption of fibrinogen or γ-globulin [48–56]. The ability of albumin to inhibit platelet adhesion has been utilized in the preparation of artificial surfaces with improved blood compatibility [1,57]. The close relationship between fibrinogen and platelets supports the possibility that fibrinogen deposition on artificial surfaces is dependent on platelet adhesion and is associated with specific receptors on adherent platelets [58]. Further aspects of the importance of fibrinogen adsorption are the replacement of adsorbed fibrinogen by high-molecular-weight kininogen (HMWK) [59], a protein involved in the activation of the intrinsic coagulation, and the possible interaction of fibrinogen with leucocytes [60]. It is understandable that the timing of fibrinogen deposition and of its removal from artificial surfaces by blood is believed to have important clinical implications [61]. The adsorption of γ-globulin on artificial surfaces promotes platelet adhesion and release [62] and may be followed by leucocyte adhesion [63].

Studies on protein adsorption require to extend beyond albumin, fibrinogen and γ-globulin in order to provide improved information on the composition of the adsorbed protein layer and the possible influence of trace proteins [44]. An example of a protein for further study is fibronectin [60], which can be adsorbed onto artificial surfaces from plasma [56,64]. Although fibronectin may not be involved in platelet adhesion and aggregation [65,66], it has a possible participation in the adhesion of leucocytes [61]. It is also important to bear in mind the reactivity of proteins in the clinical situation. The adsorption of fibrinogen serves as an example. A rapid decrease in fibrinogen levels *in vitro* contrasts with *in vivo* haemodialysis where consistent fibrinogen levels represent the outcome of fibrinogen conversion into degradation products and the production of new fibrinogen [67].

With respect to the blood coagulation factors, activation of the intrinsic pathway is initiated by the contact Factor XII, Factor XI, HMWK and prekallikrein [68]. The adsorption of HMWK leads to the formation of a complex with kallikrein. Activation of Factor XII by kallikrein establishes a feedback mechanism, which ensures the autoactivation on or near the artificial surface. HMWK also forms a complex with Factor XI, making Factor XI available to Factor XIIa and enabling the progression of the coagulation cascade [1]. Therefore, Factor XII has a critical role in the contact-phase activation.

Platelet adhesion and aggregation are inevitable consequences of the contact of blood with an artificial surface [69,70] and platelet adhesion is strongly influenced by protein adsorption. The possession of saccharide chains by fibrinogen and γ-globulin is believed to be a factor in the promotion of platelet adhesion [62,71,72], with the mechanism similar to that proposed for the platelet–collagen reaction in damaged blood vessels [73]. Platelet adhesion to protein-coated surfaces leads to a change in platelet shape, the coalescence of platelets into an irregular monolayer and, with increasing platelet adhesion, the formation of mounds in which erythrocytes and leucocytes are trapped in fibrin [74]. The adhesion of platelets to an artificial surface is followed by the platelet-release reaction [29] taking place in the adhering platelets and then platelet aggregation occurring on the surface [75]. Platelet constituents relevant to blood–biomaterial interactions include β-thromboglobulin, serotonin, platelet factor 4, ADP, thromboxane B_2 (TxB_2) and thrombospondin [1]. Platelet numbers may fall significantly.

As thrombus formation on the artificial surface proceeds, an interaction between platelets and the intrinsic pathway occurs [76]. Initiation of the intrinsic coagulation results from procoagulants liberated from platelets [77,78] or from Factor XII activation due to platelets stimulated by released ADP. Thrombin formation as a consequence of intrinsic pathway activation induces the rapid production of a fibrin monolayer on an artificial surface, thereby enhancing platelet adhesion and aggregation [79,80], and thrombin generation induces the platelet release reaction [81–83]. The end result is platelet and clotting-factor consumption.

Erythrocytes also adhere to the adsorbed protein layer [76] and influence protein adsorption [84,85], either by a membrane-related effect or by an effect due to the competitive adsorption of released haemoglobin. Erythrocytes promote platelet adhesion on an artificial surface by reducing the adsorption of platelet-protective proteins or by depositing an adhesive substance [44], and if haemolysis occurs the platelet release reaction is induced and ADP is also released [86].

In the interactions between a biomaterial and blood, the influence of leucocytes contrasts strongly with the mainly passive role of the erythrocytes [60]. Leucocytes are attracted to the thrombus, contribute to platelet recruitment and fibrin formation and participate in fibrinolysis. Leucocytes adhere to artificial surfaces [87], with preferential adsorption of polymorphonuclear leucocytes or granulocytes in comparison to lymphocytes [88–90]. Evidence of a direct role for leucocytes in thrombus formation, due to granulocyte adhesion and its influence on platelet aggregation [91], is supported by granulocyte possession of endogenous proaggregating activity [92] and procoagulant activity [93,94]. An important feature of leucocyte alterations in blood–biomaterial interactions is the possibility of a change in cell function, since leucocyte damage resulting from blood–biomaterial contact [87] leads to an impairment in phagocytic activity and a diminished ability to combat infection [4]. Leucocyte alterations may also result in the release of noxious humoral substances, such as superoxide and other free radicals, leucotrienes, interleukins and tumour necrosis factor [17].

A focus of biomaterials research has been investigations into the relationship between leucocytes and complement activation. This is particularly relevant for extracorporeal applications [17,95]. Activation of complement components mediates the chemotactic, adhesive and phagocytic responses of polymorphonuclear leucocytes in the inflammatory process, with the anaphylatoxins C3a, C4a and C5a of particular interest. The adhesion of leucocytes to artificial surfaces may also be mediated by complement activation [96].

Finally, if it is accepted that the different systems are involved in the response of blood to a biomaterial function in an integrated manner, it is necessary to take into account fibrinolysis and fibrinolytic activity. Measurement of the levels of fibrin degradation products demonstrates that blood–biomaterial contact induces fibrinolytic activity.

Antithrombotic agents

For clinical purposes, it is necessary to use an antithrombotic agent in association with all biomaterials and consequently it is important to consider the interaction of both biomaterial and antithrombotic agent. In the overall relationship between blood, biomaterial and antithrombotic agent, a more compatible response can result from alteration to the biomaterial, the antithrombotic agent or both [97].

Antithrombotic agents are used to prevent or remove thrombus and the three main types relevant to extracorporeal situations are anticoagulants, platelet aggregation inhibitors (antiplatelet agents) and plasminogen activators.

The most widely used antithrombotic agent in extracorporeal situations is the anticoagulant heparin, which operates by potentiating the influence of antithrombin III. By forming a complex with antithrombin III, heparin catalyses the action of antithrombin III on thrombin [98], thereby inhibiting thrombin, the aggregation of platelets by thrombin, the thrombin-mediated conversion of fibrinogen to fibrin, and Factors Xa, IXa, XIa and XIIa. Possible alternatives to heparin are low-molecular-weight heparin (LMWH) [99], which has a more specific action, and recombinant hirudin [100], which acts directly on thrombin. It is possible that for a given biomaterial, an improved blood response can be obtained by replacing heparin with LMWH [101] or hirudin [102]. As an alternative to the administration of heparin, procedures are available for the ionic or covalent attachment of heparin to biomaterial surfaces [1,57,103]. Careful laboratory monitoring of heparin is essential to prevent haemorrhagic consequences.

Platelet aggregation inhibitors (e.g. aspirin, dipyridamole) may be used as a replacement for heparin or in association with heparin. With biomaterials, such agents have been used in immobilized form [104–106] or controlled release form [107,108].

Fibrinolytic therapy can be achieved by the administration of the plasminogen activators urokinase and streptokinase. The binding of urokinase to biomaterials has been reported [109–111]. These drugs are usually used to remove thrombus which has formed and is interfering with the function of the device. Bleeding may result from systemic actions.

Blood reaction and disease states

The response of blood to an artificial surface is influenced by the disease state. This influence is illustrated in Fig. 12.2, which compares scanning electron micrographs of platelets. Figure 12.2(a) is a scanning electron micrograph of a platelet on poly(ethylene terephthalate) film, where the micrograph was obtained with the platelet-rich plasma of a healthy donor. Striking features of such platelets are the number and length of the pseudopodia, making apparent the likelihood of platelet interaction and aggregate formation. Figure 12.2(b) is a scanning electron micrograph obtained again for poly(ethylene terephthalate) film but with the platelet derived from the platelet-rich plasma of a uraemic patient. Most of the

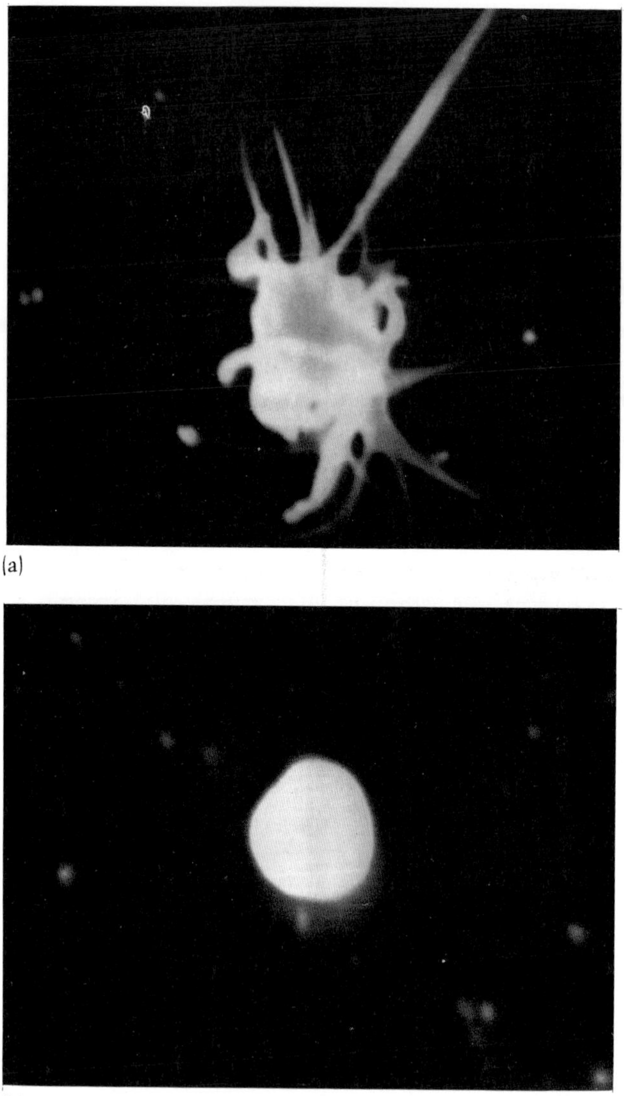

(a)

(b)

Fig. 12.2 Scanning electron micrograph of platelets derived from platelet-rich plasma after deposition on a poly(ethylene terephthalate) surface. (a) Platelet from healthy donor; (b) platelet from uraemic patient.

uraemic patient's platelets demonstrated this unreactive pattern, which has been shown to correlate with deficient platelet function, as represented by induced platelet aggregation with ADP or collagen, and with a bleeding tendency [97].

As indicated previously, such a bleeding tendency may be enhanced by the presence of antithrombotic agents, for example in an individual response to heparin [112]. A change in blood status may also result from the introduction of a new drug therapy, such as the use of recombinant erythropoietin in the treatment of chronic renal failure [113].

Factors relevant to mode of application

Other factors contributing to the blood response relate to the clinical application [114]. These are the exposure time of blood to the biomaterial and the extent of trauma to particular blood components, e.g. the platelet response in blood–biomaterial contact is influenced by diffusion [115] and shear forces [116], with the shear rate and contact time critical factors for platelet adhesion [117]. The metabolism of erythrocyte membranes can undergo significant changes during blood–biomaterial contact, with shear-induced haemolysis likely [4]. Leucocytes display an apparent similarity to platelets with respect to sensitivity to mechanical trauma [118] and shear stress influences leucocyte damage and aggregation [119].

Haemodialysis and related procedures

Membrane-based haemodialysis is now an established technique for the treatment of chronic renal failure. Since its clinical introduction, haemodialysis has been dominated by the use of regenerated cellulose membranes and despite numerous attempts at replacement [120], cellulose membranes remain the most commonly used.

Haemodialysis, using dialysis and ultrafiltration, removes solutes predominantly by diffusion, with a minor contribution coming from convective solute transfer during the removal of water by ultrafiltration. Haemofiltration utilizes membranes with water permeability and solute molecular weight cut-off greater than those of haemodialysis membranes in order to purify blood by a combination of ultrafiltration and convective solute transport. High-flux haemodialysis describes the procedure where membrane solute and water permeability exceed those of conventional haemodialysis membranes but are not comparable to those of haemofiltration membranes and there is no requirement to compensate for fluid loss. However, haemodialysis remains the most widely used procedure.

In haemodialysis, high-flux haemodialysis or haemofiltration, the nature of the membrane influences not only permeability but also the blood response. The interest in improved blood compatibility has been stimulated by studies of coagulopathies and the neutropenia known to occur with cellulose membranes [121] resulting from leucocyte activation and complement activation [122–126].

Blood interaction with dialysis membranes

Protein adsorption during blood–dialysis membrane contact is inevitable and the adsorbed protein layer affects subsequent reactions. *In vitro* and *in vivo* studies have demonstrated that cellulose, modified cellulose and synthetic membranes all adsorb protein from plasma, but in different patterns [127–129]. Albumin adsorption is a general feature [127], fibrinogen adsorption *in vivo* may be followed by conversion to fibrin [129] and the levels of fibronectin appear higher with haemodialysis than with haemofiltration [130].

In haemodialysis, interest has been focused not only on the role of platelets in the mechanism of haemostasis but also in the involvement of platelets in immunological and inflammatory reactions [131]. The sequestration of platelet aggregates during haemodialysis may be a major contributing factor in the haemodialysis-induced acute phenomenon of leucopenia [132] and platelet interactions with the complement system may include activation of platelets by complement components and activation of complement components by platelets [131]. Platelet activation has been confirmed for cellulose and non-cellulose membranes by the detection of increased levels of β-thromboglobulin, platelet factor 4 and TxB_2 [133,134]. Investigations into the association between platelet reactions and complement activation are likely to continue, although the relevance of animal models may be limited [16,134] because of species-related differences for platelet–biomaterial reactions [135] and the presence of C3b receptors on the platelets of some animals but not on those of humans [136].

When blood contacts artificial surfaces during haemodialysis, there is complement activation and cellular reactions [137,138]. Complement activation can take place in the dialyser [139], with the liberation of C3a and C5a. The release of C5a is particularly important, since it is a potent mediator of granulocyte responses, including chemotaxis, adherence, aggregation, degranulation and toxic oxygen-radical production [140]. While C5a normally contributes to host defence by promoting leucocyte accumulation and activation at local sites of inflammation, systemic or intravascular complement activation and C5a formation are believed to induce diffuse granulocyte activation and damage to multiple organ systems [137].

Therefore, haemodialysis can cause complement activation [122], transient leucopenia [121], increased granulocyte adherence [141], enhanced release of granular enzymes [142], a fall in arterial oxygen pressure with intrapulmonary sequestration of leucocytes [122] and an alteration to granulocyte oxidative metabolism [143]. Other possible consequences of haemodialysis are the release of eicosanoids [144], the production of platelet activating factor [145], depressed natural killer function of lymphocytes [146], activation of monocytes with the production of interleukin-1 [147,148], the induction of tumour necrosis factor [149] and reduced phagocytosis [150]. Activation of intrinsic coagulation by contact activation [151–153] and activation of the fibrinolytic system [154] (Fig. 12.3), in association with the bleeding tendency found in renal failure, plus the presence of an antithrombotic agent, often produce a risk of haemorrhage.

Characteristics of membranes

Membrane structure is categorized as cellulose, synthetic or modified cellulose [126,155,156].

Complement activation by cellulose membranes has been attributed to the presence of hydroxyl groups and activation via the alternative pathway [157], which is consistent with the known influence of polysaccharide structures on the complement system. Clinical investigation [139,158–163] has demonstrated that complement activation and leucopenia are reduced when cellulose membranes are replaced by membranes derived from synthetic polymers, such as polyacrylonitrile, poly(methyl methacrylate) and polysulphone. This reduced influence of synthetic membranes is generally true for other leucocyte alterations but a poly(methyl methacrylate) membrane inducing less complement activation and leucopenia than cellulose causes a greater release of granulocyte elastase [164]. The low complement activation with synthetic membranes could result from minimal generation of C3a and C5a or from adsorption of complement proteins on synthetic membrane surfaces [165–166].

Modification of cellulose by the partial substitution of hydroxyl groups reduces complement activation and leucopenia, with the effect of modification dependent on both the degree of substitution and the nature of the modifying group. In comparison to modification with

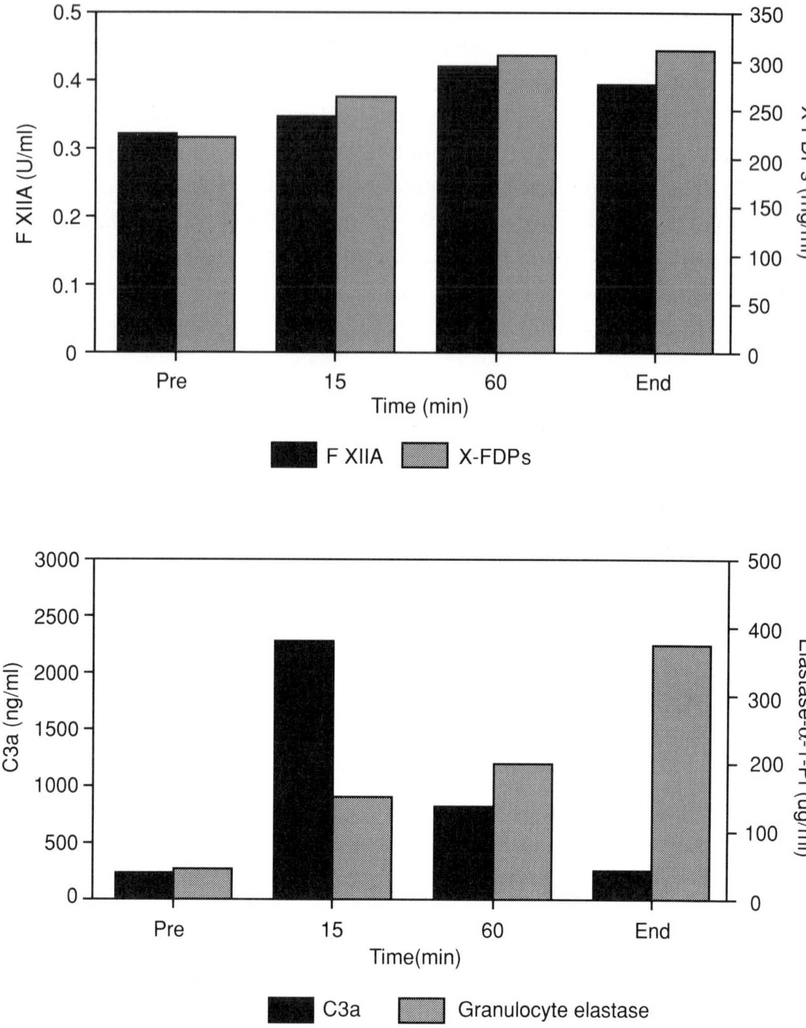

Fig. 12.3 Typical changes in blood components as a result of haemodialysis with a regenerated cellulose membrane. FxiiA, factor xii-like activity; X-FDPs, fibrin degradation products.

acetate groups, a much greater reduction in complement activation and low degrees of substitution are achieved by modification with diethylaminocthyl groups [167–169]. Modified cellulose membranes offer the potential of improved compatibility at a lower cost than synthetic membranes.

Cellulose membranes remain the first choice for routine haemodialysis, with cost an undoubted factor. The situation might alter because of increased evidence from biocompatibility evaluation, such as the link between haemodialysis with cellulose membranes and reduced phagocytic ability [150]. Additionally, since compatibility cannot be isolated from permeability, interest in alternative membranes could come from a renewed focus on the uraemic toxins [14] or on specific substances such as β_2-microglobulin [170], a protein implicated in the pathogenesis of a new type of amyloidosis [171].

Antithrombotic agents in haemodialysis

The prothrombotic effect of most membranes used in haemodialysis, high-flux haemodialysis or haemofiltration is such that these procedures normally require heparin. However, in the treatment of patients already with a high bleeding risk, it is possible to perform so-called 'heparin-free' haemodialysis [172–174]. This involves the use of a high blood flow, frequent saline flushes through the blood inlet line, or continuous saline infusion.

Although widely used in haemodialysis, there are potential disadvantages associated with heparin, such as a risk of haemorrhage [175] and adverse effects on platelets [176,177]. Therefore, there is interest in replacing standard heparin with LMWH [178,179]. Other possibilities are the use of antiplatelet agents such as prostacyclin (PGI_2) or stable PGI_2 analogues, either alone [180], or in combination with 'low-dose' heparin [181]. Advantages have been suggested for the application of the antiplatelet agent piracetam [182] and nafomostat mesilate, a multi-enzyme inhibitor acting against the coagulation and complement systems, has been evaluated [167,183].

Finally, the relationship between blood, the biomaterial and the antithrombotic agent [97] suggests that the combination of new membranes and alternative anticoagulants [184] is a suitable objective.

Disease state

Blood–biomaterial interactions during the treatment of chronic renal failure are influenced by the state of blood components (Fig. 12.2). When the blood is markedly altered with the use of recombinant erythropoietin, a corresponding change in the blood response to artificial surfaces might be expected.

An important aspect of the treatment of chronic renal failure is the large variability between patients with respect to parameters used to monitor the blood response. This has been found for measurements of Factor XII activity and crosslinked fibrin degradation products [67].

Mode of application

The importance of the mode of application to the well-being of the uraemic patient has been emphasized [114]. Potential advantages of high-flux haemodialysis and haemofiltration over haemodialysis can be offset by difficulties in operation. The more permeable membranes in high-flux haemodialysis may permit contamination by back-diffusion of substances from non-sterile dialysate [185], while the supply of sterile physiological solution is essential in haemofiltration. Although the focus in the procedures is understandably on the membrane, it must not be forgotten that the membrane is utilized in a device and the device forms one component in an extracorporeal circuit. Consequently, consideration of the clinical performance covers not only blood–membrane interactions but also the selection of blood tubing [186] and potential hazards from toxicity [187] and sterilization procedures [188,189].

Membrane plasma separation

The utilization of membranes with much greater solute permeability than those of haemodialysis or haemofiltration enables the blood cellular elements to be separated from plasma in membrane plasma separation or membrane plasmapheresis. Although not nearly as commonly used as haemodialysis, the options of subjecting the separated plasma to exchange, filtration or sorption have enabled membrane plasma separation to extend blood purification into areas inappropriate to haemodialysis and related procedures. Therapeutic membrane plasmapheresis has a specialized role and a more general application of membrane plasma separation may prove to be in blood transfusion in relation to plasma donation [193].

If membrane plasma separation is considered in terms of the scheme shown in Fig. 12.1, it can be appreciated that since it has been applied to renal, hepatic and haematological disorders, alterations in blood factors have an important influence. Similarly, the different processes available for treatment of plasma ensure that the application can also contribute significantly to the blood response. An important feature is that the transmembrane pressure must be lower than that for haemodialysis and much lower than that for haemofiltration in order to avoid an unacceptable decrease in membrane permeability resulting from protein adsorption. Bearing in mind the relevance of the blood condition and the mode of application, the focus in membrane plasmapheresis can be directed towards membranes and anticoagulants.

Membranes

From knowledge of blood–biomaterial interactions and extracorporeal blood circulation, it is not unexpected that membrane plasma separation induces blood cellular and humoral alterations similar to those discussed for haemodialysis [194–198], with the membrane nature a contributory factor.

Available membranes are derived from cellulose acetate, polypropylene, polyethylene, polyvinyl alcohol and polyvinyl chloride.

Anticoagulants

The selection of an anticoagulant for membrane plasmapheresis involves heparin and citrate [199,200]. Heparin is the most common, with a recommendation for strict dosage control [199]. Citrate has been used in centrifugal plasmapheresis, primarily in the blood transfusion area, and can be used alone or in combination with heparin [200]. The linking of membrane structure to anticoagulant selection is again important.

Cardiopulmonary bypass

The application of cardiopulmonary bypass involves the use of devices in cardiothoracic surgery, where the heart and lungs are bypassed via an extracorporeal circuit which oxygenates the blood and pumps the oxygenated blood round the circulation. The objective of extracorporeal circulation is to provide suitable conditions for intracardiac operations, while maintaining essential physiological tissue and organ perfusion and oxygenation for limited periods of time, with complete return of functional integrity of all parameters of homoeostasis after the procedure [201]. This objective is attained by placement of a gas-exchange device in the extracorporeal circuit.

The changes in blood constituents during cardiopulmonary bypass are a consequence of a complex extracorporeal process and blood compatibility may be influenced by materials, device design, operating procedure and the nature of antithrombotic agent [202]. In this respect, the relationship between cardiopulmonary bypass and the blood response can be illustrated (Fig. 12.1). Prior to a description of the alteration of blood components, it is appropriate to consider the utilization of biomaterials and the nature of the process.

Biomaterial utilization

There are two basic types of gas-exchange device utilized in extracorporeal circuits, viz. direct contact devices and membrane-based devices. Generally, in direct contact devices, oxygen is bubbled directly through blood which is then debubbled through a settling or filtering chamber, whereas in membrane-based devices, a gas-exchange membrane is interposed between the gas and blood phases [203].

Direct contact or bubble oxygenators have been widely used because of ease of assembly and priming and relatively low cost. However, the traumatic mode of operation has been associated with damage to blood elements and their consumption, microemboli formation and protein denaturation [204–206].

The utilization of membrane oxygenators was promoted by the view that an improved physiological response would be obtained with devices operating on the same principle as the human lung. The presence of a permeable membrane between blood and gas phases eliminates direct blood–gas contact [207]. Evidence [208] that membrane-based devices were less traumatic to the blood than direct-contact devices encouraged such device design and development [209] and the clinical application of membrane oxygenators for prolonged extracorporeal circulation [206,210], where the less traumatic influence on blood constituents was advantageous [211,212]. Membranes may be classified into three categories [213]. These are (i) homogeneous (polysiloxane or silicone rubber), (ii) microporous (derived from hydrophobic polymers such as polypropylene and polytetrafluoroethylene), and (iii) composites of types (i) and (ii).

Nature of process

Cardiopulmonary bypass procedures create severe alterations in haemostasis [214]. In addition to the surgical operation, the blood response is influenced by temperature gradients, mechanical trauma, mode of blood flow and drug administration [215,216].

The composition of the solution used to prime the circuit may contribute to haematological problems [217]. Primes have included heparinized homologous blood, acid citrate dextrose blood, saline, saline-like solutions, dextrose solution and dextran solution [210,218]. An all blood prime provides normal haematocrit and oxygen-carrying capacity but leads to increased viscosity, haemolysis and the risk of transfusion reaction or hepatitis [219]. The haemodilution caused by non-blood primes has been reported to induce no serious haematological derangement [220] and may offer benefits with respect to reduced blood viscosity and haemolysis [221].

The production of particulate or gaseous microemboli is an important consideration in cardiopulmonary bypass [222] and attention has been drawn to the role of microemboli in producing an alteration in cerebral function [223–225]. Causes of organ dysfunction following open-heart surgery [202] include particulate emboli of aggregated blood elements, denatured proteins, fat, calcium and antifoam substances. This problem of microemboli production during cardiopulmonary bypass has led to the use of filters [222].

These responses during bypass can be altered by the use of pulsatile flow and, in the clinical application of prolonged extracorporeal membrane oxygenation (ECMO), there are potential advantages in substituting the normal venoarterial mode of perfusion by arteriovenous perfusion.

Blood response

Study of artificial surfaces in contact with blood [1] emphasizes that protein adsorption is inevitable with cardiopulmonary bypass, although interest has focused more on protein denaturation and emboli formation [217,226]. In membrane-based devices, there is a reduction in protein denaturation and the tendency to form microaggregates, with the pattern of protein adsorption influenced by the nature of the membrane.

During cardiopulmonary bypass, contact of blood with gaseous or solid surfaces may induce a fall in platelet count [227], the formation of circulating platelet aggregates [228], a loss of platelet sensitivity to activating agents [229,230] and the release of platelet contents [231,232].

While there is strong evidence [217] of a decrease in platelet count during cardiopulmonary bypass, the fall could result not only from platelet adhesion but also from platelet aggregates [219,223,234] or a platelet sequestration [234]. Significant thrombocytopenia was observed in early studies [214] but not detected in subsequent investigations [235–237].

The loss of platelet function has been considered the most significant haematological consequence of cardiopulmonary bypass with bubble and membrane systems [238]. There is an inhibition of platelets during bypass, which persists after cessation of the procedure. It is not clear whether the restoration of platelet function after bypass is due to the recovery of previously inhibited platelets or to the formation of new platelets. The most profound platelet alterations appear to take place immediately following contact of blood with the artificial surfaces of the extracorporeal circuit and consequences of this contact are prolonged bleeding time and increased blood loss. Data on reduced platelet damage with membrane oxygenators [239–245] support the view [246] that the membrane oxygenator is less traumatic to blood elements and while this view has been challenged [238], there is evidence of different mechanisms of platelet activation by membrane and bubble oxygenators [247,248].

Studies of coagulation factor deficiencies have produced a variety of results, which may reflect differences in surgical technique and preoperative medication, the selection of pulsatile or non-pulsatile flow and the application of direct contact or membrane-based devices. Protein adsorption is induced by blood contact and although coagulation factors are not selectively adsorbed, decreased levels of Factors II, V, VII, VIII, IX and X have been regularly reported [230]. The determination of Factor XII activity during cardiopulmonary bypass has revealed a gradual increase, which was significant throughout the procedure [249] and remained high in the postoperative period, gradually decreasing over 7 days [250].

Studies of factors influencing erythrocyte destruction in artificial organs [251,252] demonstrated the haemolytic effect of the shear forces and haemolysis in areas of high shear stresses, cavitation and turbulence. Comparisons have shown lower levels of erythrocyte damage with membrane oxygenators [246,253,254].

There is an activation of leucocytes during cardiopulmonary bypass and a decrease in numbers with the onset of extracorporeal circulation [219,255]. This decrease, which takes place with both bubble and membrane oxygenators, may be explained partly on the basis of dilution but aggregation and embolization may also occur [217,219]. Sequestration of leucocytes in the lungs has been reported [256] and aggregated leucocytes have been identified in the lungs of dogs following cardiopulmonary bypass [257]. During bypass, there is the release of active substances from leucocytes, either in response to activation or from cytolysis [258]. Intrapulmonary leucocyte sequestration with release of proteolytic enzymes, such as granulocyte elastase, and generation of oxygen free radicals has been implicated in the mechanism of acute lung injury in the adult respiratory distress syndrome (ARDS) [259–263]. The release of granulocyte elastase is gradual throughout bypass [249,264,265] and levels remain elevated at the end of the procedure, with this postoperative elevation dependent on the period of bypass [250]. While the leucocyte count returns to normal, there is a reduced phagocytic function during and after bypass [266,267]. It has been reported [255] that leucocyte behaviour during cardiopulmonary bypass is influenced by a plasma factor in a manner similar to the influence of the complement component C5a on leucocytes during haemodialysis, i.e. activation of neutrophils and alteration of their shape and motility [268,269].

Complement activation is considered an important component of the pathological events by which sepsis and trauma activate common humoral cascades leading to pulmonary membrane damage [270]. There has been controversy [271] over whether the reduction of complement haemolytic activity was due to consumption through activation [272], denaturation [273] or interference with haemolytic activity by polyanions such as heparin [274]. Complement activation during cardiopulmonary bypass [275] has been confirmed in bubble and membrane oxygenators [271] and is probably unrelated to pulsatile flow [276]. The evidence [270] indicates that the extracorporeal circulation itself activates complement and might increase damage in already affected lungs. During cardiopulmonary bypass, contact of blood with artificial surfaces leads to the release of the anaphylatoxins C3a and C5a [275] and similar rates of complement activation have been found with bubble or membrane oxygenators [277]. Comparison has been made with haemodialysis, where it has been demonstrated [278] that the sharp and profound leucopenia observed [121] is mediated by C5a [122]. Interaction with leucocytes leads to modification and activation of these cells, which are then trapped in the lung microvasculature [268] and this leucoembolization is believed to induce some of the cardiac and lung complications of haemodialysis [122]. The same pathogenesis may be involved in the clinical consequences of cardiopulmonary bypass, in particular the 'postperfusion syndrome' or multiorgan failure seen after uneventful bypass [275,279–281].

Activation of the fibrinolytic system during and after cardiopulmonary bypass has been reported [237,282]. Fibrinolytic activity, as measured by crosslinked fibrin degradation products, has been shown to increase steadily during bypass and remain elevated postoperatively [250].

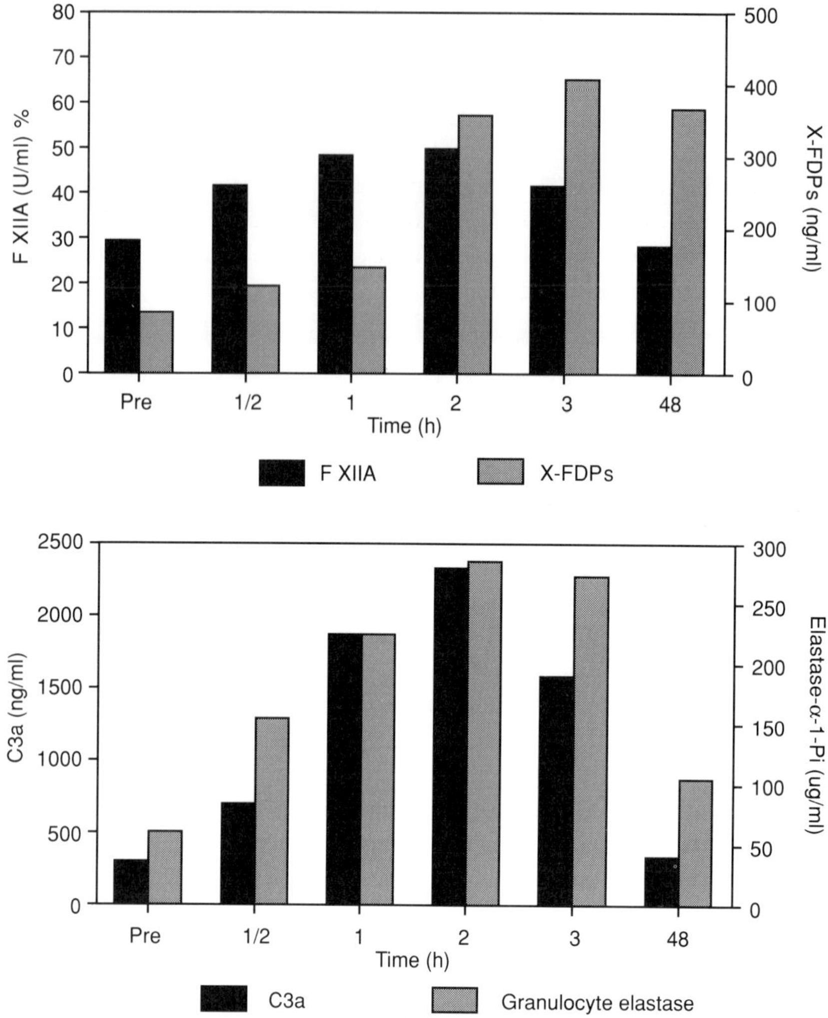

Fig. 12.4 Typical changes in blood components as a result of cardiopulmonary bypass with a bubble oxygenator. FXIIA, factor XII-like activity; X-FDPs, fibrin degradation products.

Typical changes in blood constituents as a result of cardiopulmonary bypass with a bubble oxygenator are presented in Fig. 12.4.

Modification of the blood response

Normal clinical cardiopulmonary bypass requires the use of heparin. Extracorporeal circulation using high heparin dosage has been linked to the induction of platelet damage, with reduced platelet count and impaired function, and prolonged bleeding [283]. The possibility exists for replacing heparin with LMWH [98] or platelet aggregation inhibitors [283–285]. Other approaches include the use of a synthetic complement inhibitor [286], aprotonin as a kallikrein inhibitor [287], an inhibitor for leucocyte sequestration [288] and a platelet-preserving agent [289].

The blood response can also be modified by the coating of surfaces in the circuit with albumin [290], an albumin–heparin complex [291] or by the attachment of heparin [292,295].

Artificial heart valves

The routine replacement of diseased or malfunctioning human heart valves is well established [296]. While early valves were often the result of surgical innovation, progress has resulted from developments in both the design of artificial valves and the materials used. Artificial heart valves are normally classified into two categories—mechanical and tissue.

1 *Mechanical heart valves* [297] offer advantages of consistency of manufacture and long-term durability, but are offset by the unnatural form, the risk of embolism and thrombosis and the requirement for long-term anticoagulant therapy. If the blood response is considered as in Fig. 12.1, there is a continuing need for an anticoagulant or the combination of an anticoagulant and an antiplatelet agent [1].

2 *Tissue valves* [298] are generally produced from animal tissue treated with glutaraldehyde. In comparison to mechanical valves, tissue valves offer a more natural form and function and there is no need for long-term anticoagulant therapy. The disadvantages are an unproven long-term durability, difficulty in achieving consistency of manufacture and *in vivo* calcification.

Artificial heart and assist devices

With the artificial heart, there are problems of thrombus formation [289,300], and bleeding associated with use of anticoagulants. In addition, current designs involving an external power source, the presence of heart valves and the risk of infection remain clinical problems [301]. Such difficulties have forced a reappraisal of the role of an artificial heart as a bridge to transplantation and led to the development of assist devices. However, with such devices, consumption of clotting factors with the production of emboli is a major problem [302]. The blood

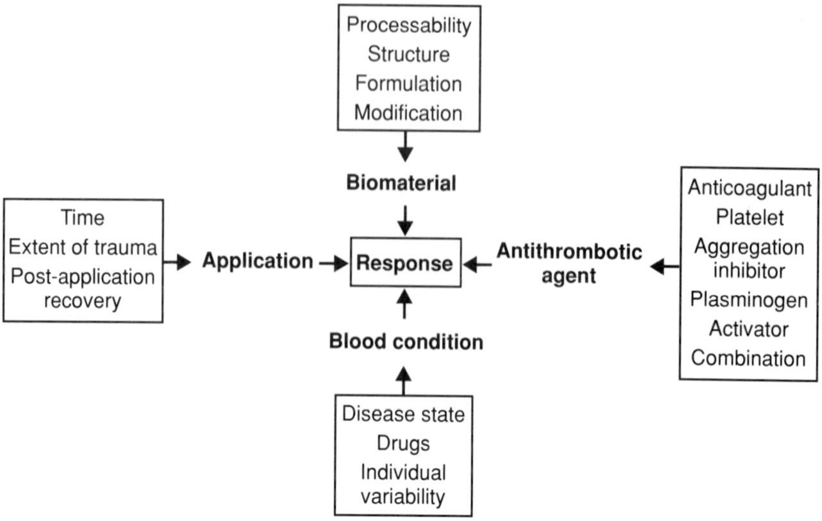

Fig. 12.5 Possibilities for altering the factors influencing the response of blood in the clinical application of biomaterials.

response is influenced by the biomaterials utilized, the nature of the mechanical pumping and the anticoagulant used [303].

Summary

There is no doubt that interest in improving the response of blood to biomaterials will continue and that this interest will cover the four features influencing the response (Fig. 12.5). Therefore, approaches can be anticipated on novel biomaterials [304,305], novel methods of biomaterial modification [103,301,307], the application of agents to control the response [308–310] an improved understanding of the relationship between the blood condition and the biomaterial [16,311] and an appreciation of the role of the application [312,313].

References

1 Forbes, C.D. and Courtney, J.M. Thrombosis and artificial surfaces. In: *Haemostasis and Thrombosis* (Eds Bloom, A.L. & Thomas, D.P.), pp. 902–921. Churchill Livingstone, Edinburgh (1987).

2 Forbes, C.D., Courtney, J.M., Saniabadi, A.R. and Morrice, L.M.A. Thrombus formation in artificial organs. In: *Progress in Bioengineering* (Eds Paul, J.P.,

Barbenel, J.C., Courtney, J.M. & Kenedi, R.M.), pp. 13–20. Adam Hilger, Bristol (1989).

3 Williams, D.J. (Ed.) *Definitions in Biomaterials*. Elsevier, Amsterdam (1987).

4 Bruck, S.D. *Properties of Biomaterials in the Physiological Environment*. CRC Press, Boca Raton (1980).

5 Szycher, M. (Ed.) *Biocompatible Polymers, Metals, and Composites*. Technomic, Lancaster, PA (1983).

6 Paul, J.P., Gaylor, J.D.S., Courtney, J.M. and Gilchrist, T. (Eds) *Biomaterials in Artificial Organs*. Macmillan, London (1984).

7 Hastings, G.W. and Ducheyne, P. (Eds) *Macromolecular Biomaterials*. CRC Press, Boca Raton (1984).

8 Nosé, Y., Kjellstrand, C. and Ivanovich, P. (Eds) *Progress in Artificial Organs—1985*. ISAO Press, Cleveland, OH (1986).

9 Barbenel, J.C., Fisher, A.C., Gaylor, J.D.S. *et al.* (Eds) *Blood Flow in Artificial Organs and Cardiovascular Prostheses*. Clarendon Press, Oxford (1989).

10 Paul, J.P., Rappelsberger, P. and Schütz, P.W. (Eds) *The Influence of New Technologies on Medical Practice*. Verlag für medizinische Wissenschaften Wilhelm Maudrich, Vienna (1991).

11 Didisheim, P., Olsen, D.B., Farrer, D.J. *et al.* (1989) Infections and thromboembolism with implantable cardiovascular devices. *Trans. Am. Soc. Artif. Intern. Organs*, **35**, 54–70.

12 Kambic, H.E. and Nosé, Y. Biomaterials for blood pumps. In: *Blood Compatible Materials and Devices* (Eds Sharma, C.P. & Szycher, M.), pp. 141–152. Technomic, Lancaster, PA (1991).

13 Nosé, Y. (1988) Long term compatibility of artificial kidneys. *Artif. Organs*, **12**, 1.

14 Ringoir, S. and Vanholder, R. (1990) New trends in dialysis. *Contrib. Nephrol.*, **82**, 102–106.

15 Andrade, J.D., Coleman, D.L., Didisheim, P. *et al.* (1981) Blood–materials interactions—20 years of frustration. *Trans. Am. Soc. Artif. Intern. Organs*, **27**, 659–662.

16 Murabayashi, S. and Nosé, Y. (1986) Biocompatibility: bioengineering aspects. *Artif. Organs*, **10**, 114–121.

17 Ringoir, S. and Vanholder, R. (1986) An introduction to biocompatibility. *Artif. Organs*, **10**, 20–27.

18 Vanholder, R. and Ringoir, S. (1989) Bioincompatibility: an overview. *Int. J. Artif. Organs*, **12**, 356–365.

19 Nosé, Y. (1991) What is blood compatibility? *Artif. Organs*, **15**, 1.

20 Ogston, D. *The Physiology of Hemostasis*. Croom Helm, London (1983).

21 Spaet, T.H. and Gaynor, E. (1970) Vascular endothelial damage and thrombosis. *Adv. Cardiol.*, **4**, 47–66.

22 Danon, D. and Skutelsky, E. (1976) Endothelial surface charge and its possible relationship to thrombogenesis. *Ann. NY Acad. Sci.*, **275**, 47–63.

23 Mason, R.G., Sharp, D.E., Chuang, H.Y.K. and Mohammad, S.F. (1977) The endothelium: roles in thrombosis and hemostasis. *Arch. Pathol. Lab. Med.*, **101**, 61–64.

24 Mason, R.G., Mohammad, S.F., Saba, H.J. *et al.* (1979) Functions of endothelium. *Pathobiol. Ann.*, **9**, 1–48.

25 Cazenave, J.P., Dejana, E., Kinlough-Rathbone, R. *et al.* (1979) Platelet interactions with the endothelium and the subendothelium: the role of thrombin and prostacyclin. *Haemostasis*, **8**, 183–192.
26 Weiss, H.J., Tschopp, T.B., Baumgartner, H.R. *et al.* (1974) Decreased adhesion of giant (Bernard–Soulier) platelets to endothelium. Further implications on the role of the von Willebrand factor in hemostasis. *Am. J. Med.*, **57**, 920–925.
27 Sakariassen, K.S., Bolhuis, P.A. and Sixma, J.J. (1979) Human blood platelet adhesion to artery subendothelium is mediated by Factor VIII–von Willebrand factor bound to the subendothelium. *Nature*, **279**, 636–638.
28 Nurden, A.T. and Caen, J.P. (1979) The different glycoprotein abnormalities in thromboasthenic and Bernard–Soulier platelets. *Semin. Hematol.*, **16**, 234–250.
29 Holmsen, H., Day, H.J. and Stormorken, J. (1969) The blood platelet release reaction. *Scand. J. Haematol.* (Suppl), **8**, 1–26.
30 McNicol, G.P. and Douglas, A.S. The fibrinolytic enzyme system. In: *Human Blood Coagulation, Haemostasis and Thrombosis* (Ed. Biggs, R.), 2nd edn, pp. 399–435. Blackwell Scientific Publications, Oxford (1976).
31 Collen, D. (1980) On the regulation and control of fibrinolysis. *Thromb. Haemost.*, **43**, 77–89.
32 Herzlinger, G.A. Activation of complement by polymers in contact with blood. In: *Biocompatible Polymers, Metals, and Composites* (Ed. Szycher, M.), pp. 89–101. Technomic, Lancaster, PA (1983).
33 Moncada, S., Higgs, E.A. and Vane, J.R. (1977) Human arterial and venous tissues generate prostacyclin (prostaglandin X), a potent inhibitor of platelet aggregation. *Lancet*, **i**, 18–20.
34 Lollar, P. and Owen, W.G. (1980). Clearance of thrombin from circulation in rabbits by high-affinity binding sites on endothelium: possible role in the inactivation of thrombin by antithrombin III. *J. Clin. Invest.*, **66**, 1222–1230.
35 Loskutoff, D.J. and Edgington, T.S. (1981) An inhibitor of plasminogen activator in rabbit endothelial cells. *J. Biol. Chem.*, **256**, 4142–4145.
36 Thorgeirsson, G. and Robertson, A.L. Jr. (1978) The vascular endothelium—pathobiologic significance. *Am. J. Pathol.*, **93**, 803–848.
37 Bagnall, R.D. (1978) Adsorption of plasma proteins on hydrophobic surfaces. II. Fibrinogen and fibrinogen-containing protein mixtures. *J. Biomed. Mater. Res.*, **12**, 203–217.
38 Chan, B.M.C. and Brash, J.L. (1981) Adsorption of fibrinogen on glass: reversibility aspects. *J. Coll. Int. Sci.*, **82**, 217–225.
39 Vroman, L., Adams, A.L., Klings, M. *et al.* (1977) Reactions of formed elements of blood with plasma proteins at interfaces. *Ann. NY Acad. Sci.*, **283**, 65–76.
40 Gendrau, R.M., Winters, S., Leininger, R.I. *et al.* (1981) Fourier transform infrared spectroscopy of protein adsorption from whole blood: *ex vivo* dog studies. *Appl. Spectrosc.*, **35**, 353–357.
41 Baier, R.E., Loeb, G.I. and Wallace, G.T. (1971) Role of an artificial boundary in modifying blood proteins. *Fed. Proc.*, **30**, 1523–1538.
42 Lyman, D.J., Metcalf, L.C., Albo, D. Jr. *et al.* (1974) The effect of chemical-structure and surface properties of synthetic polymers on the coagulation of blood. III. *In vivo* adsorption of proteins on polymer surfaces. *Trans. Am. Soc. Artif. Intern. Organs*, **20**, 474–478.

43 Baier, R.E. (1977) The organization of blood components near interfaces. *Ann. NY Acad. Sci.*, **283**, 17–36.

44 Brash, J.L. Protein adsorption and blood interactions. In: *Biocompatible Polymers, Metals, and Composites* (Ed. Szycher, M.), pp. 35–52. Technomic, Lancaster, PA (1983).

45 Klinkmann, H. The role of biomaterials in the application of artificial organs. In: *Biomaterials in Artificial Organs* (Eds Paul, J.P., Gaylor, J.D.S., Courtney, J.M. & Gilchrist, T.), pp. 1–8. Macmillan, London (1984).

46 Lee, W.H. Jr and Hairston, P. (1971) Structural effects on blood proteins at the gas–blood interface. *Fed. Proc.*, **30**, 1615–1620.

47 Ihlenfeld, J.V. and Cooper, S.L. (1979) Transient *in vivo* protein adsorption onto polymeric biomaterials. *J. Biomed. Mater. Res.*, **13**, 577–591.

48 Packham, M.A., Evans, G., Glynn, M.F. and Mustard, J.F. (1969) The effect of plasma proteins on the interaction of platelets with glass surfaces. *J. Lab. Clin. Med.*, **73**, 686–697.

49 Zucker, M.B. and Vroman, L. (1969) Platelet adhesion by fibrinogen adsorbed onto glass. *Proc. Soc. Exp. Biol. Med.*, **131**, 318–320.

50 Salzman, E.W., Merrill, E.W., Binder, A. *et al.* (1969) Protein–platelet interaction on heparinized surfaces. *J. Biomed. Mater. Res.*, **3**, 69–81.

51 Lyman, D.J., Klein, K.G., Brash, J.L. and Fritzinger, B.K. (1970) The interaction of platelets with polymer surfaces. *Thromb. Diathes. Haemorrh.*, **23**, 120–128.

52 Jenkins, C.S.P., Packham, M.A., Guccione, M.A. and Mustard, J.F. (1973) Modification of platelet adherence to protein-coated surfaces. *J. Lab. Clin. Med.*, **81**, 280–290.

53 Whicher, S.J. and Brash, J.L. (1978) Platelet–foreign surface interactions: release of granule constituents from adherent platelets. *J. Biomed. Mater. Res.*, **12**, 181–201.

54 Neumann, A.W., Moscarello, M.A., Zingg, W. *et al.* (1979) Platelet adhesion from human blood to bare and protein coated polymer surfaces. *J. Polym. Sci. Polym. Symp.*, **66**, 391–398.

55 Adams, G.A. and Feuerstein, I.A. (1980) Visual fluorescent and radio-isotopic evaluation of platelet accumulation and embolization. *Trans. Am. Soc. Artif. Intern. Organs*, **26**, 17–22.

56 Absolom, D.R., Zingg, W., Policova, Z. and Neumann, A.W. (1983) Determination of the surface tension of protein coated materials by means of the advancing solidification front technique. *Trans. Am. Soc. Artif. Intern. Organs*, **29**, 146–151.

57 Fougnot, C., Labarre, D., Jozefonwicz, J. and Jozefowicz, M. Modifications to polymer surfaces to improve blood compatibility. In: *Macromolecular Biomaterials* (Eds Hastings, G.W. & Ducheyne, P.), pp. 215–238. CRC Press, Boca Raton (1984).

58 Young, B.R., Lambrecht, L.K., Albrecht, R.M. *et al.* (1983) Platelet–protein interactions at blood–polymer interfaces in the canine test model. *Trans. Am. Soc. Artif. Intern. Organs*, **29**, 442–446.

59 Vroman, L., Adams, A.L., Fischer, G.C. and Munoz, P.C. (1980) Interaction of high molecular weight kininogen, Factor XII, and fibrinogen in plasma at interfaces. *Blood*, **55**, 156–159.

60 Szycher, M. Thrombosis, hemostasis, and thrombolysis at prosthetic interfaces. In: *Biocompatible Polymers, Metals, and Composites* (Ed. Szycher, M.), pp. 1–33. Technomic, Lancaster, PA (1983).
61 Vroman, L. Protein/surface interaction. In: *Biocompatible Polymers, Metals, and Composites* (Ed. Szycher, M.), pp. 81–88. Technomic, Lancaster, PA (1983).
62 Evans, G. and Mustard, J.F. (1968) Platelet–surface reaction and thrombosis. *Surgery*, **64**, 273–280.
63 Adams, A.L., Fischer, G.C. and Vroman, L. (1978) The complexity of blood at simple interfaces. *J. Coll. Int. Sci.*, **65**, 468–478.
64 Grinnell, F. and Feld, M.K. (1981) Adsorption characteristics of plasma fibronectin in relationship to biological activity. *J. Biomed. Mater. Res.*, **15**, 363–381.
65 Harfenist, E.J., Izzotti, M.J., Packham, M.A. and Mustard, J.F. (1980) Plasma fibronectin is not involved in ADP-induced aggregation of rabbit platelets. *Thromb. Haemost.*, **44**, 108.
66 Sochynsky, R.A., Boughton, B.J., Burnes, J. *et al.* (1980) The effect of human fibronectin on platelet collagen adhesion. *Thromb. Res.*, **18**, 521–533.
67 Courtney, J.M., Irvine, L., Jones, C. *et al.* Compatibility aspects of biomaterials for artificial organs and assist devices. In: *The Influence of New Technologies on Medical Practice* (Eds Paul, J.P., Rappelsberger, P. & Schütz, P.W.), pp. 154–162. Verlag für medizinische Wissenschaften Wilhelm Maudrich, Vienna (1991).
68 Griffin, J.H. and Cochrane, C.G. (1979) Recent advances in the understanding of contact activation reactions. *Semin. Thromb. Hemost.*, **5**, 254–273.
69 Mason, R.G. (1972) The interaction of blood hemostatic elements with artificial surfaces. *Prog. Hemost. Thromb.*, **1**, 141–164.
70 Mason, R.G., Mohammad, S.F., Chuang, H.Y.K. and Richardson, P.D. (1976) The adhesion of platelets to subendothelium, collagen and artificial surfaces. *Semin. Thromb. Hemost.*, **3**, 98–116.
71 Kim, S.W., Lee, R.G., Oster, H. *et al.* (1974) Platelet adhesion to polymer surfaces. *Trans. Am. Soc. Artif. Intern. Organs*, **20**, 449–455.
72 Lee, R.G. and Kim, S.W. (1974) The role of carbohydrate in platelet adhesion to foreign surfaces. *J. Biomed. Mater. Res.*, **8**, 393–398.
73 Jamieson, G.A. Role of glycoproteins in platelet function. In: *Erythrocytes, Thrombocytes, Leukocytes: Recent Advances in Membrane and Metabolic Research* (Eds Gerlach, E., Moser, K., Deutsch, E. & Willmanns, W.), pp. 209–232. Thieme, Stuttgart (1973).
74 Salzman, E.W., Lindon, J., Brier, D. and Merrill, E.W. (1977) Surface-induced platelet adhesion, aggregation and release. *Ann. NY Acad. Sci.*, **283**, 114–127.
75 Baumgartner, H.R., Muggli, R., Tschopp, T.B. and Turitto, V.T. (1976) Platelet adhesion, release and aggregation in flowing blood: effects of surface properties and platelet function. *Thromb. Haemost.*, **35**, 124–138.
76 Feijen, J. Thrombogenesis caused by blood–foreign surface interaction. In: *Artificial Organs* (Eds Kenedi, R.M., Courtney, J.M., Gaylor, J.D.S. & Gilchrist, T.), pp. 235–247. Macmillan, London (1977).
77 Walsh, P.N. Platelet–coagulant protein interactions. In: *Hemostasis and Thrombosis: Basic Principles and Clinical Practice* (Eds Colman, R.W., Hirsh, J., Marder, V.J. & Salzman, E.W.), pp. 404–420. Lippincott, Philadelphia (1982).
78 Needleman, S.W. and Hook, J.C. Platelets and leukocytes. In: *Hemostasis and*

Thrombosis: Basic Principles and Clinical Practice (Eds Colman, R.W., Hirsh, J., Marder, V.J. & Salzman, E.W.), pp. 716–725. Lippincott, Philadelphia (1982).

79 Waugh, D.F. and Baughman, D.J. (1969) Thrombin adsorption and possible relations to thrombus formation. *J. Biomed. Mater. Res.*, **3**, 145–164.

80 Chuang, H.Y.K., Crowther, P.E., Mohammad, S.F. and Mason, R.G. (1979) Interactions of thrombin and antithrombin III with artificial surfaces. *Thromb. Res.*, **14**, 273–282.

81 Shuman, M.A. and Levine, S.P. (1980) Relationship between secretion of platelet factor 4 and thrombin generation during *in vitro* blood clotting. *J. Clin. Invest.*, **65**, 307–313.

82 Patrono, C., Ciabattoni, G., Pinca, E. *et al.* (1980) Low dose aspirin and inhibition of thromboxane B_2 production in healthy subjects. *Thromb. Res.*, **17**, 317–327.

83 Philips, D.R., Jennings, L.K. and Prasanna, H.R. (1980) Ca^{2+}-mediated association of glycoprotein G (thrombin-sensitive protein, thrombospondin) with human blood. *J. Biol. Chem.*, **255**, 11629–11632.

84 Brash, J.L. and Uniyal, S. (1976) Adsorption of albumin and fibrinogen to polyethylene in presence of red cells. *Trans. Am. Soc. Artif. Intern. Organs*, **22**, 253–259.

85 Uniyal, S., Brash, J.L. and Degterev, I.A. (1982) Influence of red blood cells and their components on protein adsorption. *Am. Chem. Soc. Adv. Chem.*, **199**, 277–292.

86 Stormorken, H. (1971) Platelets, thrombosis and hemolysis. *Fed. Proc.*, **30**, 1551–1555.

87 Kusserow, B., Larrow, R. and Nichols, J. (1971) Perfusion- and surface induced injury in leucocytes. *Fed. Proc.*, **30**, 1516–1520.

88 Wright, D.G., Kauffman, J.C., Terpstra, G.K. *et al.* (1978) Mobilization and exocytosis of specific (secondary) granules by human neutrophils during adherence to nylon wool in filtration leukapheresis (FL). *Blood*, **52**, 770–782.

89 Lederman, D.M., Cumming, R.D., Petschek, H.E. *et al.* (1978) The effect of temperature on the interaction of platelets and leukocytes with materials exposed to flowing blood. *Trans. Am. Soc. Artif. Intern. Organs*, **24**, 557–560.

90 Absolom, D.R., Neumann, A.W., Zingg, W. and van Oss, C.J. (1979) Thermodynamic studies of cellular adhesion. *Trans. Am. Soc. Artif. Intern. Organs*, **25**, 152–156.

91 Cumming, R.D. (1980) Important factors affecting initial blood–material interactions. *Trans. Am. Soc. Artif. Intern. Organs*, **26**, 304–308.

92 Harrison, M.J., Emmons, P.R. and Mitchell, J.R. (1966) The effect of white cells on platelet aggregation. *Thromb. Diathes. Haemorrh.*, **16**, 105–121.

93 Niemetz, J. (1972) Coagulant activity of leukocytes. Tissue factor activity. *J. Clin. Invest.*, **51**, 307–313.

94 Saba, H.I., Herion, J.C., Walker, R.I. and Roberts, H.R. (1973) The procoagulant activity of granulocytes. *Proc. Soc. Exp. Biol. Med.*, **142**, 614–620.

95 Farrell, P.C. Biocompatibility aspects of extracorporeal circulation. In: *Biomaterials in Artificial Organs* (Eds Paul, J.P., Gaylor, J.D.S., Courtney, J.M. & Gilchrist, T.), pp. 342–350. Macmillan, London (1984).

96 Herzlinger, G.A. and Cumming, R.D. (1980) Role of complement activation in

cell adhesion to polymer blood contact surfaces. *Trans. Am. Soc. Artif. Intern. Organs*, **26**, 165–170.

97 Courtney, J.M., Irvine, L., Jones, C. *et al.* Biomaterials in medicine—a bioengineering perspective. *Int. J. Artif. Organs.* In press.

98 Rosenberg, R.D. Heparin–antithrombin system. In: *Hemostasis and Thrombosis: Basic Principles and Clinical Practice* (Eds Colman, R.W., Hirsh, J., Marder, V.J. & Salzman, E.W.), pp. 962–985. Lippincott, Philadelphia (1982).

99 Thomas, D.P. (1986) Current status of low molecular weight heparin. *Thromb. Haemost.*, **56**, 241–242.

100 Talbot, M.D., Ambler, J., Butler, K.D. *et al.* (1989) Recombinant desulphatohirudin (CGP 39393) anticoagulant and antithrombotic properties *in vivo*. *Thromb. Haemost.*, **61**, 71–80.

101 Courtney, J.M., Travers, M., Douglas, J.T. *et al.* Blood–membrane interactions: *in vitro* evaluation of the influence of membrane structure and antithrombotic agents. In: *Blood Flow in Artificial Organs and Cardiovascular Prostheses* (Eds Barbenel, J.C., Fischer, A.C., Gaylor, J.D.S., Angerson, W.J. & Sheldon, C.D.), pp. 104–112. Clarendon Press, Oxford (1989).

102 Robertson, L.M., Courtney, J.M., Irvine, L. *et al.* (1990) Modification of the blood compatibility of hemodialysis membranes. *Artif. Organs*, **14** (Suppl. 2), 41–43.

103 Engbers, G.H. and Feijen, J. (1991) Current techniques to improve the blood compatibility of biomaterial surfaces. *Int. J. Artif. Organs*, **14**, 199–215.

104 Grode, G.A., Pitman, J., Crowley, J.P. *et al.* (1974) Surface-immobilized prostaglandin as a platelet protective agent. *Trans. Am. Soc. Artif. Intern. Organs*, **20**, 38–41.

105 Marconi, W., Bartoli, F., Mantovani, E. *et al.* (1979) Development of new antithrombotic surfaces by employing platelet antiaggregating agents: preparation and characterization. *Trans. Am. Soc. Artif. Intern. Organs*, **25**, 280–285.

106 Ebert, C.D., Lees, E.S. and Kim, S.W. (1982) The antiplatelet activity of immobilized prostacyclin. *J. Biomed. Mater. Res.*, **16**, 629–638.

107 McRea, J.C. and Kim, S.W. (1978) Characterization of controlled release of prostaglandin from polymer matrices for thrombus prevention. *Trans. Am. Soc. Artif. Intern. Organs*, **24**, 746–752.

108 McRea, J.C., Ebert, C.D. and Kim, S.W. (1981) Prostaglandin releasing polymers —stability and efficacy. *Trans. Am. Soc. Artif. Intern. Organs*, **27**, 511–516.

109 Kusserow, B.K., Larrow, R.W. and Nichols, J.E. (1973) The surface bonded, covalently crosslinked urokinase surface. *Trans. Am. Soc. Artif. Intern. Organs*, **19**, 8–12.

110 Sugitachi, A., Tanaka, M., Kawahara, T. and Takagi, K. (1980) Antithrombogenicity of UK-immobilized polymer surfaces. *Trans. Am. Soc. Artif. Intern. Organs*, **26**, 274–278.

111 Ohshiro, T. and Kosaki, G. (1980) Urokinase immobilized on medical polymeric materials: fundamental and clinical studies. *Artif. Organs*, **4**, 58–64.

112 Teien, A.N. Assay of heparin using Factor Xa and a chromogenic substrate. In: *Chromogenic Peptide Substrates: Chemistry and Clinical Usage* (Eds Scully, M.F. & Kakkar, V.V.), pp. 196–204. Churchill Livingstone, Edinburgh (1979).

113 Esbach, J.W. (1989) The anaemia of chronic renal failure: pathophysiology and the effects of recombinant erythropoietin. *Kidney Int.*, **35**, 134–148.

114 Klinkmann, H., Falkenhagen, D. and Courtney, J.M. Clinical relevance of biocompatibility—the material cannot be divorced from the device. In: *Uremia Therapy* (Ed. Gurland, H.J.), pp. 125–138. Springer-Verlag, Berlin (1987).

115 Feuerstein, I.A., Brophy, J.M. and Brash, J.L. (1975) Platelet transport and adhesion to reconstituted collagen and artificial surfaces. *Trans. Am. Soc. Artif. Intern. Organs*, **21**, 427–434.

116 Richardson, P.D., Mohammad, S.F. and Mason, R.G. (1977) Flow chamber studies of platelet adhesion at controlled, spatially varied shear rates. *Proc. Eur. Soc. Artif. Organs*, **4**, 175–188.

117 Rieger, H. (1980) Dependency of platelet aggregation (PA) *in vitro* on different shear rates. *Thromb. Haemost.*, **44**, 166 (Abstract).

118 Dewitz, T.S., Hung, T.C., Martin, R.R. and McIntire, L.V. (1977) Mechanical trauma in leukocytes. *J. Lab. Clin. Med.*, **90**, 728–736.

119 Dewitz, T.S., Martin, R.R., Solis, R.T. *et al.* (1978). Microaggregate formation in whole blood exposed to shear stress. *Microvascular Res.*, **16**, 263–271.

120 Courtney, J.M., Gaylor, J.D.S., Klinkmann, H. and Holtz, M. Polymer membranes. In: *Macromolecular Biomaterials* (Eds Hastings, G.W. & Ducheyne, P.), pp. 143–180. CRC Press, Boca Raton (1984).

121 Kaplow, L.S. and Goffinet, J.A. (1968) Profound neutropenia during the early phase of hemodialysis. *JAMA*, **203**, 1135–1137.

122 Craddock, P.R., Fehr, J., Dalmasso, A.P. *et al.* (1977) Hemodialysis leukopenia. Pulmonary vascular leukostasis resulting from complement activation by dialyzer cellophane membranes. *J. Clin. Invest.*, **59**, 879–888.

123 Jacob, H.S., Craddock, P.R., Hammerschmidt, D.E. and Moldow, C.F. (1980) Complement-induced granulocyte activation. An unsuspected mechanism of disease. *New Engl. J. Med.*, **302**, 789–794.

124 Hakim, R.M. (1986) Clinical sequelae of complement activation in hemodialysis. *Clin. Nephrol.*, **26**, S9–S12.

125 Klinkmann, H., Falkenhagen, D. and Courtney, J.M. (1987) Biomaterials and biocompatibility in hemodialysis. *Contrib. Nephrol.*, **55**, 231–249.

126 Courtney, J.M., Irvine, L. and Travers, M. Hemodialysis membranes. In: *Concise Encyclopedia of Medical and Dental Materials* (Ed. Williams, D.), pp. 212–219. Pergamon, Oxford (1990).

127 Kuwahara, T., Markert, M. and Wauters, J.P. (1989) Proteins adsorbed on hemodialysis membranes modulate neutrophil activation. *Artif. Organs*, **13**, 427–431.

128 Panichi, V., Bianchi, A.M., Parrini, M. *et al.* (1989) Biocompatibility evaluation of five dialysis membranes: protein layer and anaphylatoxins generation. *Int. J. Artif. Organs*, **12**, 579.

129 McLaughlin, K.M., Travers, M., Simpson, K. *et al.* (1989) The assessment of fibrinogen and fibrinolysis during hemodialysis. *Int. J. Artif. Organs*, **12**, 587 (Abstract).

130 Pertosa, G., Pastore, A. and Schena, F.P. (1989) Influence of different dialyzer membranes on plasma fibronectin levels in hemodialyzed patients. *Int. J. Artif. Organs*, **12**, 36–40.

131 Henson, P.M. and Ginsberg, M.H. Immunological reactions of platelets. In: *Platelets in Biology and Pathology—2* (Ed. Gordon, J.L.), pp. 265–308. Elsevier, Amsterdam (1981).

132 Woods, H.F. (1980) The use of antiplatelet agents during hemodialysis. *Dial. Transplant.*, **9**, 957–960.
133 Adler, A.J. and Berlyne, G.M. (1981) β-Thromboglobulin and platelet factor-4 levels during hemodialysis with polyacrylonitrile. *Am. Soc. Artif. Int. Organs J.*, **4**, 100–102.
134 Mahiout, A., Meinhold, H., Kessel, M. *et al.* (1987) Dialyzer membranes: effect of surface area and chemical modification of cellulose on complement and platelet activation. *Artif. Organs*, **11**, 149–154.
135 Grabowski, E.F., Didisheim, P., Lewis, C.J. *et al.* (1977) Platelet adhesion to foreign surfaces under controlled conditions of whole blood flow: human vs. dog, calf, sheep, macaque, and baboon. *Trans. Am. Soc. Artif. Intern. Organs*, **23**, 141–149.
136 Henson, P.M. (1969) The adhesion of leukocytes and platelets induced by fixed IgG antibody or complement. *Immunology*, **16**, 107–121.
137 Chenoweth, D.E. (1986) Complement activation produced by biomaterials. *Trans. Am. Soc. Artif. Intern. Organs*, **32**, 226–232.
138 Kazatchkine, M.D. and Carreno, M.P. (1987) Activation of the complement system at the interface between blood and artificial surfaces. *Biomaterials*, **9**, 30–35.
139 Chenoweth, D.E., Cheung, A.K. and Henderson, L.W. (1983) Anaphylatoxin formation during hemodialysis: effects of different dialyzer membranes. *Kidney Int.*, **24**, 764–769.
140 Chenoweth, D.E. and Hugli, T.E. (1980) Human C5a and C5a analogs as probes of the neutrophil C5a receptor. *Mol. Immunol.*, **17**, 151–161.
141 Aljama, P., Martin-Malo, A., Perez, R. *et al.* (1985) Granulocyte adherence changes during hemodialysis. *Contrib. Nephrol.*, **46**, 75–82.
142 Schaefer, R.M., Heidland, A. and Hörl, W.H. (1985) Release of leukocyte elastase during hemodialysis. Effect of different dialysis membranes. *Contrib. Nephrol.*, **46**, 109–117.
143 Kolb, G., Fischer, W., Müller, T. *et al.* (1989) Granulocyte-related bioincompatibility of hemodialysis: Inhibition of oxidative metabolism, degranulation reaction, enzyme release and leukocyte sequestration in the lung. *Int. J. Artif. Organs*, **12**, 294–298.
144 Schultze, G., Wagner, K., Neumayer, H.-H. *et al.* (1987) Effect of dialyzer membranes on *in vitro* generation of eicosanoids. *Int. J. Artif. Organs*, **10**, 275–278.
145 Tetta, C., Segoloni, G., Pacitti, A. *et al.* (1989) The production of platelet-activating factor during hemodialysis. *Int. J. Artif. Organs*, **12**, 766–772.
146 Kay, N.E. and Raij, L. (1987) Differential effect of hemodialysis membranes on human lymphocyte natural killer function. *Artif. Organs*, **11**, 165–167.
147 Bingel, M., Lonnemann, G., Shaldon, S. *et al.* (1986) Human interleukin-1 production during hemodialysis. *Nephron*, **43**, 161–163.
148 Lonnemann, G., Bingel, M., Koch, K.M. *et al.* (1987) Plasma interleukin-1 activity in humans undergoing hemodialysis with regenerated cellulosic membranes. *Lymphokine Res.*, **6**, 63–70.
149 Lonnemann, G., van der Meer, J.W.M., Cannon, J.G. *et al.* (1987) Induction of tumor necrosis factor during extracorporeal blood purification. *New Engl. J. Med.*, **317**, 963–964.

150 Vanholder, R., Ringoir, S., Dhondt, A. and Hakim, R. (1991) Phagocytosis in uremic and hemodialysis patients: a prospective and cross sectional study. *Kidney Int.*, **39**, 320–327.

151 Stratta, P., Canavese, C., Mangiarotti, G. *et al.* (1981) Heparin is unable to prevent contact activation by three different membranes. *Proc. Eur. Dial. Transplant. Assoc.*, **18**, 269–274.

152 Wardle, E.N. and Piercy, D.A. (1982) Studies of contact activation of blood in haemodialysis. *J. Clin. Pathol.*, **25**, 1045–1049.

153 Vaziri, N.D., Toohey, J.A., Alikhani, S. and Hung, E. (1984) Effect of hemodialysis on contact group of coagulation factors, platelets, and leukocytes. *Am. J. Med.*, **77**, 437–441.

154 Kurz, H., Lerner, R.G., Weseley, S. and Nelson, J.C. (1985) Changes in fibrinolytic activity during the course of a single hemodialysis session. *Clin. Nephrol.*, **24**, 1–4.

155 Henderson, L.W., Cheung, A.K. and Chenoweth, D.E. (1983) Choosing a membrane. *Am. J. Kidney Dis.*, **3**, 5–20.

156 Baurmeister, U., Vienken, J., Ansorge, W. and Luttrell, A. (1989) Cellulosic versus synthetic membranes: a reasonable comparison? *Artif. Organs*, **13**, 52–57.

157 Chenoweth, D.E. (1984) Complement activation during hemodialysis: clinical observations, proposed mechanisms and theoretical implications. *Artif. Organs*, **8**, 281–287.

158 Ivanovich, P., Chenoweth, D.E., Schmidt, R. *et al.* (1983) Symptoms and activation of granulocytes and complement with two dialysis membranes. *Kidney Int.*, **24**, 758–763.

159 Hakim, R.M., Fearon, D.T. and Lazarus, J.M. (1984) Biocompatibility of dialysis membranes: effects of chronic complement activation. *Kidney Int.*, **26**, 194–200.

160 Akizawa, T., Sekiguchi, T., Nakayama, F. *et al.* Complement activation during hemodialysis: effects of membrane materials and anticoagulants. In: *Progress in Artificial Organs—1985* (Eds Nosé, Y., Kjellstrand, C. & Ivanovich, P.), pp. 1169–1173. ISAO Press, Cleveland (1986).

161 Wegmüller, E., Montandon, A., Nydegger, U. and Descoeudres, C. (1986) Biocompatibility of different hemodialysis membranes: activation of complement and leukopenia. *Int. J. Artif. Organs*, **9**, 85–92.

162 Amato, M., Salvadori, M., Bergesio, F. *et al.* (1988) Aspects of biocompatibility of two different dialysis membranes: cuprophane and polysulfone. *Int. J. Artif. Organs*, **11**, 175–180.

163 Moll, S., De Moerloose, P., Rieber, G. *et al.* (1990) Comparison of two hemodialysis membranes, polyacrylonitrile and cellulose acetate, on complement and coagulation systems. *Int. J. Artif. Organs*, **13**, 273–279.

164 Schaefer, R.M., Heidland, A. and Hörl, W.H. Leukocyte elastase—a new marker of biocompatibility in hemodialysis. In: *Progress in Artificial Organs—1985* (Eds Nosé, Y., Kjellstrand, C. & Ivanovich, P.), pp. 966–968. ISAO Press, Cleveland (1986).

165 Cheung, A.K. (1989) Adsorption of unactivated complement proteins by hemodialysis membranes. *Am. J. Kidney Dis.*, **14**, 472–477.

166 Kandus, A., Ponikvar, R., Drinovec, J. *et al.* (1990) Anaphylatoxins C3a and C5a

adsorption on acrylonitrile membrane of hollow-fiber and plate dialyzer—an *in vivo* study. *Int. J. Artif. Organs*, **13**, 176–180.

167 Akizawa, T., Kitaoka, T., Koshikawa, S. *et al.* (1986) Development of a regenerated cellulose noncomplement activating membrane for hemodialysis. *Trans. Am. Soc. Artif. Intern. Organs*, **32**, 76–79.

168 Bosch, T., Schmidt, B., Spencer, P.C. *et al.* (1987) *Ex vivo* biocompatibility evaluation of a new modified cellulose membrane. *Artif. Organs*, **11**, 144–148.

169 Lucchi, L., Bonucchi, D., Acerbi, M.A. *et al.* (1989) Improved biocompatibility by modified cellulosic membranes: the case of Hemophan. *Artif. Organs*, **13**, 417–421.

170 Zingraff, J., Beyne, P., Urena, P. *et al.* (1988) Influence of hemodialysis membranes on β_2-microglobulin kinetics: *in vivo* and *in vitro* studies. *Nephrol. Dial. Transp.*, **3**, 284–290.

171 Houglustaine, D., Waier, M., Michielsen, P. *et al.* (1986) Haemodialysis membranes, serum β_2-microglobulin, and dialysis amyloidosis. *Lancet*, **ii**, 1211.

172 Ivanovich, P., Xu, C.G., Kwaan, H.C. and Hathiwala, S. (1983) Studies of coagulation and platelet functions in heparin-free hemodialysis. *Nephron*, **33**, 116–120.

173 Caruana, R.J., Raja, R.M., Bush, J.V. *et al.* (1987) Heparin-free dialysis: comparative data and results in high-risk patients. *Kidney Int.*, **31**, 1351–1355.

174 Preuschof, L., Keller, F., Seemann, J. and Offermann, G. (1988) Heparin-free hemodialysis with prophylactic change of dialyser and blood lines. *Int. J. Artif. Organs*, **11**, 255–258.

175 Leonard, C.D., Weil, E. and Scribner, B.H. (1969) Subdural haematomas in patients undergoing haemodialysis. *Lancet*, **ii**, 239–240.

176 Lindsay, R.M., Rourke, J.T.B., Reid, B.D. *et al.* (1977) The role of heparin on platelet retention by acrylonitrile copolymer dialysis membranes. *J. Lab. Clin. Med.*, **89**, 724–734.

177 Kelton, J.C. (1986) Heparin-induced thrombocytopenia. *Haemostasis*, **16**, 173–186.

178 Bambauer, R., Rücker, S., Weber, U. and Köhler, M. (1990) Comparison of low molecular weight heparin and standard heparin in hemodialysis. *Trans. Am. Soc. Artif. Intern. Organs*, **36**, M646–M649.

179 von Bonsdorff, M., Stiekema, J., Harjanne, A. and Alapiessa, U. (1990) A new low molecular weight heparinoid Org 10172 as anticoagulant in hemodialysis. *Int. J. Artif. Organs*, **13**, 103–108.

180 Zusman, R.M., Rubin, R.H., Cato, A.E. *et al.* (1981) Hemodialysis using prostacyclin instead of heparin as the sole antithrombotic agent. *New Engl. J. Med.*, **304**, 934–939.

181 Maurin, N. (1988) The *in vitro* bleeding time while using a stable prostacyclin analogue during hemodialysis. *Int. J. Artif. Organs*, **11**, 243–248.

182 Grekas, D., Alivanis, P., Karamouzis, M. *et al.* (1989) A pilot study of piracetam in Cuprophan hemodialysis. *Artif. Organs*, **13**, 422–426.

183 Akizawa, T., Sato, M., Kitaoka, T. *et al.* (1985) Usefulness of multienzyme inhibitor, nafomostat mesilate, in high bleeding risk hemodialysis. *Proc. Eur. Dial. Transplant. Assoc.*, **22**, 334–338.

184 Ward, R.A., Schmidt, B. and Gurland, H.J. (1990) Low-dose heparinization can be

used with DEAE cellulose hemodialysis membranes. *Trans. Am. Soc. Artif. Intern. Organs*, **36**, M321–M324.

185 Man, N., Ciancioni, C., Faivre, J. *et al.* (1988) Dialysis-associated adverse reactions with high-flux membranes and microbial contamination of liquid bicarbonate concentrate. *Contrib. Nephrol.*, **62**, 24–34.

186 Blass, C.R., Jones, C., Courtney, J.M. (1992) Biomaterials for blood tubing: the application of plasticised poly(vinyl chloride). *Int. J. Artif. Organs*, **15**, 200–203.

187 Kjellstrand, C.M., Alfrey, A.C., Eaton, J.W. *et al.* (1978) Toxicity of materials and medications used in dialysis. *Trans. Am. Soc. Artif. Intern. Organs*, **24**, 764–769.

188 Dolovich, J., Marshall, C.P., Smith, E.K.M. *et al.* (1984) Allergy to ethylene oxide in chronic hemodialysis patients. *Artif. Organs*, **8**, 334–337.

189 Nicholls, A. (1986) Ethylene oxide and anaphylaxis during haemodialysis. *Br. Med. J.*, **292**, 1221–1222.

190 Sieberth, H.G. (Ed.) *Plasma Exchange: Plasmapheresis—Plasma Separation.* Schattauer Verlag, Stuttgart (1980).

191 Nosé, Y., Malchesky, P.S. and Smith, J.W. (Eds) *Plasmapheresis: New Trends in Therapeutic Applications.* ISAO Press, Cleveland (1983).

192 Lysaght, M.J. and Gurland, H.J. Principles and practice of membrane plasmapheresis. In: *Biomaterials in Artificial Organs* (Eds Paul, J.P., Gaylor, J.D.S., Courtney, J.M. & Gilchrist, T.), pp. 9–16. Macmillan, London (1984).

193 Gurland, H.J. Therapeutic plasmapheresis: the road not yet taken. In: *Uremia Therapy* (Ed. Gurland, H.J.), pp. 64–71. Springer-Verlag, Berlin (1987).

194 McLeod, B.C., Viernes, A. and Sassetti, R.J. (1983) Complement metabolism during membrane plasma separation. *Artif. Organs*, **7**, 443–449.

195 Takaoka, T., Goldcamp, J., Abe, Y. *et al.* (1984) Biocompatibility of membrane plasma separation. *Trans. Am. Soc. Artif. Intern. Organs*, **30**, 347–352.

196 Omokawa, S., Malchesky, P.S., Sakamoto, H. *et al.* (1986) Changes in interleukin-1 during membrane plasmapheresis. *Trans. Am. Soc. Artif. Intern. Organs*, **32**, 392–396.

197 Omokawa, S., Suzuki, T., Dustoor, M.M. *et al.* (1987) Humoral, cellular and hemodynamic changes induced by blood–material interaction in membrane plasmapheresis. *Trans. Am. Soc. Artif. Intern. Organs*, **33**, 112–117.

198 Omokawa, S., Malchesky, P.S., Suzuki, T. *et al.* (1989) Surface area effects on efficiency and biocompatibility in experimental membrane plasmapheresis. *Artif. Organs*, **13**, 78–86.

199 Frasca, G.M., Buscaroli, A., Borgnino, L.C. and Vangelista, A. (1988) Optimization of heparin anticoagulation during membrane plasma separation. *Int. J. Artif. Organs*, **11**, 313–316.

200 Omokawa, S., Malchesky, P.S., Yamashita, M. *et al.* (1990) Effect of anticoagulant on biocompatibility in membrane plasmapheresis. *Int. J. Artif. Organs*, **13**, 768–777.

201 Ionescu, M.I., Tandon, A.P., Roesler, M.F. and Mary, D.A.S. Blood loss following extracorporeal circulation for heart valve surgery. In: *Techniques in Extracorporeal Circulation* (Ed. Ionescu, M.I.), 2nd edn, pp. 345–367. Butterworths, London (1981).

202 Courtney, J.M., Irvine, L., Gaylor, J.D.S. *et al.* Blood compatibility in cardio-

pulmonary bypass. In: *Cardiovascular Biomaterials* (Ed. Hastings, G.W.), pp. 37–79. Springer-Verlag, London (1992).

203 Gaylor, J.D.S. Artificial organs. In: *A Textbook of Biomedical Engineering* (Ed. Kenedi, R.M.), pp. 115–158. Blackie, Glasgow (1980).

204 Kayser, K.L. (1974) Blood–gas interface oxygenators versus membrane oxygenators: what are the proved differences? *Ann. Thorac. Surg.*, **17**, 459–463.

205 Peirce, E.C. II (1974) Is the blood–gas interface of clinical importance? *Ann. Thorac. Surg.*, **17**, 526–529.

206 Bartlett, R.H. and Gazzaniga, A.B. (1978) Extracorporeal circulation for cardiopulmonary failure. *Curr. Probl. Surg.*, **15**, 1–96.

207 Bramson, M.L., Osborn, J.J. and Gerbode, F. The membrane lung. In: *Techniques in Extracorporeal Circulation* (Ed. Ionescu, M.I.), 2nd edn, pp. 63–82. Butterworths, London (1981).

208 Lee, W.H. Jr, Krumhaar, D., Derry, G. *et al.* (1961) Comparison of the effects of membrane and non-membrane oxygenators on the biochemical and biophysical characteristics of blood. *Surg. Forum*, **12**, 200–202.

209 Drinker, P.A. (1972) Progress in membrane oxygenator design. *Anaesthesiology*, **37**, 242–260.

210 Zapol, W.M. and Qvist, J. (Eds) *Artificial Lungs for Acute Respiratory Failure.* Academic Press, New York (1975).

211 Solis, R.T., Kennedy, P.S., Beall, A.C. Jr *et al.* (1975) Cardiopulmonary bypass: microembolization and platelet aggregation. *Circulation*, **52**, 103–108.

212 Beall, A.C. Jr, Solis, R.T., Kakvan, M. *et al.* (1976) Clinical experience with the Teflon disposable membrane oxygenator. *Ann. Thorac. Surg.*, **21**, 144–150.

213 Courtney, J.M. and Gaylor, J.D.S. Artificial membranes. In: *Physics in Medicine and Biology Encyclopedia. Medical Physics, Bioengineering and Biophysics* (Ed. McAinsh, T.F.), pp. 22–26. Pergamon Press, Oxford (1985).

214 Bick, R.L. Alterations of hemostasis associated with surgery, cardiopulmonary bypass surgery, and prosthetic devices. In: *Disorders of Hemostasis* (Eds Ratnoff, O.D. & Forbes, C.D.), pp. 379–409. Grune & Stratton, New York (1984).

215 Edmunds, L.H. Jr and Stephenson, L.W. Cardiopulmonary bypass for open heart surgery. In: *Thoracic and Cardiovascular Surgery* (Eds Glen, W.W.L., Baue, A.E. & Lindskog, B.S.), pp. 1091–1106. Appleton-Century-Crofts, New York (1982).

216 Edmunds, L.H. Jr. (1982) Pulseless cardiopulmonary bypass. *J. Thorac. Cardiovasc. Surg.*, **84**, 800–804.

217 de Leval, M.R., Hill, J.D. and Mielke, C.H. Haematological aspects of extracorporeal circulation. In: *Techniques in Extracorporeal Circulation* (Ed. Ionescu, M.I.), 2nd edn, pp. 369–389. Butterworths, London (1981).

218 Edie, R.N., Haubert, S.M. and Malm, J.R. The use of haemodilution and a non-haemic prime for cardiopulmonary bypass. In: *Techniques in Extracorporeal Circulation* (Ed. Ionescu, M.I.), 2nd edn, pp. 179–198. Butterworths, London (1981).

219 Bartlett, R.H. and Gazzaniga, A.B. Physiology and pathophysiology of extracorporeal circulation. In: *Techniques in Extracorporeal Circulation* (Ed. Ionescu, M.I.), 2nd edn, pp. 1–43. Butterworths, London (1981).

220 Hara, M., Maris, M. Crumpler, J. *et al.* (1967) Effect of various priming solutions upon red cell mass, plasma volume, and extracellular fluid volume of dogs

following haemodilution technique of extracorporeal circulation. *J. Thorac. Cardiovasc. Surg.*, **53**, 353–359.

221 Peirce, E.C. II. *Extracorporeal Circulation for Open-Heart Surgery.* Thomas, Springfield (1969).

222 Pearson, D.T. Cardiotomy reservoirs and blood filters. In: *Techniques in Extracorporeal Circulation* (Ed. Ionescu, M.I.), 2nd edn, pp. 155–178. Butterworths, London (1981).

223 Allardyce, D.B., Yoshida, S.H. and Ashmore, P.G. (1966) The importance of microembolism in the pathogenesis of organ dysfunction caused by prolonged use of the pump oxygenator. *J. Thorac. Cardiovasc. Surg.*, **52**, 706–715.

224 Patterson, R.H. and Kessler, J. (1969) Microemboli during cardiopulmonary bypass detected by ultrasound. *Surg. Gynec. Obstet.*, **129**, 505–510.

225 Solis, R.T., Noon, G.P., Beall, A.C. and DeBakey, M.E. (1974) Particulate microembolism during cardiac operation. *Ann. Thorac. Surg.*, **17**, 332–344.

226 Lee, W.H. Jr, Krumhaar, D., Fonkalsrud, E.W. *et al.* (1961) Denaturation of plasma proteins as a cause of morbidity and death after intracardiac operations. *Surgery*, **50**, 29–39.

227 Salzmann, E.W. (1963) Blood platelets and extracorporeal circulation. *Transfusion*, **3**, 274–277.

228 Dutton, R.C., Edmunds, L.H. Jr, Hutchison, J.C. and Roe, B.B. (1974) Platelet aggregate emboli produced in patients during cardiopulmonary bypass with membrane and bubble oxygenators. *J. Thorac. Cardiovasc. Surg.*, **67**, 258–265.

229 McKenna, R., Bachman, F., Whittaker, B. *et al.* (1975) The hemostatic mechanism after open-heart surgery. II. Frequency of abnormal platelet functions during and after extracorporeal circulation. *J. Thorac. Cardiovasc. Surg.*, **70**, 298–308.

230 Harker, L.A., Malpass, T.W., Branson, H.E. *et al.* (1980) Mechanism of abnormal bleeding in patients undergoing cardiopulmonary bypass: acquired transient platelet dysfunction associated with selective α-granule release. *Blood*, **56**, 824–834.

231 Davies, G.C., Sobel, M. and Salzman, E.W. (1980) Elevated plasma fibrinopeptide A and thromboxane B_2 levels during cardiopulmonary bypass. *Circulation*, **61**, 808–814.

232 Addonizio, V.P. Jr, Smith, J.B., Strauss, J.F. III *et al.* (1980) Thromboxane synthesis and platelet secretion during cardiopulmonary bypass with a bubble oxygenator. *J. Thorac. Cardiovasc. Surg.*, **79**, 91–96.

233 Dutton, R.C. and Edmunds, L.H. Jr. (1973) Measurement of emboli in extracorporeal perfusion systems. *J. Thorac. Cardiovasc. Surg.*, **65**, 523–530.

234 de Leval, M., Hill, J.D., Mielke, H. *et al.* (1972) Platelet kinetics during extracorporeal circulation. *Trans. Am. Soc. Artif. Intern. Organs*, **18**, 355–358.

235 de Vries, S.I., van Creveld, S., Groen, P. *et al.* (1961) Studies on the coagulation of the blood in patients treated with extracorporeal circulation. *Thromb. Diathes. Haemorrh.*, **5**, 426–446.

236 Müller, N., Popov-Cenic, S., Buttner, W. *et al.* (1975) Studies of fibrinolytic and coagulation factors during open heart surgery. II. Postoperative bleeding tendency and changes in the coagulation system. *Thromb. Res.*, **7**, 589–598.

237 Bick, R., Schmalhorst, W., Crawford, L. *et al.* (1975) The hemorrhagic diathesis created by cardiopulmonary bypass. *Am. J. Clin. Pathol.*, **63**, 588.

238 Edmunds, L.H. Jr, Ellison, N., Colman, R.W. *et al.* (1982) Platelet function during cardiac operation. Comparison of membrane and bubble oxygenators. *J. Thorac. Cardiovasc. Surg.*, **83**, 805–812.

239 Liddicoat, J.E., Bekassy, S.M., Beall, A.C. Jr. *et al.* (1975) Membrane vs. bubble oxygenator: clinical comparison. *Ann. Surg.*, **181**, 747–753.

240 Siderys, H., Herod, G.T., Halbrook, H. *et al.* (1975) A comparison of membrane and bubble oxygenation as used in cardiopulmonary bypass. *J. Thorac. Cardiovasc. Surg.*, **69**, 708–712.

241 Wright, J.S., Fisk, G.C., Torda, T.A. *et al.* (1975) Some advantages of the membrane oxygenator for open-heart surgery. *J. Thorac. Cardiovasc. Surg.*, **69**, 884–890.

242 Mortensen, J.D. (1977) Evaluation of tests for blood damage produced by oxygenators. *Trans. Am. Soc. Artif. Intern. Organs*, **23**, 747–755.

243 Clark, R.E., Beauchamp, R.A., Magrath, R.A. *et al.* (1979) Comparison of bubble and membrane oxygenators in short and long perfusions. *J. Thorac. Cardiovasc. Surg.*, **78**, 655–666.

244 De Jong, J.C.F., Smit Sibinga, C. Th. and Wildevuur Ch., R.H. (1979) Platelet behaviour in extracorporeal circulation. *Transfusion*, **19**, 72–80.

245 Peterson, K.A., Dewanjee, M.K. and Kaye, M.P. (1982) Fate of indium 111-labelled platelets during cardiopulmonary bypass performed with membrane and bubble oxygenators. *J. Thorac. Cardiovasc. Surg.*, **84**, 39–43.

246 Peirce, E.C. II. (1980) The membrane versus bubble oxygenator controversy. *Ann. Thorac. Surg.*, **29**, 497–499.

247 Addonizio, V.P. Jr, Strauss, J.F. III., Colman, R.W. and Edmunds, L.H. Jr. (1979) Effects of prostaglandin E_1 on platelet loss during *in vivo* and *in vitro* extracorporeal circulation with a bubble oxygenator. *J. Thorac. Cardiovasc. Surg.*, **77**, 119–126.

248 Addonizio, V.P. Jr, Macarak, E.J., Niewiarowski, S. *et al.* (1979) Preservation of human platelets with prostaglandin E_1 during *in vitro* simulation of cardiopulmonary bypass. *Circ. Res.*, **44**, 350–357.

249 Irvine, L., Sundaram, S., Courtney, J.M. *et al.* (1991) Monitoring of Factor XII activity and granulocyte elastase release during cardiopulmonary bypass. *Trans. Am. Soc. Artif. Intern. Organs*, **37**, 569–571.

250 Sundaram, S., Irvine, L., Courtney, J.M. *et al.* (1992) Patterns of blood response during cardiopulmonary bypass. *Int. J. Artif. Organs*, **15**, 243–248.

251 Bernstein, E.F., Blackshear, P.L. Jr and Keller, K.H. (1967) Factors influencing erythrocyte destruction in artificial organs. *Am. J. Surg.*, **114**, 126–138.

252 Bernstein, E.F., Indeglia, R.A., Shea, M.A. and Varco, R.L. (1967) Sublethal damage to the red blood cell from pumping. *Circulation*, **35** (Suppl. 1), 226–233.

253 Chopra, P.S., Dufek, J.H., Kroncke, G.M. *et al.* (1973) Clinical comparison of the General Electric–Peirce membrane lung and bubble oxygenator for prolonged cardiopulmonary bypass. *Surgery*, **74**, 874–879.

254 Alon, L., Turrina, M. and Gattiker, R. (1979) Membrane and bubble oxygenator: a clinical comparison in patients undergoing aortocoronary bypass procedures. *Herz*, **4**, 56–62.

255 Pranger, R.L., Mook, P.H., Elstrodt, J.M. *et al.* (1980) Improved tissue perfusion (PO_2 histograms) in extracorporeal circulation using membrane instead of bubble oxygenators. *J. Thorac. Cardiovasc. Surg.*, **79**, 513–522.

256 Timmes, J.J. and Wilson, J.W. (1973) Microcirculatory considerations in extracorporeal oxygenation. *NY State J. Med.*, **73**, 2337–2346.

257 Ratliff, N.B., Young, W.G. Jr, Hackel, D.B. *et al.* (1973) Pulmonary injury secondary to extracorporeal circulation: an ultrastructural study. *J. Thorac. Cardiovasc. Surg.*, **65**, 425–432.

258 Edmunds, L.H. Jr and Addonizio, V.P. Jr. Platelet physiology during cardiopulmonary bypass. In: *Pathophysiology and Techniques of Cardiopulmonary Bypass* (Ed. Utley, J.R.), pp. 106–119. Williams & Wilkins, Baltimore (1981).

259 Hohn, D.C., Meyers, A.J., Gherini, S.T. *et al.* (1980) Production of acute pulmonary injury by leukocytes and activated complement. *Surgery*, **88**, 48–58.

260 Del Maestro, R.F., Thaw, H.H., Bjork, J. *et al.* (1980) Free radicals as mediators of tissue injury. *Acta Physiol. Scand.*, **492** (Suppl.), 43–57.

261 Westaby, S., Fleming, J. and Royston, D. (1985) Acute lung injury during cardiopulmonary bypass, the role of neutrophil sequestration and lipid peroxidation. *Trans. Am. Soc. Artif. Intern. Organs*, **31**, 604–608.

262 Royston, D., Fleming, J.S., Westaby, S. *et al.* (1985) Neutrophil kinetics and oxidative injury associated with cardiopulmonary bypass. *Thorax*, **40**, 240 (Abstract).

263 Royston, D., Fleming, J.S., Braude, S. *et al.* (1986) Lung injury following cardiopulmonary bypass; the potential role of oxidant-free radicals. *Life Support Systems* **4**, 151–154.

264 Wolf, B., Zeplin, H.E., Reinards, R. *et al.* Elastase: a sensitive indicator for granulocyte lesions by extracorporeal oxygenators. In: *Progress in Artificial Organs–1985* (Eds Nosé, Y., Kjellstrand, C. & Ivanovich, P.), pp. 575–578. ISAO Press, Cleveland (1986).

265 Riegel, W., Spillner, G., Schlosser, V. and Hörl, W.H. (1988) Plasma levels of main granulocyte components during cardiopulmonary bypass. *J. Thorac. Cardiovasc. Surg.*, **95**, 1014–1019.

266 Kusserow, B. and Larrow, R. (1968) Studies of leukocyte responses to prolonged blood pumping—effects upon phagocytic capability and total white cell count. *Trans. Am. Soc. Artif. Intern. Organs*, **14**, 261–263.

267 Silva, J. Jr, Hoeksema, H. and Fekety, F.R. Jr. (1974) Transient defects in phagocytic functions during cardiopulmonary bypass. *J. Thorac. Cardiovasc. Surg.*, **67**, 175–183.

268 Hammerschmidt, D.E., Stroncek, D.F., Bowers, T.K. *et al.* (1981) Complement activation and neutropenia during bypass. *J. Thorac. Cardiovasc. Surg.*, **81**, 370–377.

269 Kirklin, J.K., Westaby, S., Blackstone, E.H. *et al.* (1983) Complement and the damaging effects of cardiopulmonary bypass. *J. Thorac. Cardiovasc. Surg.*, **86**, 845–857.

270 Wildevuur, Ch. R.H. and Oeveren, W.V. (1986) Artificial lung: current problems. *Life Support Systems*, (Suppl. 1) 130–135.

271 Collett, B., Alhaq, A., Abdullah, N.B. *et al.* (1984) Pathways to complement activation during cardiopulmonary bypass. *Br. Med. J.*, **289**, 1251–1254.

272 Parker, D.J., Cantrell, J.W., Karp, R.B. *et al.* (1972) Changes in serum complement and immunoglobulins following cardiopulmonary bypass. *Surgery*, **71**, 824–827.

273 Boralessa, H., Shifferli, J.A., Zaimi, F. *et al.* (1982) Perioperative changes in complement associated with cardiopulmonary bypass. *Br. J. Anaesth.*, **54**, 1047–1052.

274 Rent, R., Ertel, N., Eisenstein, R. and Gewurz, H. (1975) Complement activation

by interaction of polyanions and polycations. *J. Immunol.*, **114**, 120–124.
275 Chenoweth, D.E., Cooper, S.W., Hugli, T.E. *et al.* (1981) Complement activation during cardiopulmonary bypass: evidence for generation of C3a and C5a anaphylatoxins. *New Engl. J. Med.*, **304**, 497–503.
276 Boscoe, M.J., Yewdall, V.M.A., Thompson, M.A. and Cameron, J.S. (1983) Complement activation during cardiopulmonary bypass: quantitative study of effects of methylprednisolone and pulsatile flow. *Br. Med. J.*, **287**, 1747–1750.
277 Kazatchkine, M.D. (1986) Alterations in host defence mechanism associated with cardiopulmonary bypass. *Life Support Systems*, (Suppl. 1), 144–152.
278 Craddock, P.R., Fehr, J., Brigham, K.L. *et al.* (1977) Complement and leukocyte-mediated pulmonary dysfunction in hemodialysis. *New Engl. J. Med.*, **296**, 769–774.
279 Haslam, P.L., Townsend, P.J. and Branthwaite, M.A. (1980) Complement during cardiopulmonary bypass. *Anaesthesia*, **35**, 22–26.
280 Westaby, S. (1983) Complement and the damaging effects of cardiopulmonary bypass. *Thorax*, **38**, 321–325.
281 Wysocki, H., Ponizyński, A., Wierusz-Wysocka, B. *et al.* (1982) Cardiopulmonary bypass-induced complement activation. Evidence for C5a participation. *Int. J. Artif. Organs*, **5**, 305–308.
282 Gomes, M.R. and McGoon, D. (1970) Bleeding patterns after open-heart surgery. *J. Thorac. Cardiovasc. Surg.*, **60**, 87–97.
283 Takahama, T., Kanai, F., Iizuka, I. *et al.* (1984) Application of a new prostaglandin I_2 analogue (APS-306) on cardiopulmonary bypass. *Trans. Am. Soc. Artif. Intern. Organs*, **30**, 44–48.
284 Rådegran, K., Arén, C. and Teger-Nilsson, A.-C. (1982) Prostacyclin infusion during extracorporeal circulation for coronary bypass. *J. Thorac. Cardiovasc. Surg.*, **83**, 205–211.
285 Faichney, A., Davidson, K.G., Wheatley, D.J. *et al.* (1982) Prostacyclin in cardiopulmonary bypass. *J. Thorac. Cardiovasc. Surg.*, **84**, 601–608.
286 Miyamoto, H., Hirose, H., Matsuda, H. *et al.* (1985) Analysis of complement activation profile during cardiopulmonary bypass and its inhibition by FUT-175. *Trans. Am. Soc. Artif. Intern. Organs*, **31**, 508–510.
287 Heller, W., Fuhrer, G., Gallimore, M.J. *et al.* Changes in the kallikrein–kinin-system after different dose regimen of aprotonin during cardiopulmonary bypass operation. In: *Kinins V Part B. Advances in Experimental Medicine and Biology* (Eds Abe, K., Moriya, H. & Fujii, S.), Vol. 247B, pp. 43–48. Plenum, New York (1989).
288 Ohtani, M., Matsuda, H., Shirakura, R. *et al.* (1988) Attenuation of pulmonary leukocyte sequestration during extracorporeal circulation by a new c-AMP phosphodiesterase inhibitor. *Trans. Am. Soc. Artif. Intern. Organs*, **34**, 761–764.
289 Tatsumi, E., Matsuda, T., Takano, H. *et al.* (1988) A synthetic tetrapeptide as a novel platelet-preserving agent during cardiopulmonary bypass. *Trans. Am. Soc. Artif. Intern. Organs*, **34**, 813–816.
290 Addonizio, V.P. Jr, Macarak, E.J., Nicolau, K.C. *et al.* (1979) Effects of prostacyclin and albumin on platelet loss during an *in vitro* simulation of extracorporeal circulation. *Blood*, **53**, 1033–1042.
291 Whittlesey, G.C., Kundu, S.K., Salley, S.O. *et al.* (1988) Is heparin necessary for

extracorporeal circulation? *Trans. Am. Soc. Artif. Intern. Organs*, **34**, 823–826.

292 Cottonaro, C.N., Roohk, H.V., Bartlett, R.H. *et al.* (1982) A new non-thrombogenic surface. *Trans. Am. Soc. Artif. Intern. Organs*, **28**, 478–481.

293 Bindslev, L., Eklund, L., Norlander, O. *et al.* (1987) Treatment of acute respiratory failure by extracorporeal carbon dioxide elimination performed with surface heparinized artificial lung. *Anesthesiology*, **67**, 117–120.

294 Mottaghy, K., Oedekoven, B., Pöppel, K. *et al.* (1989) Heparin free long-term extracorporeal circulation using bioactive surfaces. *Trans. Am. Soc. Artif. Intern. Organs*, **35**, 635–637.

295 Nilsson, L., Storm, K.E., Thelim, S. *et al.* (1990) Heparin-coated equipment reduces complement activation during cardiopulmonary bypass in the pig. *Artif. Organs*, **14**, 46–48.

296 Black, M.M., Drury, P.J. and Tindale, W.B. (1983) Twenty-five years of heart valve substitutes: a review. *J. Roy. Soc. Med.*, **76**, 667–680.

297 Dellsperger, K.C. and Chandran, K.B. Prosthetic heart valves. In: *Blood Compatible Materials and Devices* (Eds Sharma, C.P. & Szycher, M.), pp. 153–165. Technomic, Lancaster, PA (1991).

298 Lee, J.M. and Boughner, D.R. Bioprosthetic heart valves: tissue mechanics and implications for design. In: *Blood Compatible Materials and Devices* (Eds Sharma, C.P. & Szycher, M.), pp. 167–188. Technomic, Lancaster, PA (1991).

299 Klinkmann, H. Progress in artificial organs. In: *Progress in Bioengineering* (Eds Paul, J.P., Barbenel, J.C., Courtney, J.M. & Kenedi, R.M.), pp. 7–12. Adam Hilger, Bristol (1989).

300 Falkenhagen, D. Some aspects of new developments in biomedical technology. In: *The Influence of New Technologies on Medical Practice* (Eds Paul, J.P., Rappelsberger, P. & Schütz, P.W.), pp. 99–109. Verlag für medizinische Wissenschaften Wilhelm Maudrich, Vienna (1991).

301 Burns, G.L. and Olsen, D.B. (1989) Immune response changes with blood pump use in calves. *Trans. Am. Soc. Artif. Intern. Organs*, **35**, 700–702.

302 Solen, K.A., Mohammad, S.F., Reynolds, L.O. *et al.* (1989) Characterization of blood microemboli associated with *ex vivo* left ventricular assist devices in a bovine model. *Trans. Am. Soc. Artif. Intern. Organs*, **35**, 370–372.

303 Taenaka, Y., Matsuda, T., Takano, H. *et al.* Influences of ventricular assist device pumping on blood coagulation. *Trans. Am. Soc. Artif. Intern. Organs*, **35**, 396–398.

304 Rosen, J.J. (1988) The role of biomaterials science in the next generation of artificial organ technology. *Trans. Am. Soc. Artif. Intern. Organs*, **34**, 163–167.

305 Mujais, S.K. (1988) New membranes: the promise of ingenuity. *Int. J. Artif. Organs*, **11**, 219–222.

306 Mohammad, S.F. and Olsen, D.B. (1986) Reduced platelet adhesion and activation of coagulation factors on polyurethane treated with albumin-IgG complex. *Trans. Am. Soc. Artif. Intern. Organs*, **32**, 323–326.

307 Greisler, H.P., Klosak, J.J., Steinam, S. *et al.* (1989) Platelet interactions with heparin binding growth factor and fibronectin. *Trans. Am. Soc. Artif. Intern. Organs*, **35**, 561–563.

308 Chandy, T. and Sharma, C.P. (1988) Changes in albumin/platelet interaction with an artificial surface—due to antibiotics, pyridoxal phosphate, and lympho-

cytes. *Artif. Organs*, **12**, 143–151.

309 Takahama, T., Kanai, F., Hiraishi, M. *et al.* (1990) Combined administration of protease inhibitor and thromboxane A_2 synthetase inhibitor for anticoagulation of a left ventricle assist device. *Trans. Am. Soc. Artif. Intern. Organs*, **36**, M141–M144.

310 Teraoka, S., Takahashi, K., Suzuki, T. *et al.* (1990) Non-heparin hemodialysis with oral administration of newly developed antiplatelet agent. *Trans. Am. Soc. Artif. Intern. Organs*, **36**, M212–M215.

311 Takemoto, Y., Matsuda, T., Kishimoto, T. *et al.* (1989) Molecular understanding of cellular adhesion on artificial surfaces. *Trans. Am. Soc. Artif. Intern. Organs*, **35**, 354–356.

312 Schoen, F.J., Clagett, G.P., Hill, J.D. *et al.* (1987) The biocompatibility of artificial organs. *Trans. Am. Soc. Artif. Intern. Organs*, **33**, 824–833.

313 Lundin, A.P. (1988) The pathology of hemodialysis as seen in the long-surviving patient: consequences of hemodialysis to the human body. *Artif. Organs*, **12**, 122–123.

Part 3
Management

Chapter 13
Effects of haemorrhage

IAN S. GRANT AND CHARLES P.J. MORTON

The principal effects of haemorrhage stem from the impairment of oxygen delivery to organs and tissues. Following major haemorrhage a number of compensatory mechanisms are activated which mitigate the effects of blood loss for a short period but, if unchecked, haemorrhage rapidly leads to a state of hypovolaemic shock. The shock state should not be defined in haemodynamic terms alone, but rather in terms of oxygen supply to and oxygen utilization by the tissues, since it is the inadequacy of oxygen supply and possibly also reperfusion of ischaemic tissue that leads to functional and structural disturbances.

While the various shock syndromes (hypovolaemic; distributive; cardiogenic) can be defined at an early clinical stage by haemodynamic measurements, in late shock the pathophysiological changes present are similar and independent of aetiology. End-stage shock in turn inevitably leads to the syndrome of multiple organ failure and carries an extremely poor prognosis. Thus optimization of outcome in the bleeding patient requires an early recognition of hypovolaemia, prompt and appropriate restoration of circulating volume, successful haemostasis and continuous monitoring and, if necessary, support of organ function.

Consequences of whole blood loss

Haemorrhage results in the loss of all constituents of whole blood: red and white blood cells, platelets, clotting factors, proteins, water and electrolytes. Loss of red blood cells reduces oxygen-carrying capacity while loss of circulating fluid volume results in a reduction of cardiac output, compounding the overall reduction in tissue oxygen delivery.

Effects on oxygen transport

Oxygen delivery ($D\text{O}_2$) is the product of arterial oxygen content ($Ca\text{O}_2$) and cardiac output (CO). Since CO varies according to the size of the patient, it is usually indexed for body surface area (CI). The Do_2 measurements are thus likewise indexed and expressed in units of ml/min/m^2. Oxygen content depends on haemoglobin concentration and its percentage oxygen saturation. Oxygen carriage is affected not just by a reduction in haemoglobin concentration but also by the affinity of oxygen for haemoglobin. Acidosis shifts the oxygen dissociation curve to the right, improving tissue oxygen release but a reduction in 2,3-diphosphoglycerate (DPG) has the opposite effect and may affect oxygen availability to the tissues. To measure overall body oxygen consumption (Vo_2) in clinical practice requires the sampling of mixed venous blood from the distal lumen of a pulmonary artery catheter and an oximeter to measure the mixed venous oxygen saturation (Svo_2). Vo_2 is then measured using the reverse Fick equation (Fig. 13.1).

$$\begin{aligned} Do_2 &= \mathrm{CI} \times Cao_2 \times 10\,\mathrm{ml/min/m^2} \\ Vo_2 &= \mathrm{CI} \times C(\mathrm{a}-\mathrm{v})\mathrm{o}_2 \times 10\,\mathrm{ml/min/m^2} \\ Cao_2 &= \mathrm{Hb} \times Sao_2 \times 1.39 + Pao_2\ (\mathrm{kPa}) \times 0.02\,\mathrm{ml/100\,ml} \end{aligned}$$

Clearly, in the vast majority of bleeding patients adequacy of cardiorespiratory function, and in particular oxygen delivery, can be gauged from basic clinical signs—respiratory rate, heart rate, blood pressure, urinary output and mental status. Nevertheless, the more invasive precise monitoring of oxygen transport variables in critically ill patients involving the use of arterial and pulmonary artery catheters has improved our understanding of the pathophysiology of shock and modified our approach to therapy. For example, in patients with trauma or haemorrhage who are at risk of developing the adult respiratory distress syndrome (ARDS), those who developed ARDS had greater reductions in blood volume and Do_2 than those who did not [1]. Furthermore, in a broad group of critically ill surgical patients, non-survivors had a lower CI and Do_2 than survivors [2]. A reduced Do_2 in such patients is associated with a reduction in tissue oxygen consumption, as a result of impaired control of oxygen utilization. Implementation of a goal-directed therapy regimen with the aim of achieving supranormal values of CI, Do_2 and Vo_2 appears to reduce mortality markedly [3].

Following major trauma, and thus by inference other stressful situations such as major haemorrhage, oxygen consumption increases markedly at the expense of an increased oxygen extraction ratio and decreased Svo_2 [4]. An Svo_2 as low as 50% means that blood returning to the heart from some tissues has a much lower saturation, and thus cells at the venous end of the microcirculation are receiving blood from

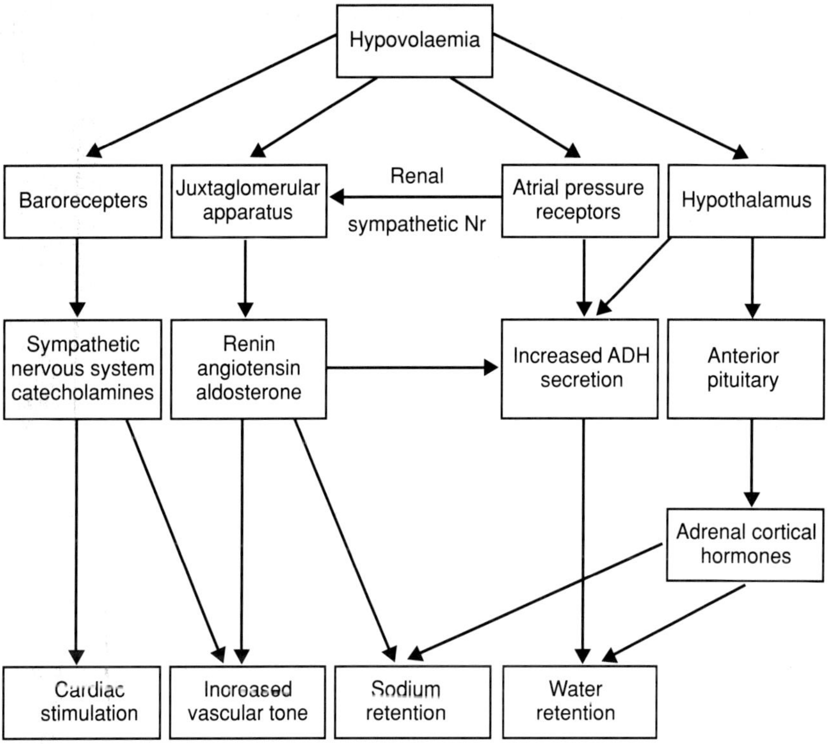

Fig. 13.1 Homoeostatic responses to haemorrhage.

which almost all extractable oxygen has already been removed. This results in anaerobiasis and lactic acidosis. Therapy to increase $D\text{O}_2$, consisting of oxygen, and fluid resuscitation with colloid and blood, results in a reduction in the oxygen extraction ratio and elevation of $S\text{vO}_2$ with benefits to tissue oxygenation.

Water and electrolyte losses

Water and electrolyte losses from the circulation are to some extent replenished both by fluid shift from the extravascular compartment and by salt and water retention. A total body fluid deficit remains however, and this justifies the inclusion of some crystalloid in resuscitation infusion regimens. Interstitial fluid losses amounting to 25% of overt blood loss [5].

Other losses

Unless haemorrhage requires transfusion of more than one blood volume (8–10 units in an adult male) the loss and/or dilution of platelets and clotting factors is unlikely to be associated with a haemostatic problem in patients without underlying medical problems [6]. Coagulopathy associated with haemorrhage may, however, occur due to the effects of hypoxia, especially on the liver, tissue damage and sepsis as well as coexisting liver or bone-marrow disorder.

White blood cells in the circulation represent only a small fraction of the total number in the body as they are stored sixfold in the bone marrow and 12-fold in the tissues, and thus their loss from haemorrhage is relatively insignificant.

Homoeostatic responses to bleeding

Many integrated physiological mechanisms have evolved in man, with the aim of limiting blood loss and maintaining perfusion of vital organs (Fig. 13.1). These compensatory mechanisms are activated rapidly and may successfully maintain blood pressure and perfusion for a limited period. If bleeding is self-limiting or is controlled at an early stage, the body's homoeostatic mechanisms can in time achieve restoration of circulating volume and replenishment of lost blood constituents. Nevertheless, certain of the body's responses appear inappropriate and may adversely affect outcome.

Limitation of blood loss

Haemostasis has been discussed already in Chapter 1.

Limitation of the fall in cardiac output and maintenance of perfusion pressure

Provision of adequate blood flow and oxygen delivery to tissues demands the maintenance of a relatively constant perfusion pressure. In the face of blood loss the sympathetic nervous system is activated in an attempt to maintain an adequate pressure by means of arteriolar constriction, usually at the expense of blood flow.

Blood loss causes reductions in capacitance volume, venous return and both right and left end-diastolic volumes, which in turn lead to a fall in cardiac output. A fall in blood pressure is detected by the baroreceptors of the carotid sinuses and aortic arch and results in decreased afferent impulses passing to the medullary vasomotor centre. An increase in sympathetic discharge follows, with a number of effects:

1 Arteriolar constriction brings about an increase in overall systemic vascular resistance and hence blood pressure. Constriction occurs predominantly, at least initially in skin, muscle and splanchnic beds, redistributing blood flow to maintain brain, heart and renal perfusion. Regional tissue perfusion may be adversely affected in an attempt to maintain blood pressure and vital-organ perfusion.

2 Constriction of venous capacitance vessels leads to an increase in venous return and maintenance of filling pressures and cardiac output.

3 There is an increase in myocardial contractility and heart rate, the latter in part due to decreased parasympathetic discharge in an attempt to maintain cardiac output.

The effects of the increased sympathetic discharge are augmented by secretion of adrenaline and noradrenaline from the adrenal medulla. These cause further constriction in poorly innervated vessels as well as causing anxiety and restlessness.

Baroreceptor regulation is maximal within the limits of normal blood pressure. As pressure falls further, peripheral chemoreceptors in the carotid and aortic bodies are stimulated by a local reduction in oxygen tension secondary to decreased perfusion, resulting in a similar sympathetic pressor response and hyperventilation.

Although the neurohumeral responses described above typically produce tachycardia in response to blood loss, this is not invariable. Studies of venesection in human volunteers and animals reported an initial increase in heart rate and peripheral resistance, but as blood loss proceeded to >30% of total volume, both heart rate and resistance fell in some subjects [7,8]. This lack of a tachycardic response has also been observed in patients with massive haemorrhage of varying aetiology, and has been attributed variously to stimulation of pressure receptors in the ventricles with vagal reflex activity, and to an endogenous opioid mechanism [9]. Thus it may be, especially in cases of occult major bleeding, that heart rate is not a good guide to the extent of haemorrhage.

Regulation of organ blood flow

Blood flow to the various organs and tissues of the body is regulated to meet changing demand. Changes in metabolism and blood flow are coupled by variation in arteriolar tone; accumulation of metabolic waste products generally leads to vasodilatation and increased flow. This process of autoregulation varies in speed and efficiency between and within organs, but relies on the maintenance of an adequate overall perfusion pressure.

The cerebral, coronary and renal circulations have efficient autoregulatory systems and can preserve a constant blood flow by varying local arteriolar tone within a range of blood pressure (mean perfusion pressure 60–130 mmHg for cerebral circulation). In contrast, skin, muscle and splanchnic circulations are sacrificed in situations of severe blood loss by adrenergic-mediated constriction to maintain overall perfusion pressure.

Other emergency mechanisms exist to maintain blood pressure during severe blood loss. These include angiotensin II, a very powerful constrictor of arterioles of skin, kidney and splanchnic beds, and antidiuretic hormone (ADH) which augments splanchnic vasoconstriction induced by catecholamines and angiotensin II. Whereas baroreceptor-mediated vasoconstriction occurs within seconds, the renin–angiotensin system takes around 20 min to produce vasoconstriction.

Maintenance of circulating volume

Circulating volume is maintained within normal limits by a system involving low-pressure receptors in the artria innervated by the vagus nerve, and the secretion of renin, aldosterone and ADH. In severe haemorrhage, decreased stimulation of the atrial receptors is transmitted by the vagus to the brainstem. This leads to increased renal sympathetic activity, posterior pituitary secretion of ADH and, through the anterior pituitary–adrenal axis, an increase in adrenocorticoid secretion. Underperfusion of the juxtaglomerular apparatus causes release of renin, initiating the production of angiotensin II. As well as being a powerful vasoconstrictor, angiotensin promotes (active) salt and (passive) water retention both by direct effect on the kidney and by stimulation of aldosterone secretion from the adrenal cortex. The overall effect is of oliguria, salt and water retention, reducing further fluid loss from the circulation.

Mobilization of fluid from other body compartments

The movement of fluid between intravascular and extravascular compartments depends upon the relationship between hydrostatic and oncotic pressures across the capillary wall as well as on capillary permeability. Arteriolar constriction following haemorrhage leads to a reduction in capillary hydrostatic pressure and thus alters the balance towards a net movement of fluid into the circulation. Thus losses from the circulation are gradually replenished, but at the expense of the interstitial and intracellular compartments. Intracellular dehydration is the stimulant for the thirst that is often experienced with severe blood loss. Following experimental haemorrhage of 10–20% of total blood volume over 20–40 min, transcapillary fluid shift restored circulating volume to normal within 30–40 h [10]. Salt and water retention and increased intake then restores the interstitial compartment within a few days. Transcapillary fluid shifts later on in shock are discussed below.

Increased erythropoiesis occurs within 24 h of major haemorrhage, although new red cells do not appear in the circulation until 5 days later. Plasma proteins are in equilibrium with tissue proteins in a constant process of synthesis and degradation, but following haemorrhage there is evidence of increased albumin synthesis.

Consequences of continued untreated haemorrhage

As previously stated, the major consequence of haemorrhage is a reduction in tissue oxygenation. Lack of oxygen has devastating effects on cell metabolism, ultimately leading to cellular destruction. The final common metabolic pathway, the citric acid cycle and cytochrome C oxidase system situated in cell mitochondria, is involved in the production of adenosine triphosphate (ATP), the principal high-energy phosphate compound in the body, and the main source of biological energy. When ATP is split into adenosine diphosphate (ADP) and inorganic phosphate, the high-energy bond holding the third phosphate releases its energy. Aerobic metabolism is the most efficient way of producing ATP for a given quantity of glucose. Anaerobic metabolism involving the conversion of pyruvate to lactate is much less efficient in terms of ATP production.

Aerobic metabolism

Glucose $\rightarrow$ Pyruvic acid $\rightarrow Co_2 + H_2O + 38$ ATP

Anaerobic metabolism

Glucose $\rightarrow$ Pyruvic acid $\rightarrow$ Lactic acid $+ 2$ ATP

To achieve production of the large amounts of ATP required under hypoxic conditions, much greater amounts of glucose are required than can be consumed. ATP depletion therefore occurs. Furthermore, there is an accumulation of lactic acid, with resultant acidosis. Oxidative phosphorylation ceases and anaerobic metabolism ensues when the mitochondrial P_{O_2} falls to around 0.13 kPa, although this critical level may differ from one tissue to another.

The first consequence of ATP depletion at a cellular level is derangement of the energy-dependent ATPases leading to dysfunction of cell-membrane channels [11,12]. Sodium, calcium and water enter the cells while potassium escapes down concentration gradients, and cell swelling occurs. Intracellular membranes such as the sarcoplasmic reticulum are also disrupted, leading to loss of regulation of intracellular movement of calcium ions and ultimately to cell death [13].

As endothelial cells become hypoxic, anaerobic metabolism yields lactic acid, which along with kinins, histamine and other vasoactive substances such as prostaglandins, has dilating effects on arterioles. Venules remain more resistant to dilatation and capillary hydrostatic pressure rises, leading to fluid loss into the interstitial and intracellular compartments. This loss is aggravated by increased capillary permeability caused by vasoactive mediators such as histamine released from mast cells and kinins produced by proteolytic enzyme action. This clinical picture of vasodilatation producing hypotension and capillary leakage causing hypovolaemia is compounded by myocardial depression caused by hypoxia, acidosis and myocardial depressant factor, a peptide released from hypoxic pancreas. It is the typical picture of septic shock but is the end result of all shock states, no matter what the initial aetiology. One further factor in its development may well be gut ischaemia and endotoxin translocation from the bowel with subsequent Kupffer-cell activation and mediator release.

Mediators of shock

The area of mediator release in shock is an extremely complex one and knowledge in this field is continually evolving [14,15]. A number of cell groups are particularly involved, namely granulocytes, lymphocytes, macrophages, platelets and vascular endothelial cells, and a number of biochemical cascade reactions occur activated by proteolytic enzymes released from hypoxic or activated cells (Fig. 13.2):

- Complement system.
- Arachidonic acid cascade.
- Coagulation cascade.
- Fibrinolytic system.
- Kallikrein–kinin system.

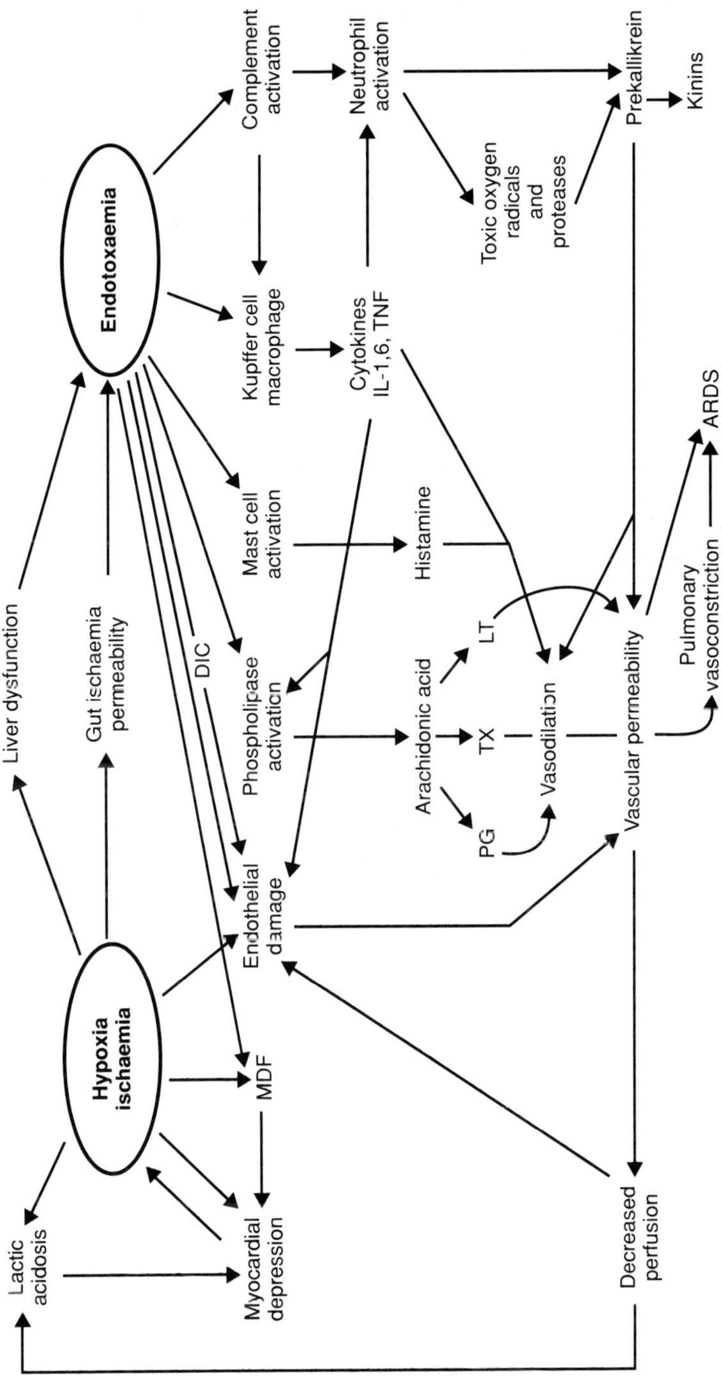

Fig. 13.2 Effect of hypoxia/ischaemia in end-stage shock and role of endotoxin.

Release of lysosomal enzymes from hypoxic cells occurs particularly in the liver and pancreas, which are supplied by the vulnerable splanchnic circulation [13]. Proteolytic action leads to the production of kinins and complement factors C3a and C5a, as well as histamine being released. Endotoxin escaping into the systemic circulation in combination with C3a and C5a leads to activation and adherence of granulocytes to the capillary endothelium; this is most clearly demonstrated in the pulmonary circulation in ARDS [16]. Granulocytes then release proteolytic enzymes such as elastase, collagenase and cathepsin G. Elastase in particular appears to be essential for neutrophil-induced endothelial injury, and its plasma level appears to be related to the severity of the disease process. Granulocytes also release toxic oxygen radicals and arachidonic acid metabolites.

Phospholipase A_2 acts on phospholipid in destabilized hypoxic cell membranes to produce arachidonic acid, which undergoes cyclo-oxygenation to form prostaglandins such as PGE_1, PGE_2, prostacyclin and thromboxane A_2, or lipoxygenation to form the leucotrienes. The vasodilator prostaglandins contribute to systemic vasodilatation and capillary permeability, while thromboxane A_2 causes pulmonary vasoconstriction and the leucotrienes contribute to the pulmonary capillary leak of ARDS.

The role of the macrophage in the pathogenesis of multiple organ failure appears to be particularly important. The liver Kupffer cells, which constitute 70% of all macrophages, are stimulated by endotoxin to release cytokines such as interleukin-1 (IL-1), tumour necrosis factor (TNF) and IL-6, which are associated with many of the features of multiple organ failure such as hypotension, vasodilatation, tachycardia and pyrexia. The cytokines may be mediators of many of the effects of endotoxin such as complement system and granulocyte activation. In addition, macrophages, which may also be activated by C5a and granulocytes, release proteolytic enzymes, PGE_2 and toxic oxygen radicals.

The effect of haemorrhage on organ systems

Respiratory system

In the early stages of haemorrhagic shock hyperventilation occurs both as a result of the action of catecholamines on the CNS and the stimulation of peripheral and central chemoreceptors by hypoxia and acidosis, respectively. Hypoxaemia may be an early feature due to increased intrapulmonary shunting, while the low mixed venous oxygen saturation consequent upon the reduced cardiac output further exacerbates arterial hypoxaemia.

Adult respiratory distress syndrome

Prolonged uncorrected haemorrhage is one of the principal conditions associated with the development of ARDS. The term 'ARDS' is used to describe a condition of acute respiratory failure with severe hypoxaemia refractory to high inspired oxygen concentrations and requiring ventilatory support. Other features are diffuse infiltrates on chest X-ray, reduced pulmonary compliance and a pulmonary artery wedge pressure of <18 mmHg to exclude cardiogenic pulmonary oedema. Only a minority of patients with a predisposing factor actually develop ARDS, around 5% in the case of patients with haemorrhagic shock [17]. Mortality may be depressingly high and varies depending upon the predisposing condition, with a rate of 45% associated with massive blood loss and transfusion [17]. Death is rarely due directly to respiratory failure (15% of patients), and is more commonly the result of sepsis syndrome and multiple organ failure [18].

Studies of the cardiorespiratory patterns of patients with trauma or haemorrhage who are at risk of developing ARDS showed that those who developed the syndrome had greater reductions of blood volume, red-cell mass and Do_2, and a higher pulmonary vascular resistance than those who did not [1]. Non-survival from ARDS was likewise associated with greater blood volume deficits. The precise mechanism of the development of ARDS is unclear. Protein-rich interstitial and alveolar oedema is associated with inflammatory cell infiltration and subsequent fibrosis. Type-II pneumocytes proliferate and hyaline membrane deposition occurs. Oedema results from pulmonary capillary endothelial damage leading to increased permeability and fluid leak. Crucial in the development of increased permeability is the sequestration of granulocytes in the pulmonary capillaries and their adhesion to endothelial cells [16]. Endotoxin, in combination with activated complement C3a, appears to be at least one mechanism involved in the process. Endotoxaemia in the context of haemorrhagic shock is most likely due to gut ischaemia and bacterial translocation [19]. The role of cytokines released from macrophages in response to endotoxin is not clear, but they may be the principal mediators present.

Avoidance of ARDS in patients with massive haemorrhage would appear to depend upon prompt and adequate resuscitation to ensure correction of blood volume deficit and attain a high level of oxygen delivery and consumption, and to avoid gut and liver ischaemia which might lead to endotoxaemia.

Liver and gastrointestinal tract

The liver and gut are particularly at risk of ischaemic injury in hypovolaemic shock, as a direct result of splanchnic vasoconstriction. It has been shown in animal experiments that relatively mild hypovolaemia (10% of blood volume lost over 2 h) can result in a 40% reduction in splanchnic blood flow even though virtually no change occurs in blood pressure or heart rate [20]. Furthermore, the splanchnic circulation, unlike cerebral, coronary or renal circulations, has a very limited ability to autoregulate its flow in the face of hypotension: flow is essentially pressure dependent. In addition the liver receives 80% of its blood flow and 50% of its oxygen requirements from the portal vein, and is vulnerable to a reduction in portal venous oxygen saturation—the inevitable result of an overall fall in splanchnic blood flow. Extremely low hepatic venous saturations may occur, and centrilobular hepatocyte necrosis is the ultimate result of severe hypoxia.

Mucosal ischaemia may be the prime factor responsible for gastric stress ulceration; a low intramural pH indicative of ischaemia appears to be associated with ulceration [21]. Gastric intramural pH may now be measured relatively easily using measurements of $P\text{CO}_2$ from a gastric tonometer and arterial bicarbonate concentration [21].

Systemic endotoxaemia has been demonstrated both in trauma and in burns patients [22,23] as well as in experimental haemorrhagic shock [24]. It results both from failure of the gut mucosal barrier to the passage of endotoxin and failure of the hepatic Kupffer-cell filter [24]. While ischaemia would appear to be the main cause, reperfusion injury may also be involved. Kupffer-cell activation by endotoxin may lead to the release of cytokines such as IL-1, IL-6 and tumour necrosis factor (TNF), which produce the clinical picture attributed to endotoxaemia even in the absence of systemic endotoxaemia. Whether directly or indirectly, endotoxin contributes to the development of multiple organ failure.

Kidneys

The kidneys are second only to the brain in their ability to autoregulate their blood supply. The lower limit of autoregulation is a systolic arterial pressure of 80 mmHg, below which renal blood flow decreases in line with blood pressure. In a state of renal hypoperfusion there is a reduction in glomerular filtration rate and in sodium excretion. Intrarenal shunting of blood flow from cortex to medulla occurs, and renal hypoxia occurs principally in the cortex and outer medulla.

The neuroendocrine response to hypovolaemic shock exacerbates renal ischaemia since the activation of the sympathetic nervous system and release of catecholamines, renin, angiotensin II and arginine vasopressin are all associated with vasoconstriction and sodium retention. These in turn stimulate renal synthesis of eicosanoids, such as thromboxane A_2 which is also vasoconstrictive, as well as vasodilator prostaglandins such as PGE_2 and prostacyclin (PGI_2) [26].

The conventional view of acute renal failure is one of acute tubular necrosis with backflow of filtrate, possibly in combination with tubular obstruction. It is now recognized that there is often an absence of significant structural damage and oliguria is the result of a primary filtration failure due to disturbed renal haemodynamics. There may be a 60–80% decrease in renal cortical blood flow with intense preglomerular vasoconstriction.

Differentiation of prerenal from renal failure may be made from measurement of plasma and urinary osmolality and sodium, urea and creatinine concentrations (Table 13.1). In practice this distinction may not be an absolute one.

In uncomplicated haemorrhagic shock acute renal failure should not develop, although prerenal uraemia may occur. The development of end-stage unresponsive shock associated with endothelial damage and hepatosplanchnic ischaemia may well lead to acute renal failure as a component of multiple organ failure.

Management of acute renal failure in the context of haemorrhagic shock is based on early aggressive volume resuscitation to achieve a

Table 13.1 Urinary measurements in prerenal and renal failure

Parameter	Prerenal	Renal
Specific gravity	High > 1.020	1.010–1.012
Sodium	Low < 20 mmol/l	High > 40 mmol/l
U : P urea ratio	High > 20	Low < 10
U : P creatinine ratio	High > 40	Low < 10
U : P osmolality ratio	High > 2.1	Low < 1.2

U, urine; P, plasma.

normal or above normal blood volume, a high cardiac index ≥4.5 l/min/m^2) and $D\text{O}_2$ ≥600 ml/min/m^2) and a normal blood pressure (mean arterial pressure of 80 mmHg). In many cases this may be achieved using central venous pressure (CVP) and urine output monitoring, but in other cases pulmonary artery catheterization and full cardiorespiratory monitoring may be required. The value of dopaminergic agents is still controversial. A dopamine infusion will often achieve a diuresis; even when used in low dose this may be in part due to its inotropic, pressor, diuretic and natriuretic actions [27]. It is important to stress that in acute renal failure, dopamine should not be infused blindly; it is much more important to monitor haemodynamics and oxygen transport and to use the appropriate vasoactive agents (which may include dopamine) to achieve the above therapeutic goals, and to use dopamine or its newer analogue, dopexamine, as an adjuvant agent. Frusemide appears to have beneficial actions firstly by increasing renal cortical blood flow, an effect mediated by vasodilator prostaglandins, and secondly by reducing the oxygen-expensive fluid reabsorption in the ascending limb of the loop of Henle [28].

The brain

Under normal conditions, mean cerebral blood flow is approximately 50 ml/100 g/min with a mean oxygen consumption of approximately 3.6 ml/100 g/min. During episodes of hypovolaemia, local autoregulation preserves cerebral blood flow preferentially over other regional circulations until mean arterial pressure has dropped to approximately 60 mmHg. As cerebral blood flow drops to 25 ml/100 g/min EEG (electroencephalograph) changes occur (increase in slow delta-wave activity). At 20 ml/100 g/min, cell membranes start to fail and potassium leaks from the cells. At this point cerebral impulse propagation is affected. These changes may be reversed if blood flow is promptly restored by resuscitation. Irreversible changes occur at a cerebral blood flow of 10 ml/100 g/min with calcium influx into the cells, enzyme dysfunction and organ destruction, as occurs elsewhere in the body. Clinically, increasing cerebral hypoxia is seen with confusion, altered consciousness level, convulsions, coma and finally death.

In the management of the bleeding patient, the most important factor for cerebral protection is maintenance of oxygenation and an adequate perfusion pressure.

Clinical considerations

The clinical presentation of the bleeding patient depends upon the site of bleeding. Very often haemorrhage is clinically obvious, as for example obstetric-, gastrointestinal- or trauma-related haemorrhage. However, internal haemorrhage into soft tissues, pelvis, retroperitoneal or thoracic spaces may be quite insidious and pass unnoticed, for example after blunt abdominal trauma. The classic symptoms and signs of haemorrhagic shock reflect both the effect of blood loss and the compensatory mechanisms (Table 13.2). Tachycardia may be exacerbated by pain and anxiety. Hypotension may not occur until up to 25–30% of blood loss has occurred, the pressure being maintained by intense vasoconstriction until sudden decompensation occurs. This is particularly true in young previously fit patients. Thus blood pressure should always be considered in conjunction with peripheral perfusion. Core–peripheral temperature gradient is a useful measure of circulating volume in bleeding patients, although it has been largely discarded as an index of cardiac output or vascular resistance in other contexts. Sweating, pallor and tachypnoea are common accompanying signs; light-headedness indicates mild cerebral ischaemia; collapse and cyanosis indicate a profound fall in cardiac output.

Clinical signs in the bleeding patient should be augmented by monitoring of cardiovascular, respiratory and renal function. As well as the frequent measurement of heart rate, respiratory rate and blood pressure, ECG (electrocardiograph) monitoring and measurement of core–peripheral temperature gradient is useful. Cuff blood pressures may be extremely unreliable in severely shocked patients, and blood pressure is more accurately measured directly using intra-arterial cannulation [29]. The femoral route is most appropriate in such cases. Pulse oximetry, although theoretically attractive, is not practical in situations where there is poor peripheral blood flow; misleadingly low values of SaO_2 may be obtained, or no signal at all. In any event, high-flow oxygen is essential in patients with major bleeding.

If 20% blood volume replacement (1 litre in adults) leads to no improvement in vital signs, central venous monitoring is essential, the internal jugular vein being the preferred route of access. CVP is determined not merely by circulating blood volume; other factors affecting its value include venous tone, right-heart function and intrathoracic pressure. In severe haemorrhage, venous tone is markedly increased due to sympathetic stimulation, and thus capacitance volume is markedly

Table 13.2 Classification of hypovolaemic shock according to blood loss. (From [5] with permission)

Parameter	Class I	Class II	Class III	Class IV
Blood loss:				
Percentage	<15	15–30	30–40	>40
Volume (ml)	750	800–1500	1500–2000	>2000
Blood pressure:				
Systolic	Unchanged	Normal	Reduced	Very low
Diastolic	Unchanged	Raised	Reduced	Very low or unrecordable
Pulse (beats/min)	Slight tachycardia	100–120	120 (thready)	>120 (Very thready)
Capillary refill	Normal	Slow (>2 s)	Slow (>2 s)	Undetectable
Respiratory rate	Normal	Normal	Tachypnoea (>20/min)	Tachypnoea (>20/min)
Urinary flow rate (ml/h)	>30	20–30	10–20	0–10
Extremities	Colour normal	Pale	Pale	Pale and cold
Complexion	Normal	Pale	Pale	Ashen
Mental state	Alert	Anxious or agressive	Anxious, agressive, or drowsy	Drowsy, confused, or unconscious

decreased with a resultant maintenance of CVP. In late shock, hypoxia can cause pulmonary vasoconstriction and hypertension and thus raise right-heart pressures and CVP. Intrathoracic pressure increases associated with positive pressure ventilation also raise CVP. Although its value must be interpreted with care, nevertheless CVP is useful in the differential diagnosis of shock occurring following major surgery, where there may be doubt in differentiating a haemorrhagic from septic or cardiogenic aetiology. In addition, serial CVP measurements are essential for titration of fluid replacement.

Pulmonary artery catheterization is not normally required in haemorrhagic shock. However, if shock is prolonged and uncorrected or if evidence of organ dysfunction occurs such as ARDS or acute renal failure, the pulmonary artery flotation catheter provides vital information, including the pulmonary artery wedge pressure as an index of left ventricular filling, mixed venous oxygen content, cardiac output, oxygen delivery and consumption.

Urine output must be continuously monitored, necessitating catheterization. Serial hydrogen-ion concentrations and blood gases allow assessment of tissue oxygenation, a metabolic acidosis indicating the possibility of anaerobic metabolism which can be confirmed by blood lactate estimation. Serial blood lactate levels are a good index of response to therapy in shock. Serial haemoglobin or haematocrit estimations are also essential, as are electrolyte estimations during fluid and blood replacement.

Clinical management of bleeding patients requires a broad understanding of the consequences of haemorrhage, and the application of physiological principles with the broad aim of rapidly restoring tissue oxygen delivery and thus minimizing the adverse consequences of hypoxia and organ failure.

References

1 Shoemaker, W.C., Appel, P., Czer, L.S.C. *et al.* (1980) Pathogenesis of respiratory failure (ARDS) after haemorrhage and trauma. *Crit. Care Med.*, **8**, 504–512.

2 Bland, R.D., Shoemaker, W.C., Abraham, E. and Cobo, J.C. (1985) Haemodynamic and oxygen transport patterns in surviving and non-surviving post-operative patients. *Crit. Care Med.*, **13**, 85–90.

3 Shoemaker, W.C., Appel, P.L. and Kram, H.B. (1988) Prospective trial of supranormal values of survivors as therapeutic goals in high risk surgical patients. *Chest*, **94**, 1176–1186.

4 Edwards, J.D. Oxygen transport following major trauma. In: *Update in Intensive*

Care and Emergency Medicine, 5 (Ed. Vincent, J.L.), pp. 25–31. Springer-Verlag, Berlin (1988).

5 Baskett P.J.F. (1990) Management of hypovolaemic shock. *Br. Med. J.*, **300**, 1453–1457.

6 McLelland, D.B.L. (Ed.) *Handbook of Transfusion Medicine*. HMSO, London (1989).

7 Barcroft, H., Edholm, O.G., McMichael, J. and Sharpey-Schafer, E.P. (1944) Post haemorrhagic fainting. Study by cardiac output and forearm blood flow. *Lancet*, **i**, 489–491.

8 Little, R.A. (1988) 8th Fitt's Lecture: Heart rate changes after haemorrhage and injury—a reappraisal. *J. Trauma*, **29**(7), 903–906.

9 Van Leeuwen, A.F., Evans, R.G., Ludbrook, J. (1989) Haemodynamic responses to acute blood loss: new roles for the heart, brain and endogenous opioids. *Anaesth. Intensive Care*, **17**, 312–319.

10 Moore, F.D. (1965) The effects of haemorrhage on body composition. *New Engl. J. Med.*, **273**, 567–577.

11 Cunningham, J.N., Shires, G.T. and Wagner, Y. (1971) Cellular transport defects in haemorrhagic shock. *Surgery*, **70**, 215–222.

12 Shires, G.R., Cunningham, J.N., Baker, C.R.F. *et al.* (1972) Alterations in cellular membrane functions during shock in primates. *Ann. Surg.*, **176**, 288–295.

13 Marzella, L.L. and Trump, B.F. Cell injury and its meaning in shock and resuscitation. In: *Trauma, Emergency Surgery and Critical Care* (Ed. Siegel, J.H.), pp. 33–36. Churchill Livingstone, New York (1987).

14 Hack, O.F. and Thijs, L. The orchestra of mediators in the pathogenesis of septic shock. In: *Update in Intensive Care and Emergency Medicine*, 14 (Ed. Vincent, J.L.), pp. 232–246. Springer-Verlag, Berlin (1991).

15 Fong, Y., Moldawer, L.L., Shires, G.T. and Lowry, S.F. (1990) The biologic characteristics of cytokines and their implication in surgical injury. *Surg. Gynec. Obstet.*, **170**, 363–378.

16 Parsons, P.E., Worthen, G.S., Moore, E.E. *et al.* (1989) The association of circulating endotoxin with the development of the adult respiratory distress syndrome. *Am. Rev. Resp. Dis.*, **140**, 294–301.

17 Fowler, A.A., Hamman, R.F., Good, J.T. *et al.* (1983) Adult respiratory distress syndrome: risk with common predispositions. *Ann. Intern. Med.*, **98**, 593–597.

18 Montgomery, B., Stager, M.A., Carrico, J. and Hudson, L.D. (1985) Causes of mortality in patients with adult respiratory distress syndrome. *Am. Rev. Resp. Dis.*, **132**, 485–489.

19 Ramsey, G. and Runcie, C. Hepatic dysfunction in shock. In: *Update in Intensive Care and Emergency Medicine*, 8 (Ed. Vincent, J.L.), pp. 368–375. Springer-Verlag, Berlin (1989).

20 Gilmour, D.G., Aitkenhead, A.R., Hothersall, A.P. and Ledingham, I.McA. (1980) The effect of hypovolaemia on colon blood flow in the dog. *Br. J. Surg.*, **67**, 82–84.

21 Fiddian-Green, R.G., McGough, E., Pittenger, G. and Rothman, E. (1983) Predictive value of intramural pH and other risk factors for massive bleeding from stress ulceration. *Gastroenterology*, **85**, 613–620.

22 Rush, B.F., Sori, A.J., Murphy, T.F. *et al.* (1988) Endotoxemia and bacteremia during hemorrhagic shock. *Ann. Surg.*, **207**, 549–554.

23 Ziegler, T.R., Smith, R.J., O'Dwyer, S.T. *et al.* (1988) Increased intestinal per-

meability associated with infection in burn patients. *Arch Surg.*, **123**, 1313–1319.

24 Koziol, J.M., Rush, B.F., Smith, S.M. and Machiedo, G.W. (1988) Occurrence of bacteraemia during and after haemorrhagic shock. *J. Trauma*, **28**, 10–16.

25 Ramsey, G., Newman, P.M., McArtney, A.C. and Ledingham, I.McA. Endotoxaemia in multiple organ failure due to sepsis. In: *Bacterial Endotoxins: Pathophysiological Effects, Clinical Significance and Pharmacological Control*, (Eds Levin, J. *et al.*), pp. 237–246. A.R. Liss, New York (1980).

26 Cumming, A.D. Renal function in septic shock. In: *Update in Intensive Care and Emergency Medicine*, 8 (Ed. Vincent, J.L.), pp. 348–357. Springer-Verlag, Berlin (1989).

27 Lokhandwale, M.F. and Hedge, S.S. (1990) Cardiovascular dopamine receptors: role of renal dopamine and dopamine receptors in sodium excretion. *Pharmacol. Toxicol.*, **66**, 237–243.

28 Mackay, I.G., Muir, A.L. and Watson, M.L. (1984) Contribution of prostaglandins to the systemic and renal vascular response to frusemide in normal man. *Br. J. Clin. Pharmacol.*, **17**, 513–519.

29 Gurman, G.M. and Kriemerman, S. (1985) Cannulation of big arteries in critically ill patients. *Crit. Care Med.*, **13**, 217–220.

Chapter 14
Role of the anaesthetist

JOHN E. UTTING AND SUSAN K. HAWLEY

In any situation in which surgery is contemplated on the patient who is bleeding, the anaesthetist should be immediately involved. Anaesthesia is an additional assault on the patient's powers of physiological compensation and it is the anaesthetist who will be responsible for keeping him or her in as good a condition as possible during surgery. The available antecedent history must be known and an opportunity obtained to consider possible associated medical conditions and treatments. Such factors as the integrity of the airway, the probable ease (or otherwise) of tracheal intubation and venous cannulation, and the likely amount of gastric content have to be assessed and this, if possible, before the patient enters the anaesthetic room.

Anaesthetists often have more experience of bleeding patients than other staff and should be adept, for example, at setting up intravenous infusions and monitoring progress. Finally, they may sometimes provide a sense of urgency when the approach is too casual or lethargic.

The anaesthetist who is attending the patient may have to decide who is going to give the anaesthetic and what help is required. This may require the summoning of more senior staff, the provision of additional help and the rearrangement of departmental work. *The Report of a Confidential Enquiry into Perioperative Deaths* (1988) (CEPOD) [1] showed up deficiencies in respect of the seniority of staff dealing with emergency situations: avoidable deaths occurred among emergency cases because they were dealt with, often at night, by staff who were too inexperienced and who failed to resuscitate patients adequately prior to surgery. This situation needs to be remedied urgently.

General management

The sources of bleeding in patients coming to surgery are protean but most patients must be assumed to have a 'full stomach'. This poses a serious problem which will be dealt with later, and means that tracheal intubation is nearly always indicated.

It is beyond the scope of this chapter to deal with problems which arise when the airway is compromised by trauma. If a tracheal tube cannot be passed—a rare event—the anaesthetist must attempt to keep the airway open by such means as cricothyroid puncture, trans-tracheal jet ventilation or emergency tracheostomy. Patients with cervical spine injuries present particular problems since the process of tracheal intubation can give rise to spinal-cord injury [2].

The anaesthetist must be aware that injuries may have been missed. Difficulty in inflating the patient's lungs, for example, should arouse immediate suspicion of pneumothorax or haemopneumothorax (particularly deadly, since tension is often increased by positive pressure ventilation), haemothorax by itself, inhalation of gastric content or pulmonary oedema. Arterial hypoxaemia can occur in severe shock, but declining arterial oxygen saturation despite adequate inspired tension may be due to fat embolism. Resistant hypotension, despite apparently adequate resuscitation with fluids, should alert either to the possibility of undiagnosed sources of bleeding, such as a ruptured spleen, to unsuspected head injury, or to myocardial ischaemia or depression.

Inotropic support may be required for a heart failing despite adequate fluid replacement—a matter often of crucial importance and requiring considerable judgement. Prolonged hypovolaemia may be associated with a pronounced metabolic acidosis and this will have to be at least partially corrected to restore myocardial function.

In the operating theatre the anaesthetist is involved in activities other than giving an anaesthetic. Further monitoring may have to be established, records kept and a strategy of resuscitation, which will change as events unfold, must be worked out. Fluids (blood, blood products, crystalloids, colloids, clotting factors) have to be given—often with the use of pumps. Materials for transfusion must be ordered and liaison with the laboratory established. New intravenous lines may have to be set up, blood loss estimated, giving sets changed, and so on.

The inhalation risk

Most patients who present for surgery with active bleeding must be considered to be in danger of inhaling gastric contents during the induction of anaesthesia until a cuffed tracheal tube has been inserted into the trachea, the cuff blown up and the tracheobronchial tree thus mechanically isolated from the oesophagus. This is no trivial detail: immediate death from aspiration or life-threatening pulmonary morbidity is one of the most serious threats to the patient who is bleeding and who is coming to surgery.

The risk of aspiration is obvious if the patient is bleeding from, say, stomach, oesophagus, duodenum or tonsillar bed. But after injury there is good evidence that gastric emptying can be delayed for many hours, though recent work [3] has cast some doubt on this. The opiates undeniably decrease the rate of gastric emptying.

The sequelae of inhalation can vary from, for example, the sudden obstructive death from solid matter to an infective bronchopneumonia. Inhalation of very acid content, $\leqslant$pH 2.5, is known to be especially damaging [4], even in low volumes, some 25 ml being critical, and is associated especially with obstetric patients [5]. Gastric acid aspiration causes the Mendelson syndrome [6], with the stigmata of bronchospasm, tachycardia, cyanosis and, in severe cases, respiratory and cardiovascular collapse.

The stomach cannot be reliably emptied mechanically. An 18-gauge Salem Sump nasogastric tube, with double lumen and multiple orifices, is slightly less unsatisfactory than the single-lumen tube [7], especially if the patient's position is changed with the tube *in situ*, a manoeuvre usually contraindicated in the bleeding patient. A large-bore orogastric tube may sometimes be of use but in all events solid residue, including clot, and an important volume of liquid may remain.

Pharmacological methods of solving the problem are, again, only partially successful. Metoclopramide speeds gastric emptying and inhibits vomiting. H_2-receptor antagonists, particularly ranitidine, reduce gastric acidity. Separately or together they reduce the risk of dangerous aspiration, but take time to act and are most relevant to obstetric practice. The use of non-particulate antacids to reduce the risk of acid aspiration immediately before induction of anaesthesia is again common in obstetric practice. Sodium citrate (0.3 mol/l, 15 ml) is suitable as a single oral dose in emergency situations [8]; it should be given some 15 min before induction.

All these measures from the use of gastric tubes to the exhibition of sodium citrate may be largely irrelevant to the bleeding patient. In any event they may be only partially successful and one must usually rely on the legerdemain of the anaesthetist during induction of anaesthesia.

Choice of technique

Local anaesthesia

The scope for using local analgesia in the bleeding patient is very limited. Unless the patient is normovolaemic the use of the spinal or epidural block is contraindicated, or, at least, these techniques should be used only with great caution and with a vasoconstrictor, such as ephedrine, immediately available: usually the site of bleeding makes these methods irrelevant anyway. Both cause peripheral vasodilatation (of arterioles and veins) which, in the hypovolaemic patient, can give rise to a precipitous fall in blood pressure [9,10].

General anaesthesia

Techniques are, of course, very numerous. What follows is the barest outline of a possible approach. The more relevant pharmacology of some of the agents mentioned is summarized later.

In almost all bleeding patients the passage of a tracheal tube is, as has been emphasized, mandatory. The use of a simple technique of anaesthesia, for example with a mask and airway, is of limited application.

The induction of anaesthesia is a dangerous episode, especially if the patient is hypovolaemic. Every effort must be made to make sure that he or she has an adequate circulating volume before this takes place and it is usually appropriate to increase the rate of fluid administration before and during induction.

In practice, adequate circulating volume cannot always be achieved. Indeed, when the bleeding patient is *in extremis* an endotracheal tube may be passed without any anaesthetic. Usually, though, the anaesthetist will render the patient unconscious using as small a dose as possible of an induction agent (such as etomidate or thiopentone) after making the patient breathe oxygen for 2–5 min (preoxygenation) to increase the volume of oxygen in the lung—a manoeuvre which decreases the risks of hypoxia should difficulty arise in inserting the tracheal tube. There are other ways of inducing anaesthesia, for example with low concentrations of a volatile agent in oxygen before suxamethonium is given. This may be especially relevant if the patient is very ill. Immediately after induction, the very short-acting muscle relaxant suxamethonium is given. This is the basis of the 'rapid sequence' induction.

As anaesthesia is induced precricoid pressure is applied (Sellick's manoeuvre) [11] and kept up until the tracheal tube is in place and its cuff blown up. Precricoid pressure is an expert procedure and should not be performed by the untrained. It consists of applying pressure backwards on the cricoid with the finger and thumb and should effectively prevent regurgitated material reaching the pharynx.

Anaesthesia is maintained with nitrous oxide, oxygen and usually a volatile agent. When spontaneous ventilation is resumed after the suxamethonium has worn off the anaesthetist is presented with alternative courses of action. Spontaneous ventilation may be allowed to continue, using nitrous oxide in oxygen, a volatile agent and perhaps small doses of a narcotic agent—small to avoid respiratory depression. Alternatively, a longer-acting (non-depolarizing) muscle relaxant may be administered and controlled ventilation (intermittent positive pressure ventilation—IPPV) continued, anaesthesia being typically maintained with nitrous oxide, oxygen, a volatile agent and analgesic adjuvants.

The use of a muscle relaxant in this way makes positive pressure ventilation mandatory, but it enables the operation to be performed using relatively light anaesthesia which minimizes cardiovascular depression; it also reduces the risk of respiratory depression postoperatively. In fact, in most bleeding patients, muscular relaxation is required for the performance of the surgery.

There is a tendency, in the very acute situation, to minimize the concentration of anaesthetic agent and even to give pure oxygen. This must be avoided whenever possible. Awareness during anaesthesia is a particular hazard in this sort of patient for just this reason [12].

Artificial ventilation

It would be expected that IPPV would, by increasing mean intrathoracic pressure, cause a reduction in venous return, and reduce cardiac output and arterial blood pressure. This is the case [13] and the effect is exaggerated in hypovolaemia. Here there will already be a great degree of venoconstriction and, as additional venoconstriction will be one compensatory mechanism for increased intrathoracic pressure, there may be a further fall in cardiac output, accompanied by a fall in arterial blood pressure. Deep anaesthesia, too, will make things worse [14].

In practice, with skilful IPPV, this hazard is more apparent than real. It would be wrong to avoid tracheal intubation and IPPV, even when the patient is pulseless, if ventilation is failing and the airway being lost. Here gentle pulmonary ventilation with pure oxygen using low inflation pressures together with a rapid infusion of crystalloid, colloid or blood increases the chance of survival.

Pharmacology

This abbreviated account of the pharmacology of the anaesthetic drugs and agents is intended to give the salient points related to the bleeding patient. There are many excellent accounts of the subject in standard anaesthetic textbooks.

Premedication

There are only two important reasons for giving drugs before anaesthesia—to relieve anxiety and to allay pain. The benzodiazepines are probably the most useful for the former purpose. They have only limited application in the bleeding patient; certainly they are of little use in the patient who is restless and anxious because of shock, where it is best to avoid all sedative medications.

Morphine

Of the analgesic drugs morphine, perhaps combined with an antiemetic, remains the drug of choice, and does have some anxiolytic effect. There are clear contraindications to its use (e.g. respiratory obstruction, head injury, fear that it may cloud a diagnosis) and, in hypovolaemia, it may cause a further fall in blood pressure. Morphine is usually given intramuscularly but in the bleeding patient absorption may be delayed and there is thus a temptation to repeat doses inappropriately. The intravenous injection of very small doses, with careful observation, is a useful technique, but even here the effect may take much longer than expected as the circulation may be very much slowed. In all events it must be used with great caution.

Induction agents

When general anaesthesia is used, the patient must be unconscious before a muscle relaxant is given and a tracheal tube passed. This is usually achieved with an intravenous dose of a short-acting agent after preoxygenation. Of the agents currently available thiopentone and etomidate require some mention. Ketamine may be used intramuscularly: it is radically different from the others.

Thiopentone

This drug developed a peculiarly sinister reputation in the shocked patient, even when there was good compensation [15]: precipitous falls in blood pressure, probably due mainly to venodilation [16] can occur. Indeed, it has been stated that thiopentone should not be used in the presence of blood loss. This is untrue, but the dose requirements are very much smaller than in normal patients.

Etomidate

This is a much newer drug, and is held to have a more benign effect on the cardiovascular system than thiopentone, though clinical doses do reduce arterial blood pressure, probably mainly through a decrease in peripheral vascular resistance. Many would regard it as the drug of choice in the bleeding patient.

Ketamine

This has a relatively slow onset of action. It normally increases blood pressure and pulse rate due to sympathetic and myocardial stimulation and there is little respiratory depression, so it maintains cardiovascular stability in the hypovolaemic patient [17].

In the UK ketamine is more discussed than given. In the field (e.g. for an emergency amputation), however, it may have an appreciable place.

Muscle relaxants

Immediately after induction of anaesthesia suxamethonium, which is very rapid in onset and short-acting, is usually given to facilitate rapid tracheal intubation. Thereafter, when there are some signs of recovery, a more long-acting non-depolarizing agent is given such as, for example, pancuronium (which some regard as particularly indicated), atracurium or vecuronium, and its use continued in increments or as an infusion. The action of the non-depolarizing agents may, in appropriate conditions be reversed with anticholinesterase (neostigmine), which must be accompanied by atropine or glycopyrrolate to obtund cholinergic effects.

Suxamethonium has complicated pharmacological effects. In the context of a rapid sequence induction the main points to remember are that a single dose may provoke bradycardia; that the drug causes a rise in serum potassium and this to a dangerous degree in some circumstances (e.g. massive trauma, burns); and that it raises intraocular and intracranial pressure.

Inhalational agents

Nitrous oxide

Nitrous oxide is used almost universally during general anaesthesia with muscle relaxants both in the UK and in many other places throughout the world. It is a relatively 'weak' anaesthetic but, in a non-hypoxic mixture (70%) in oxygen, keeps most patients unaware and without overt memory when used with artificial ventilation in conjunction with a muscle relaxant. The use of lower concentrations in oxygen is associated with an increased incidence of awareness [18] without causing any appreciable concomitant increase in arterial oxygen content, a fact explained by the nature of the oxygen dissociation curve. It is usual to supplement nitrous oxide with a low concentration of volatile agent and/or analgesic drugs (e.g. fentanyl, alfentanil, morphine): both reduce the risk of awareness and reflex activity but volatile agents are more useful for the former purpose and the analgesic drugs for the latter.

Nitrous oxide diffuses into air and some gas-filled body cavities faster than nitrogen diffuses out [19]. A pneumothorax, for example, will expand, but this is less important than it might seem, since a pneumothorax must be drained before anaesthesia is induced.

Volatile agents

All the three modern volatile agents—halothane, enflurane and isoflurane—depress the myocardium and cause a decrease in sympathetic activity and in the level of circulating catecholamines. They also depress the baroreceptor reflex, and isoflurane causes considerable peripheral vasodilatation. All cause hypotension but myocardial blood flow is well maintained in proportion to demand.

In practice, as low concentrations of volatile agents are used in conjunction with muscle relaxants, it matters relatively little which of the three is used as adjuvants, though halothane is currently somewhat out of favour because of the possibility of hepatic damage [20]. Isoflurane is probably the agent of choice, but many think it should be avoided when there is evidence of myocardial ischaemia because of the so-called inverse steal syndrome [21]. Many severely bleeding patients are hypoxic; not a few have concomitant myocardial disease.

Analgesic drugs

It is common, during general anaesthesia with muscle relaxants, to use supplementation with the so-called analgesic agents. These are used primarily to reduce reflex responsiveness to surgical trauma and secondly to reduce the possibility of awareness. Fentanyl, with a duration of action intermediate between morphine (long-acting) and alfentanil (short-acting) is probably the most widely used of these, often in intermittent doses given in response to a rise in blood pressure and pulse rate during surgery. It may also be given by infusion, usually after a priming dose.

Hypotension may occur and is likely to be severe in the patient who is dependent on sympathetic tone for maintenance of blood pressure, as in shock. Bradycardia, too, is common and may itself be associated with hypotension. The injudicious use of these drugs may be associated with postoperative respiratory depression.

Other drugs

The anaesthetist will frequently have to administer one or more of a great variety of drugs. Inotropic agents (e.g. dobutamine) have already been mentioned. Indeed, there may, though very infrequently, be an indication for giving peripheral vasoconstricting agents.

Fluids

The critically ill patient — one who is literally bleeding to death — requires immediate venous access and the administration of fluid as rapidly as possible, that is, under pressure. The nature of the fluid administered is of secondary importance, as is the establishment of monitoring. The patient is unlikely to succumb, in these circumstances, to haemodilution — more likely to lack of circulating volume.

In all events, adequate venous access must be firmly established before surgery. In addition to a central line one, or indeed more than one, large bore venous lines should be established and facilities for the administration of fluid under pressure must be available. Warming of fluids, especially blood, is desirable, but warming coils reduce the speed with which fluids can be administered.

Crystalloids and colloids

Much has been written on the so-called 'crystalloid/colloid' debate but no definitive solution has yet appeared (see The 'third space' below). There is a summary of the debate by Harrison and Rampton [22].

Hartmann's solution ($Na^+ = 131$; $K^+ = 5$, $Ca^{2+} = 2$, $Cl^- = 111$; HCO_3^- (as lactate) = 29 mmol/l) is similar to Ringer's lactate and is the mainstay of crystalloid administration; its composition is thus similar to extracellular fluid, though protein free. With few exceptions, glucose 5% has no place in resuscitation [23]. The lactate content of Hartmann's solution can be considered to generate bicarbonate through metabolism of lactate by the liver, but this might be inhibited in severe shock and in liver failure [24].

Like colloid solutions, Hartmann's has no oxygen-carrying capacity and dilutes clotting factors; like most colloids, except those based on blood products, it is readily available. Reactions to it are rare, a contrast to colloid solutions, in which severe reactions are uncommon but can be serious [25]. Having a low viscosity it is easy to administer; colloids in general have a somewhat higher viscosity but, again, much lower than blood—especially when it is plasma-reduced. Most colloid solutions consist, basically, of modified saline solutions with added oncotically active particles—to give colloid is usually to give sodium and chloride as well.

The crucial difference between solutions such as Hartmann's and colloid solutions is that the former pass out of the circulation rapidly and distribute themselves in proportion to the volumes of the interstitial fluid and the circulating volume (i.e. roughly in the proportion of 3 : 1). The oncotic pressure of colloid very considerably delays this process and volume is thus retained, for a variable time, in the circulation. To replace the loss of 1 litre of circulating volume would thus mean that in the order of 3 litres of Hartmann's solution would have to be administered as opposed to 1 litre of colloid. Some degree of haemodilution is permissible, perhaps desirable, but these solutions can only be used to make up for relatively minor blood losses.

Colloid solutions can be divided into blood derivatives (e.g. plasma protein solution) and artificial colloids (e.g. dextrans, modified gelatins, and hydroxyethyl starch). Some colloids (e.g. high-molecular-weight dextrans) have a higher oncotic pressure than plasma, drawing fluid in from the interstitial space—'plasma expanders'. There is a useful short summary by Twigley and Hillman [26].

Dextran 70 interferes with crossmatching, a minor disadvantage, and impairs clotting [27], but an administration of 1 g/kg is safe if haemostasis is otherwise normal [28]. This coagulation problem applies to solutions of hydroxyethyl starch too [29,30], but the effect of other solutions has not, as yet, been fully evaluated. None should be used in very large volumes, though, in practice this occurs not infrequently.

Dextran 40 has been said to be useful for its rheological features (it markedly increases flow in small vessels) in refractory shock [31] but can cause renal dysfunction in dehydrated patients and its use should be avoided in patients with organic renal insufficiency [32]. It is, in fact, little used in the UK.

Hypertonic saline

Although this is a crystalloid it is mentioned separately because its use is a recent development and must still be considered experimental. Neither of the present authors has personal experience of it.

Animal work [33] and work in patients [34] has suggested that the use of hypertonic solutions (e.g. of, say, ≥500 mmol/l) may increase chances of survival in the shocked subject. Several formulations have been investigated; as an example, Shackford and colleagues [35] used a solution of $Na^+ = 250$; $Cl^- = 180$, lactate = 63; $K^+ = 4$; and $Ca^{2+} = 3$ mmol/l.

These solutions appear to have several advantages. It is possible that they improve survival in shock as they have a beneficial effect on the circulation [36], increasing cardiac output and reducing peripheral resistance, and are associated with a lesser gain in weight in the postoperative period [37] than when large volumes of Ringer's lactate are given. They will 'draw out' water from the cellular fluid—and this is, in effect, to emphasize one of the 'natural' reactions to blood loss. They represent an interesting development.

The 'third space'

The suggestion that surgical trauma resulted in a sequestration of extracellular fluid into traumatized tissue which should be replaced by Hartmann-type solutions has been strongly criticized and the existence of such a space called into question. Certainly this 'third space' concept [38] resulted in the use of excessive volumes of crystalloid solution during surgery, a trend which even its proponents accepted as undesirable [39].

The use of very large volumes, usually of Ringer's lactate or Hartmann's solution, did not usually result in adverse effects. The reason would seem to be that pulmonary oedema is unlikely since it is pulmonary capillary pressure which mainly governs outflow from the pulmonary capillary [40] and this is low relative to the systemic circulation. This view may be simplistic: trauma is frequently followed by infection and here the general rules governing fluid egress are less clear-cut. An excessive extracellular fluid content in the systemic circulation results in considerable postoperative weight gain, but is not usually detectable as frank oedema and is generally regarded as benign, though this may not be entirely true [41] and it has been suggested, for example, that it may lead to an increased time for the gut to function adequately [35]. Even if there is true sequestration of extracellular fluid during surgery this, presumably, must eventually be mobilized.

The tendency to give relatively large volumes of crystalloid fluid (5–15 ml/kg/h) during surgery even without conspicuous blood loss preceded the hypothesis of the 'third' space. There were probably three reasons for this: (i) the surgical patient is usually mildly dehydrated; (ii) there was an obvious desire to keep up urine output; and (iii) there is a tendency for blood pressure to decline during surgery unless fluid is given. It must also be remembered that, despite what is said later, urine output *may* be considerable and must be taken into account when considering fluid balance.

Thus, though there is clearly need for moderation, the use of crystalloid solutions, usually Hartmann's, is justified as a 'background' in patients who are being severely traumatized during surgery, quite apart from the question of overt blood loss. The use of colloid solutions in place of this has the advantage that better retention of volume in the circulation and better oxygen transport is achieved [42], and this may reduce the need for infusion. Nevertheless, as has been pointed out, they have their own disadvantages.

Blood and blood products (see Chapter 16)

The best fluid replacement for blood loss is whole blood, but frequently plasma-reduced blood (packed cells) alone is available. The anaesthetist prefers fluid with a lower viscosity but cannot complain since its manufacture makes other blood products available (e.g. albumin 5%, clotting factors) which he or she may well wish to use. But plasma volume has to be made up, and the anaesthetist will generally use a mixture of artificial and human colloid and Hartmann's solution.

Blood loss in operating-theatre conditions is often considerably underestimated. This is not only because insufficient allowance is made for such factors as loss into tissues, for example after fractures of long bones, but also blood on drapes, for example, is frequently more than was thought.

Coagulation (see Chapters 3 and 16)

The most conspicuous haemostatic abnormality which occurs during massive transfusion is dilutional thrombocytopenia, and disseminated intravascular coagulation can occur in 30% of these patients. The most useful tests are the platelet count and the fibrinogen level, but the crucial factor is the presence or absence of clinical bleeding. The opinion of a haematologist should be unhesitatingly sought when there is any doubt.

Fresh frozen plasma is a source of fibrinogen but its use merely for volume replacement is debatable. In some circumstances the use of cryoprecipitate, which is a much more concentrated solution of fibrinogen, should be considered. Other clotting factors can be obtained from plasma, platelet concentrates or cryoprecipitate.

Hazards of massive transfusion

There are many hazards of massive transfusion of blood. Of these, the only ones requiring special comment are hypothermia, citrate toxicity and potassium intoxication.

Hypothermia

Hypothermia of a mild degree is common during surgery, but it may be severe during surgery for massive trauma, as large volumes of cold blood (at say 4°C) and other fluids at ambient temperature (say 25°C) are given rapidly. Cardiac arrhythmias leading to ventricular fibrillation or asystole may occur, but there are lesser difficulties, like delayed recovery, as well. Efforts should be made to warm fluids which are administered, especially blood; unfortunately heating coils materially increase the resistance of giving circuits.

Citrate intoxication

This is due to the chelating of ionized calcium, but the use of supplemental calcium salts during transfusion may itself give rise to arrhythmias [43] and is not justified. Though reduction in ionized calcium may cause prolongation of the QT interval [44] this does not usually affect cardiac function and at the end of transfusion ionized calcium levels rapidly return to normal [45] due to metabolism and excretion of citrate. Large amounts of blood (rates of 100–150 ml/min) can be used without the use of calcium [46].

Hyperpotassaemia

Hyperkalaemia is seldom of clinical importance. The potassium which has entered the plasma from the red cells in stored blood is rapidly taken up by cells, when they are warmed. Hyperpotassaemia, however, may occur especially in those with acidosis and renal failure [47]. Calcium is the physiological antidote.

Strategic implications

The kidney

During the perioperative period, and particularly during surgery itself, the anaesthetist must assume a positive role in protecting the kidney. Hypovolaemia causes intense sympathetic activity which results in renal vasoconstriction: this may, and not infrequently does, lead to acute renal failure due to tubular or even cortical necrosis.

Anaesthesia itself results in some diminution in renal function (e.g. decreased renal blood flow and glomerular filtration rate) [48] but this is transitory and unimportant compared to the effects of surgery; both are dwarfed by inadequate resuscitation. Here oliguria is the usual result, partly but not entirely due to increased secretion of vasopressin [49,50]. Breaking through this barrier is usually possible but results in a strongly positive balance for salt and water. Other hormonal responses are involved, renin and angiotensin have a definitive role, with others, for example natriuretic hormone, prostaglandins, and kallikrein–bradykinin, having an effect as yet not fully evaluated [51].

Some degree of oliguria must be expected and it is bad practice to attempt to produce a high urine flow at the expense of gross overloading. However, if a current situation and antecedent history suggest that renal damage has taken place, the anaesthetist must consider specific measures to protect the kidney.

Mannitol, an osmotic diuretic and possibly renal vasodilator, (say 1 g/kg) may be given, but repeated doses may give rise to pulmonary oedema. Alternatively, or additionally, treatment with low-dose dopamine may be instituted.

It would be useful if definitive strategies could be given for fluid replacement in the bleeding patient during surgery. This is impossible because blood loss is unpredictable: the anaesthetist is trying to hit a moving target. Even if this were not so, it would be quite impossible to obtain agreement on what should be done. What is not in debate is that the circulating volume must be kept up and the kidney especially protected. *What follows must be considered controversial.*

Though the haematocrit may be allowed to go down to 30% or even lower by dilution, the calculations on which this might be based would depend on knowing what is about to happen. Predictable and relatively small blood losses ($\leq$ 1 litre in a 70 kg man) can be replaced by crystalloid or colloid, or a mixture of both in appropriate volumes, having regard to their distribution in the body compartments. The haematocrit changes slowly and anyway is often not immediately available during surgery and, in conditions of severe bleeding tends to decline, as blood loss is frequently replaced rather more slowly than would be ideal.

If whole blood is available it should be used to replace the major part of the blood loss, and generous allowances should be made for occult loss and for loss on drapes, the floor and so on. If only plasma-reduced blood is available artificial colloids can be used initially (say 1–1.5 litres), but after that human products (e.g. albumin 5%) must be used. Attention must be given to clotting: if fresh frozen plasma is given it will, of course, be counted as plasma. Allowance should be made for 'third space' losses and these can be replaced with Hartmann's solution.

Monitoring

Some of the more important methods of monitoring are summarized in Tables 14.1 and 14.2. Observation will give useful initial information—thus in a patient who is bleeding, the concomitants of shock:

- Cold, white extremities.
- Rapid, poor-volume pulse.
- Anxiety.
- Dilated pupils.
- Restlessness and 'air hunger'.

Table 14.1 Summary of some simple non-invasive methods of monitoring the bleeding patient

Type	Detects	Advantages	Disadvantages
Clinical signs			
White/blue cold extremities with poor-capillary refill	Hypoperfusion	Simple, quick no equipment needed	Non-specific, unreliable if hypothermia present
Rapid poor-volume pulse	Hypovolaemia	Simple, quick no equipment needed	Non-specific, may be difficult to feel in shocked patient
Agitation, restlessness	Cerebral hypoperfusion or hypoxia	Observation	Non-specific
'Air hunger'	Acidosis due to hypoperfusion	Observation	Non-specific, present with other causes of metabolic acidosis
Non-invasive monitoring			
Blood pressure cuff (manual)	Blood pressure by occluding flow to limb, palpation or auscultation	Readily available Nursing staff can perform	May be difficult to palpate or auscultate in hypotension, and diastolic indistinct; needs correct size cuff
Blood pressure cuff (automatic)	As above using oscillotonometry	Automatic, built-in alarm levels measure pulse and mean pressure also	Expensive, not always available; needs correct size cuff; inaccurate at extremes of blood pressure; unable to function when pulse volume variable
ECG	Heart rate dysrhythmias; ischaemia	Widely available, easy and quick to connect by nursing staff	Prone to electrical interference from surrounding equipment; electrode contact poor on clammy patient
Pulse oximeter	Pulse rate, pulse volume, arterial oxygen saturation	Easy and quick to apply finger/ear probe	Expensive, not always available; readings unreliable with peripheral shutdown
Temperature probe (skin and central)	Skin temperature	Gives an indication of temperature, hence perfusion	Unreliable with hypothermia or peripheral vascular disease

Table 14.2 Summary of some invasive and more sophisticated methods of monitoring the bleeding patient

Type	Detects	Advantages	Disadvantages
Invasive monitoring			
Arterial line (indwelling cannula—usually radial artery)	Direct arterial blood pressure	More accurate at lower blood pressures Waveform gives indication of hypovolaemia Facilitates measurement	Requires skill and time to insert, set up and calibrate Needs transducers and appropriate monitors Long-term complications
Central venous pressure line (usually internal jugular or subclavian vein)	Central venous pressure in superior vena cava	Good indication of central venous filling pressures as aid to volume replacement Can be used with a simple gravity manometer	Requires skill and time to insert and place Influenced by tone in venous capacitance vessels Influenced by right ventricular dysfunction Risk of damage to thoracic structures Risk of air embolism Long-term complications
Pulmonary artery balloon flotation catheter (Swan–Ganz)	Pulmonary artery pressure and pulmonary capillary wedge pressure	Most accurate means of assessing volume replacement Gives indication of left ventricular function Can measure cardiac output, oxygen delivery	Requires high level of skill to insert Highly invasive; risk of arrhythmias and myocardial damage Time consuming Long-term complications Often adds little extra to CVP Use uncommon in operating theatres

call out for rapid fluid replacement. Non-invasive measurement of blood pressure is routine, easy and rapid but more elaborate techniques of monitoring, for example measurement of central venous pressure (CVP) and intra-arterial measurement of pressure, valuable though they undoubtedly are, take time to set up and may well have to be left till later.

Monitors are not infallible: a flat ECG has been interpreted as asystole when there is only disconnection from the patient. They can also distract and the amount of information may confuse the uninitiated. A malfunctioning alarm may cause attention to be diverted and the monitor, as it were, treated rather than the patient. There follows a very brief account of the three most important factors—ECG, blood pressure and central venous pressure. Urine output as a guide has already been mentioned. The pulse oximeter is also useful in detecting desaturation, but may give misleading information in severe vasoconstriction.

The electrocardiograph

This provides a useful method of determining pulse rate, and the rate can be displayed directly if an integrator is combined. It will also show the presence, and often the nature, of dysrhythmias and may detect myocardial ischaemia. A modified precardial bipolar V5 lead (cM5) is probably the most popular although it is not as sensitive to cardiac ischaemia (T-wave inversion, ST depression) as V5 proper, nor as useful in diagnosing arrhythmias as lead II.

Measurement of blood pressure

Non-invasive methods

These are usually adequate though they are by no means completely accurate. The Riva–Rocci method, using a sphygmomanometer, is still widely in use in wards but a method based on oscillometry is commonly used in theatre. The simple, manually operated oscillometer is being replaced with automatic forms based on this principle (e.g. the 'Dinamap') and these may be provided with a continuous write-out. Unfortunately they are uncomfortable on the conscious patient.

Methods based on oscillometry tend to give too high a reading when the arterial pressure is high, and underestimate when it is too low. Obesity, too, causes gross inaccuracy and in the morbidly obese bleeding patient invasive methods may be essential.

Invasive methods

Arterial pressure is measured with a cannula in an artery and a pressure transducer with electronic amplification system; this should be more accurate, but is subject to many errors and requires knowledge, skill and care to produce acceptable results. The user must be familiar with the apparatus, must be able to calibrate it accurately and must know, for example, the effects of over-damping and underdamping.

The radial artery is the most commonly used. The list of possible complications is a formidable one, ranging from haematoma formation to gangrene. The adequacy of the collateral (ulnar) circulation should be tested using the simple method described by Allen [52]. Both radial and ulnar arteries in the hand are occluded until blanching occurs; ulnar pressure is then released and the time to flushing of the hand, normally not more than 15 s, is noted. The test is unfortunately not conclusive [53].

Central venous pressure

The presence of a central venous line, via for example, internal jugular vein, subclavian vein, or peripherally through the cephalic vein, is a very useful adjunct to treatment. The results can be misleading if the catheter is misplaced: for example, should it go up the internal jugular vein and the patient's head and shoulders are elevated it will give a zero reading unless there is cardiac failure or gross hypervolaemia.

The two basic determinants of central venous pressure (CVP) are (i) cardiac function (thus it goes up in right-sided cardiac failure) and (ii) the effective circulating volume (it goes up in right-sided plethora and down in hypovolaemia). 'Effective' is an important word—CVP will go up with venoconstriction and down with venodilatation. It is important to realize that CVP is not directly related, in a linear fashion, to circulating volume—venous capacitance is involved as well.

There are two commonly used points of reference: (i) the manubriosternal angle, giving a normal reading of about zero, and (ii) the mid-axillary line giving a normal reading of 5–10 cmH_2O. Absolute values are less important than trends, and it is evident that when the circulating volume is adequate, or more than adequate, and CVP is again near normal a further infusion of, say, 250 ml of colloid will cause a rise which is sustained for some time—a test which, in practical circumstances, may be difficult to apply.

Other monitors, concerned mainly with the conduct of the anaesthetic, will not be detailed. These include equipment for measuring inspired oxygen concentration, end-tidal carbon dioxide concentration (alveolar), minute volume and peak airway pressure, all of which enable the anaesthetist to optimize patient care.

Postoperative management

In most cases, the patient will be returned to the ward, high-dependency unit or to the intensive therapy unit (ITU). Some, for example the victims of major trauma, may require positive pressure ventilation in an ITU in the immediate postoperative period.

All, however, will require adequate analgesia. It is clearly beyond the scope of this chapter to elaborate on this. Morphine is still the mainstay of postoperative analgesia, given either by intermittent injection (intramuscularly or intravenously) or by continuous intravenous infusion in a high-dependency unit or ITU (only). Epidural and spinal opiates also have a place if close supervision is practicable.

Sedulous monitoring of blood pressure, pulse rate and, except in relatively minor cases, CVP and urine output, is mandatory, as is observation of respiration, especially since the patient will be receiving opioids. Transfusion, too, may have to be continued if the patient's circulatory volume is still inadequate or if bleeding/oozing is still present.

Oxygen therapy should be routine for the first few hours and may have to be continued. A pulse oximeter is a useful tool for monitoring oxygen saturation postoperatively, but the patient on oxygen may slip into ventilatory failure (with carbon dioxide retention) with an adequate saturation if oxygen is being administered. Blood gases should be checked if this is suspected.

It is likely that the patient's body temperature will have fallen. Though pain and anxiety are the most important subjective responses after surgery, feeling cold is a most disagreeable experience and overt shivering will cause an increased oxygen consumption and may lead to hypoxaemia. Warmed blankets or special silvered hypothermia blankets are helpful.

It is good practice, when the patient is taken from theatre, fundamentally to review the situation. Further investigations may be called for—for example:

- Haemoglobin and packed-cell volume.
- Clotting profile.
- Urea and electrolytes and blood sugar.
- Blood gases.
- Chest X-ray.
- Even a full ECG may be indicated.

None, however, should be regarded as a routine necessity.

Both surgeon and anaesthetist may well be beyond their best at this stage and should welcome 'handing over' to those equally skilled, but the patient may still be critically ill and a sense of anticlimax must be avoided.

References

1 *The Report of a Confidential Enquiry into Perioperative Deaths* (Eds Buck, N., Devlin, H.B. & Lunn, J.N.). The Nuffield Provincial Hospitals Trust (1988).

2 Nicholls, B.J. and Cullen, B.F. (1988) Anesthesia for trauma. *J. Clin. Anesth.*, **1**, 115–129.

3 Marsh, R.H.K., Spencer, R. and Nimmo, W.S. (1984) Gastric emptying and drug absorption before surgery. *Br. J. Anaesth.*, **56**, 161–163.

4 Teabeaut, J.R. (1952) Aspiration of gastric contents. An experimental study. *Am. J. Pathol.*, **228**, 51–61.

5 Roberts, R.B. and Shirley, M. (1974) Aspiration during vaginal delivery. *Anesthesiology*, **40**, 317.

6 Mendelson, C.L. (1946) The aspiration of stomach contents into the lungs during obstetric anesthesia. *Am. J. Obstet. Gynec.*, **52**, 191–204.

7 Gimmon, Z. (1985) Advantageous use of Salem Sump nasogastric tube for intraoperative decompression of distended intestine. *Surg. Gynecol. Obstet.*, **161**, 69–70.

8 Lahiri, S.K., Thomas, T.A. and Hodgson, R.M.H. (1973) Single-dose antacid therapy for the prevention of Mendelson's syndrome. *Br. J. Anaesth.*, **45**, 1143–1146.

9 Kennedy, W.F., Bonica, J.J., Akamatsu, T.J. *et al.* (1968) Cardiovascular and respiratory effects of subarachnoid block in the presence of acute blood loss. *Anesthesiology*, **29**, 29–35

10 Bonica, J.J., Kennedy, W.F., Akamatsu, T.J. and Gerbershagen, H.U. (1972) Circulatory effects of peridural block: III. Effects of acute blood loss. *Anesthesiology*, **36**, 219–227.

11 Sellick, B.A. (1961) Cricoid pressure to control regurgitation of stomach contents during induction of anaesthesia. *Lancet*, **ii**, 404–406.

12 Bogetz, M.S. and Katz, J.A. (1984) Recall of surgery for major trauma. *Anesthesiology*, **61**, 6–9.

13 Cournand, A., Motley, H.L., Werko, L. and Richards, D.W. (1948) Physiological studies of the effects of intermittent positive pressure breathing on cardiac output in man. *Am. J. Physiol.*, **152**, 162–174.

14 Morgan, W.L., Binion, J.T. and Sarnoff, S.J. (1957) Circulatory depression induced by high levels of positive pressure breathing counteracted by metaraminol (Aramine). *J. Appl. Physiol.*, **10**, 26–30.

15 Halford, E.J. (1943) Critique of intravenous anesthesia in war surgery. *Anesthesiology*, **4**, 67.

16 Chamberlain, J.H., Seed, R.G.F.L. and Chung, D.C.W. (1977) Effect of thiopentone on myocardial function. *Br. J. Anaesth.*, **49**, 865–870.

17 Bond, A.C. and Davies, C.K. (1974) Ketamine and pancuronium for the shocked patient. *Anaesthesia*, **29**, 59–62.

18 Tunstall, M.E. (1979) The reduction of amnesic wakefulness during Caesarian section. *Br. J. Anaesth.*, **34**, 316–319.

19 Munson, E.S. (1974) Transfer of nitrous oxide into body air cavities. *Br. J. Anaesth.*, **46**, 202–209.

20 Stock, J.G.L. and Strunin, L. (1985) Unexplained hepatitis following halothane. *Anesthesiology*, **63**, 424–439.

21 Hobbhahn, J., Conzen, P., Forst, H. and Peter, K. (1989) Effect of inhalation anaesthetics on the myocardium. *Anaesthetist*, **38** (Suppl. 2), S561–S596.

22 Harrison, R.A. and Rampton, A.J. Colloid–crystalloid controversy. In: *Anaesthesia Review 5* (Ed. Kauffmann, L.), pp. 101–118. Churchill Livingstone, Edinburgh (1988).

23 Sieber, F.E., Smith, D.S., Traystman, R.J. and Wollman, H. (1987) Glucose: a reevaluation of its intraoperative use. *Anesthesiology*, **67**, 72–81.

24 Trinkle, J.K., Rush, B.F. and Eiseman, B. (1968) Metabolism of lactate following major blood loss. *Surgery*, **63**, 782–787.

25 Isbister, J.P. and Fisher, M.M. (1980) Adverse effects of plasma volume expanders. *Anaesth. Intensive Care*, **8**, 145–151.

26 Twigley, A.J. and Hillman, K.M. (1985) The end of the crystalloid era? *Anaesthesia*, **40**, 860–871.

27 Messmer, K.F.W. (1987) The use of plasma substitutes with special attention to their side effects. *World J. Surg.*, **11**, 69–74.

28 Gruber, U.F. (1975) Dextran and the prevention of postoperative thromboembolic complications. *Surg. Clin. North Am.*, **55**, 679–697.

29 Macintyre, E., Mackie, I.J., Ho, D., Tinker, J. *et al.* (1985) The haemostatic effects of hydroxyethyl starch (HES) used as a volume expander. *Intensive Care Med.*, **11**, 300–303.

30 Stump, D.C., Strauss, R.G., Henriksen, R.A., Petersen, R.E. and Saunders, R. (1985) Effect of hydroxyethyl starch on blood coagulation, particularly Factor VIII. *Transfusion*, **25**, 349–354.

31 Thoren, L. (1981) The dextrans—clinical data. *Dev. Biol. Stand.*, **48**, 157–167.

32 Morgan, T.O., Little, J.M. and Evans, W.A. (1966) Renal failure associated with low-molecular-weight dextran infusion. *Br. Med. J.*, **2**, 737–739.

33 Traverso, L.W., Bellamy, R.F., Hollenbach, S.J. and Witcher, L.D. (1987) Hypertonic sodium chloride solutions: effect on hemodynamics and survival after hemorrhage in swine. *J. Trauma*, **27**, 32–39.

34 de Felippe, J., Timoner, J., Velasco, I.T. *et al.* (1980) Treatment of refractory hypovolaemic shock by 7.5% sodium chloride injections. *Lancet*, **ii**, 1002–1004.

35 Shackford, S.R., Fortlage, D.A., Peters, R.M. *et al.* (1987) Serum osmolar and electrolyte changes associated with large infusions of hypertonic sodium lactate for intravascular volume expansion of patients undergoing aortic reconstruction. *Surg. Gynec. Obstet.*, **164**, 127–136.

36 Auler, J.O.C., Pereira, M.H.C., Gomide-Amaral, R.V. *et al.* Hemodynamic effects of hypertonic sodium chloride during surgical treatment of aortic aneurysms. *Surgery*, **101**, 594–601.

37 Shackford, S.R., Sise, M.J., Fridlund, P.H. *et al.* (1983) Hypertonic sodium lactate versus lactated Ringer's solution for intravenous fluid therapy in operations on the abdominal aorta. *Surgery*, **94**, 41–51.

38 Shires, T., Williams, J. and Brown, F. (1961) Acute change in extracellular fluids associated with major surgical procedures. *Ann. Surg.*, **154**, 803–810.

39 Moore, F.D. and Shires, G.T. (1967) Moderation. *Ann. Surg.*, **166**, 300–301.

40 Shires, G.T., Pietzman, A.B., Albert, S.A. *et al.* (1983) Response of extravascular lung water to intraoperative fluids. *Ann. Surg.*, **197**, 515–519.

41 Lowell, J.A., Schifferdecker, C., Driscoll, D.F. *et al.* (1990) Postoperative fluid overload: not a benign problem. *Crit. Care Med.*, **18**, 728–733.

42 Hauser, C.J., Shoemaker, W.C., Turpin, I. and Goldberg, S.J. (1980) Oxygen transport responses to colloids and crystalloids in critically ill surgical patients. *Surg. Gynec. Obstet.*, **150**, 811–816.

43 Howland, W.S. and Schweizer, O. (1965) Physiologic compensation for storage lesion of bank blood. *Anesth. Analg.*, **44**, 8–16.

44 Howland, W.S., Schweitzer, O., Carlon, G.C. and Goldiner, P.L. (1977) The cardiovascular effects of low levels of ionized calcium during massive transfusion. *Surg. Gynec. Obstet.*, **145**, 581–586.

45 Kahn, R.C., Jascott, D., Carlon, G.C. *et al.* (1979) Massive blood replacement: correlation of ionized calcium, citrate, and hydrogen ion concentration. *Anesth. Analg.*, **58**, 274–278.

46 Denlinger, J.K., Nahrwold, M.L., Gibbs, P.S. and Lecky, J.H. (1976) Hypocalcaemia during rapid blood transfusion in anaesthetized man. *Br. J. Anaesth.*, **48**, 995–999.

47 Linko, K. and Tigerstedt, I. (1984) Hyperpotassemia during massive blood transfusions. *Acta Anaesthesiol. Scand.*, **28**, 220–221.

48 Cousins, M.J. and Mazze, R.I. (1973) Anaesthesia, surgery and renal function. *Anaesth. Intensive Care*, **1**, 355–373.

49 Moran, W.H., Miltenberger, F.W., Shuayb, W.A. and Zimmermann, B. (1964) The relationship of antidiuretic hormone secretion to surgical stress. *Surgery*, **56**, 99–108.

50 Claybaugh, J.R. and Share, L. (1973) Vasopressin, renin, and cardiovascular responses to continuous slow hemorrhage. *Am. J. Physiol.*, **224**, 519–523.

51 Runciman, W.B. and Skowronski, G.A. (1984) Pathophysiology of haemorrhagic shock. *Anaesth. Intensive Care*, **12**, 193–205.

52 Allen, E.V. (1929) Thromboangitis obliterans: methods of diagnosis of chronic occlusive arterial lesions distal to the wrist with illustrative cases. *Am. J. Med. Sci.*, **178**, 237–244.

53 Slogoff, S., Keats, A.S. and Arlund, C. (1983) On the safety of radial artery cannulation. *Anesthesiology*, **59**, 42–47.

Chapter 15
Drugs used in bleeding

JOS VERMYLEN AND DANIEL BLOCKMANS

There are several reasons why patients may continue to bleed during or after a surgical intervention. However, a local surgical factor (e.g. loosening of a knot) has first to be excluded. Other possible reasons are the inadvertent transfusion of incompatible blood, or the administration of large amounts of packed cells or blood-replacing fluids. In these cases, the prevention or correction of the depletion of clotting factors and/or of platelets will restore normal haemostasis.

When surgery needs to be done on a fully heparinized patient, heparin has to be stopped 5 h previously, after which interval surgical intervention can safely be performed. In case of a very urgent surgical procedure, heparin can be neutralized by the slow intravenous administration of protamine chloride or sulphate: 10 mg of protamine neutralizes about 1000 iu of heparin. Since heparin has a longer plasma half-life than protamine, a second injection of the latter drug may be needed.

When surgery is needed for a patient who takes oral anticoagulants (vitamin K antagonists), these drugs have to be stopped 2–3 days previously, to allow the prothrombin time (PT) to reach an International Normalized Ratio (INR) below 2, at which level surgery can be safely performed. Whenever surgery is required within a shorter period of time, vitamin K can be given. After the slow intravenous administration of 10 mg of vitamin K, the PT will start to shorten in about 4 h, the time needed for hepatic synthesis of the missing vitamin K-dependent clotting factors (Factors II, VII, IX and X). After oral intake of vitamin K_1 (10 droplets, 1 mg/droplet), this rise will take about half an hour longer. In an emergency, immediate correction can be achieved by intravenous administration of a prothrombin complex concentrate. When a prolonged PT is due to vitamin K deficiency, caused by inadequate intake or by malabsorption, vitamin K_1 administration will also shorten the PT. If a prolonged PT is due to hepatocellular damage, vitamin K is of no use.

If the patient to be operated upon is known to have a specific clotting factor deficiency (e.g. haemophilia A or B), the preoperative administration of the deficient factor is the logical step to be taken. An overview of the available blood products is presented in Chapter 16. Several clotting factors, e.g. Factor VIII, are now produced by recombinant DNA technology and hence are no longer of blood origin. They probably will soon be generally available for patient treatment.

Patients with thrombocytopenia due to impaired production of platelets or with congenital thrombocytopathies will benefit from platelet transfusions, provided they have not developed isoantibodies by previous exposures to platelets. Thrombocytopenia caused by accelerated breakdown of platelets is much less responsive to platelet administration. Problems related to platelet transfusion therapy are discussed in Chapter 16.

In a number of patients, an excessive bleeding tendency cannot be overcome by the administration of a specific deficient clotting factor or of platelets, since the origin of their bleeding tendency is not understood, or due to factors which cannot be easily controlled (e.g. blood damage in extracorporeal circuits or patients with liver cirrhosis or uraemia, or drug-induced platelet dysfunction). In these patients, the use of a number of haemostatically active drugs can diminish blood loss during and following surgery. We shall especially focus on the use of the antifibrinolytic drugs tranexamic acid, ε-aminocaproic acid and aprotinin, and on the use of the vasopressin analogue, desmopressin.

Synthetic fibrinolysis inhibitors: tranexamic acid and ε-aminocaproic acid

The antifibrinolytic action of these compounds is mainly related to their reversible complex formation with the so-called 'lysine-binding sites' of human plasminogen [1]. These synthetic aminoacids block the binding of plasminogen and of the heavy chain of plasmin to fibrin via these lysine-binding sites. On a molar basis, tranexamic acid is 7–10-fold more potent than ε-aminocaproic acid (EACA) and has a longer half-life; it has therefore become the compound of choice.

Tranexamic acid

In two double-blind trials, tranexamic acid, injected intravenously half an hour before tonsillectomy, gave a significant reduction in measured blood loss when compared to placebo [2,3]. In patients undergoing prostatectomy, tranexamic acid also significantly reduces blood loss; the dosage used is 0.5–1 g intravenously 2–3 times daily, starting immediately after surgery, during the first 3 postoperative days and thereafter 1–1.5 g orally 2–3 times daily until macroscopic haematuria is no longer present [4]. An average reduction in blood loss of 70% was also noted in patients who underwent cervical conization (with or without suturing) and who received 1.5 g tranexamic acid daily for at least 12 days postoperatively [5,6].

In a recent placebo-controlled double-blind study, prophylactic tranexamic acid significantly decreased bleeding after cardiac operation (coronary artery bypass grafting or/and valve replacement) (Table 15.1). This reduced blood loss was due to inhibition of fibrinolysis, as was shown by the lower prevalence of fibrin split products in the drug group. The latter group received a 10 mg/kg infusion of tranexamic acid intravenously over a 20 min period followed by an infusion of 1 mg/kg for 10 h [7].

In a double-blind prospective randomized study in 154 patients, emergency surgery for benign bleeding lesions in the stomach and/or duodenum was significantly less frequent in patients on tranexamic acid (1 g 4-hourly for 3 days intravenously, followed by oral treatment with 1.5 g 6-hourly for another 3 days) than in patients on placebo [8].

In another prospective randomized double-blind study in patients with haemophilia needing tooth extraction, Forbes *et al.* [9] found that tranexamic acid (1 g t.i.d. for 5 days) together with replacement therapy (Factor VIII or IX), significantly reduced blood loss and transfusion requirements. These results have been confirmed by other studies. Recently, Baudo *et al.* [10] concluded that replacement therapy can even be omitted by the combination of tranexamic acid (3 × 1 g/day for 4 days) and the local application in the alveolar cavity of Tissucol, a heat-treated lyophilized human plasma fraction that contains fibrinogen in high concentration, Factor XIII and other plasma proteins.

Theoretically, the administration of antifibrinolytic drugs could facilitate the development of thrombosis. Sporadic cases have been reported; the use of antifibrinolytics is contraindicated in case of diffuse intravascular coagulation. Other side-effects of tranexamic acid are rare and rather mild—nausea, diarrhoea and an occasional orthostatic hypotension [11].

ε-Aminocaproic acid

EACA ($NH_2(CH_2)_5COOH$) is less often used than tranexamic acid, due

Table 15.1 Haemostatic agents in cardiac surgery

	Active			Placebo/control	
Study	Patient no.	Values		Patient no.	Values
Tranexamic acid					
Horrow *et al.* [7]					
12 h blood loss (ml)	18	496 ± 228	$p = 0.0057$	20	750 ± 314
Infusion of fresh frozen plasma		0/18	$p = 0.0035$		5/20
ε-Aminocaproic acid					
Vander Salm *et al.* [13]					
12 h blood loss (ml)	31	273 ± 19	$p = 0.02$	27	323 ± 2
DelRossi *et al.* [14]					
24 h blood loss (ml)	170	617 ± 44	$p < 0.05$	180	883 ± 29
Blood transfusions in first 72 h (units)		2.8 ± 2.0	$p < 0.05$		4.2 ± 2.3
Aprotinin					
Royston *et al.* [17]					
24 h drainage loss (ml)	11	286 ± 48	$p < 0.001$	11	1509 ± 388
Amount of donor blood transfused (ml)		183 ± 48	$p < 0.001$		1975 ± 520
Van Oeveren *et al.* [18]					
Postoperative blood loss (ml)	11	357	$p < 0.01$	11	674
Transfusion requirement (ml)		720	$p < 0.02$		1380

Alajmo *et al.* [19]					
Postoperative bleeding (ml)	22	486 ± 47	$p = 0.0028$	12	830 ± 17
Use of banked blood (ml)		213 ± 85			490 ± 140
Van Oeveren *et al.* [20]					
Blood loss (g haemoglobin)	30	84	$p < 0.01$	30	131
Postoperative blood transfusion					
Packed cells		0.35 ± 0.6	$p < 0.01$		1.0 ± 0.6
Fresh frozen plasma		0.35 ± 0.8	$p < 0.01$		1.0 ± 0.3
Desmopressin					
Salzman *et al.* [41]					
Operative and postoperative blood loss (primary coronary bypass grafting not occluded) (ml)	35	1317 ± 487	$p < 0.001$	33	2210 ± 1415
Rocha *et al.* [43]					
Total blood loss (ml/m^2)	50	458 ± 206	n.s.	56	536 ± 304
Intraoperative (ml/m^2)	50	131 ± 106	$p < 0.02$	50	193 ± 137
Hackmann *et al.* [44]					
Total loss after drug infusion (median and 5th–95th percentile in ml)	74	1138 (398–3238)	$p = 0.43$	76	1010 (473–3258)
Prostacyclin					
Fish *et al.* [61]					
Blood loss first 4 h (ml)	50	261 ± 159	$p < 0.02$	50	347 ± 197
Total blood loss (ml)		710 ± 351	n.s.		869 ± 498

n.s. = not significant.

to its lower potency and shorter half-life (1–2 h). It was the first representative of the plasminogen-binding blockers. The oral dose of EACA is 0.1 g/kg body weight every 6 h; intravenously a loading dose of 10 g followed by 1 g/h is needed to give the effective plasma concentration of 0.01 mol/l [4]. Due to the higher doses to be administered compared with tranexamic acid, its side-effects are more frequent—diarrhoea, dizziness, skin rash, nausea, nasal stuffiness or conjunctival suffusion [11]. As for tranexamic acid, there is always the theoretical risk of developing thrombosis, especially when other risk factors are present [12].

Vander Salm *et al.* [13] used EACA in a double-blind study vs. placebo in 60 patients undergoing elective coronary bypass surgery (5 g EACA intravenously over a 5 min period starting after being weaned from cardiopulmonary bypass, followed by EACA, 1 g/h for 6 h). They found a small but significant decrease in postoperative blood loss in the EACA treated patients (Table 15.1). Two myocardial infarctions developed in these patients, but this could have been due to chance.

The beneficial effect of the prophylactic treatment with EACA on blood loss after cardiopulmonary bypass surgery and on the need for blood transfusions was confirmed in a large placebo-controlled double-blind study on 350 patients undergoing elective surgery for coronary artery disease, repair of myocardial aneurysms, valve replacement or combined procedures [14]. The dose used was 5 g EACA intravenously prior to skin incision, followed by intravenous administration of 1 g/h for the next 6–8 h. Postoperative myocardial infarction and reoperation for bleeding were more frequent in the placebo-treated group.

EACA was also used prophylactically with success in patients with immune thrombocytopenic purpura before dental extraction and to control bleeding at other operation sites [15].

Aprotinin

Aprotinin is a serum protease inhibitor, derived from bovine lung and identical to the basic pancreatic trypsin inhibitor. It inhibits the effects of trypsin, plasma kallikrein, plasmin and chymotrypsin. It protects platelets from pathologic activation by preventing platelet aggregation elicited with thrombin and trypsin, but not with collagen [16].

In a randomized study on 22 patients undergoing repeat open heart surgery, Royston *et al.* [17] showed that the mean blood loss of patients given high doses of aprotinin (700 mg, which is 5×10^6 kallikrein inactivator units (KIU)) intravenously from the start of anaesthesia to the end of operation, was significantly lower than in the control patients (Table 15.1). Blood-transfusion requirements were eightfold higher in the control group than in the aprotinin group.

In another 22 patients undergoing elective coronary artery bypass grafting, Van Oeveren *et al.* [8] also found better preserved haemostasis postoperatively in the 11 patients who had been given aprotinin to achieve plasma concentrations of >150 KIU/ml during cardiopulmonary bypass. Significantly less blood loss in the treated group seemed to be attributable to better platelet preservation in the extracorporeal circuit (no fall in platelet count and a significantly lower generation of thromboxane).

The effectiveness in terms of decreased postoperative bleeding of high-dose aprotinin (2×10^6 KIU aprotinin at the start of anaesthesia, 500 000 KIU/h until the end of operation) in open heart surgery was confirmed by Alajmo *et al.* [19] although in this study the platelet count decreased in both groups to the same extent.

Van Oeveren *et al.* [20] stated that the first pass of blood through the extracorporeal circuit is the main cause of platelet damage, which implies that aprotinin already has to be present in sufficient amounts at that moment. Angelini *et al.* [21] however could successfully reduce life-threatening postoperative blood loss by starting aprotinin 6–14 h after termination of cardiopulmonary bypass (loading dose 2×10^6 KIU, followed by an infusion of 500 000 KIU/h for 4–6 h).

The effectiveness of aprotinin in reducing the need for blood transfusion was also suggested in patients having open heart surgery for septic endocarditis and who are at great risk for postoperative bleeding. Bidstrup *et al.* [22] found an 8–10-fold reduction in the use of bank blood compared with similar patients operated on previously at their institution.

Patients undergoing orthotopic liver transplantation, which is frequently complicated by severe coagulopathy and blood loss, also benefit from intraoperative prophylactic aprotinin administration (2×10^6 KIU); in a controlled study, the duration of surgery from time of reperfusion to wound closure was significantly shorter (40 min) and the blood loss was significantly lower, the units of red cells and of fresh frozen plasma transfused being halved [23]. This beneficial effect of aprotinin was confirmed by Mallett *et al.* [24] and seems to be due to inhibition of hyperfibrinolysis.

In peripheral vascular surgery (reconstructive surgery for aortoiliac occlusive disease), blood loss was reduced by 43% with administration of aprotinin (bolus dose of 2×10^6 KIU intravenously after induction of anaesthesia, followed by an infusion of 500 000 KIU/h, which was continued until the patient left the operating theatre) [25].

Aprotinin has few side-effects when used as a haemostatic agent; three cardiac arrests were recorded in 2000 patients receiving the drug intravenously following surgery. Occasional hypersensitivity may occur [11].

Desmopressin

Desmopressin (deamino-D-arginine vasopressin, DDAVP) is a synthetic analogue of the neurohypophyseal nonapeptide, arginine vasopressin. It has enhanced antidiuretic potency, markedly diminished pressor activity and a prolonged half-life and duration of action compared to the native hormone.

In 1974, it was shown that vasopressin, the natural hormone, produces short-term increases in plasma Factor VIII [26]. DDAVP, given intravenously to healthy volunteers and patients with moderate haemophilia and von Willebrand's disease, also increases Factor VIII and von Willebrand factor (vWF) levels [27,28]. Mannucci was the first to use DDAVP (0.3 μg/kg intravenously) in patients with moderate or mild haemophilia or von Willebrand's disease during dental extractions or major surgical procedures, and documented a factor VIII and vWF increase to approximately 3–5 times the resting levels [29].

A patient with an acquired von Willebrand's syndrome, secondary to benign monoclonal gammopathy, was given DDAVP successfully to prevent bleeding after tooth extraction [30].

Haemophilia A patients with Factor VIII levels of <10% do not benefit from DDAVP, since the posttreatment Factor VIII levels would be <30%, insufficient for haemostasis. Because of exhaustion of Factor VIII stores (and to a lesser extent vWF stores), DDAVP should not be given more frequently than once every 24–36 h. Subcutaneous DDAVP is at least as effective and more practical than intravenous DDAVP [31]; the dosages of intranasal DDAVP (3–4 μg/kg) are more than 10-fold higher than the dosages recommended for subcutaneous or intravenous use [32].

In a recent review article on the perioperative management of patients with von Willebrand's disease, Cameron and Kobrinsky [33] recommend the administration of a test infusion of DDAVP (0.3 μg/kg or 10 μg/m^2 intravenously over 20 min, 2 or 3 days preoperatively) and rechecking of the haemostatic parameters after 1 h. This is particularly true if the classification of the patient (type I, IIa, IIb or III) is not known preoperatively. If the bleeding time shortens, it can be assumed that DDAVP will be haemostatically effective in the perioperative period. DDAVP is most effective in patients with mild type I disease, has a variable effect in type IIa, is contraindicated in type IIb (since it can produce severe thrombocytopenia in these patients) and has no effect in type III.

More recently, DDAVP was used to prevent blood loss in patients with congenital and acquired platelet dysfunction, including the grey platelet syndrome, storage pool deficiency, acetylsalicylic acid intake, uraemia and liver cirrhosis [34–37]. The beneficial effect of DDAVP was less clear in patients with Glanzmann's thrombasthenia [38].

In 59 patients with the so-called vascular fragility syndrome (an isolated prolongation of the bleeding time with otherwise normal platelet counts, normal platelet aggregation and coagulation parameters including vWF, and without evidence of liver or kidney disease or exposure to antiplatelet agents), DDAVP reduced the bleeding time from 15.3 ± 3.4 min to 10.7 ± 3.9 min within 30 min following infusion [30]. There was a satisfactory arrest of acute bleeding or good control of subsequent haemostasis with surgery.

During the past few years, DDAVP has been found to reduce blood loss by about one-third in haemostatically normal patients undergoing surgery associated with major blood loss, e.g. spinal surgery for scoliosis [40] or cardiac surgery requiring cardiopulmonary bypass [41]. In the latter study, DDAVP was given at 0.3 μg/kg body weight intravenously in a 50 ml solution over 15 min when cardiopulmonary bypass had been concluded (Table 15.1). This beneficial effect was not related to a drug-induced increase in high-molecular-weight vWF multimers but rather to a rise in overall vWF concentration [42]. In another double-blind, randomized, prospective trial including 100 patients placed on cardiopulmonary bypass during surgery, Rocha *et al.* [43] only found a reduced intraoperative blood loss but the same total blood loss, using exactly the same scheme of DDAVP administration. In a third double-blind randomized placebo-controlled trial by Hackmann *et al.* [44] there was no beneficial effect of DDAVP, probably due to the fact that, in this study on 150 patients, 69% of the patients underwent primary coronary artery bypass grafting, which produces less blood loss than the complicated cardiac operations which were included in the first two studies. The futility of desmopressin in routine coronary artery bypass surgery was confirmed by other studies [45–47]. At present, a consensus has developed that DDAVP is useful in a selected group of patients: those with primary or acquired preoperative bleeding disorders, including acetylsalicylic acid ingestion, and those undergoing operations with a greater haemorrhagic risk, e.g. associated with a long cardiopulmonary bypass time [48].

Side-effects of DDAVP are mild facial flushing, transient headache, a 10–20% increase in heart rate and diastolic blood pressure. With repeated administration, there is the risk of water retention with sometimes severe hyponatraemia, due to its potent antidiuretic action. Combined with antifibrinolytic drugs, there may be an increased risk of thrombus formation.

Other drugs

A number of preparations have been claimed to improve blood clotting, and hence their use in surgery has been recommended (e.g. tissue extracts, colloidal polygalacturonic acid esters, naphthionin, aminapthone, carbazochrome, naftazone, extracts of snake venoms). Controlled studies indicating that operative blood loss is diminished are, however, lacking.

For a small number of drugs, there is more pharmacological and clinical evidence that they are haemostatically effective. These substances will briefly be discussed.

Ethamsylate

Ethamsylate (diethylamine 2,5-dihydroxybenzenesulphate) is a synthetic water-soluble drug which reduces the bleeding time in animals, normal subjects and patients with a variety of bleeding disorders, in a dose-related manner [49]. Ethamsylate has been shown to increase platelet adhesiveness to glass beads and to increase capillary resistance [50], probably by preventing the breakdown of mucopolysaccharides in the ground substance of the capillary wall. More recently, it was shown that ethamsylate inhibits the production of platelet-inhibitory prostaglandins such as PGI_2 [51]. From a clinical point of view, ethamsylate significantly reduces blood loss in primary menorrhagia [52] and periventricular haemorrhage in very-low-birthweight babies [53] but not in acute aspirin-induced gastric mucosal bleeding in healthy subjects [54]. The manufacturer also claims it to be effective in patients without bleeding tendency undergoing dental extractions, adenotonsillectomy or prostatic or proctological surgery. The recommended dose in adults is 500 mg 4 times daily. For surgery or emergency use, 750 mg should be given intravenously, followed by a further 250 mg during or at the end of operation [55].

Oestrogen–progesterone therapy

Synthetic oestrogen or oestrogen–progesterone therapy was found to be effective in preventing epistaxis in patients with hereditary haemorrhagic telangiectasia as early as 1952 [56]. In a recent double-blind placebo-controlled crossover study on 10 patients with recurrent gastrointestinal bleeding from multiple vascular malformations, a therapy regimen of 0.05 mg ethinyloestradiol plus 1 mg norethisterone daily by mouth for a 6 month period was highly effective in the prophylaxis of bleeding and in decreasing the need for blood transfusions [57]. The same authors hypothesized that the development of a thickened fibrous wall around previously abnormal blood vessels, which they could demonstrate in a patient after oestrogen–progesterone treatment, might contribute to the observed beneficial effect on bleeding [58].

Conjugated oestrogens given intravenously (total dose of 3 mg/kg body weight, divided into daily infusions of 0.6 mg/kg for 5 consecutive days) were shown to reduce the bleeding time in uraemic patients from 6 h after the first infusion onwards, with a maximum effect between days 5 and 7 and lasting for 14 days [59]. The authors concluded that, although they could not clarify the exact mechanism of action, conjugated oestrogens can be used in the treatment of bleeding associated with renal failure, especially when a longer duration of action is needed and when an immediate onset of the effect is not required, as is the case for planned non-urgent surgical procedures.

Bleeding from gastrointestinal telangiectasias in patients on haemodialysis, which is the commonest cause of gastrointestinal bleeding in this patient group, can also successfully be controlled with oral oestrogen–progesterone treatment [60].

The authors have excellent experience with oestrogen therapy in a patient with acquired von Willebrand's disease and recurrent gastrointestinal bleeding.

Conclusions

Apart from the infusion of specific blood components in the management of surgical bleeding when these are lacking, the use of haemostatic drugs is becoming recognized as beneficial in the following clinical situations:

1 *Cardiopulmonary bypass surgery.* The evidence for reduced blood loss in cardiac surgery is quite convincing for the antifibrinolytic agents tranexamic acid, EACA and aprotinin. The reduction in blood loss is not only statistically but also clinically significant, since the amount of donor blood products infused is significantly diminished. This undoubtedly is a major contribution to patient management. The reported side-effects are few, if any. Administration of antifibrinolytic agents should therefore receive careful consideration in all patients undergoing cardiopulmonary bypass surgery or when there is likelihood of excessive bleeding (re-operations, recent ingestion of aspirin, etc.). At present, there is no study directly comparing the plasminogen-binding blockers EACA and tranexamic acid to aprotinin, and it is difficult to decide which to select. On an economic basis, treatment with aprotinin costs about 35–40 times the treatment with a plasminogen-binding blocker.

2 *Orthotopic liver transplantation.* The limited studies to date clearly suggest that aprotinin significantly reduces the very important blood loss frequently associated with this intervention. Aprotinin may be preferable to tranexamic acid in this condition, which is often accompanied by disseminated intravascular coagulation; indeed, aprotinin inhibits several proteases of the haemostatic cascades, whereas tranexamic acid is a selective inhibitor of plasminogen activation and would therefore be more likely to promote diffuse deposition of fibrin in organs.

3 *Damage to mucous membranes.* Tranexamic acid is effective in reducing bleeding following tonsillectomy, prostatectomy, cervical conization or dental extractions (the latter particularly in haemophiliacs or thrombocytopenic subjects).

4 *Desmopressin.* This is mainly effective in surgical procedures performed in patients with mild haemophilia or von Willebrand's disease, or patients with a prolonged bleeding time of various origin.

References

1 Hoylaerts, M., Lijnen, H.R. and Collen, D. (1981) Studies on the mechanism of antifibrinolytic action of tranexamic acid. *Biochim. Biophys. Acta*, **673**, 75–85.

2 Castelli, G. and Vogt, E. (1977) Der Erfolg einer antifibrinolytischen Behandlung mit Tranexansaure zur Reduktion des Blutverlustes während und nach Tonsillektomien. *Schweiz. Med. Wochenschr.*, **107**, 780–784.

3 Verstraete, M., Tyberghein, J., De Greef, Y. *et al.* (1977) Double-blind trials with ethamsylate, batroxobin or tranexamic acid on blood loss after adenotonsillectomy. *Acta Clinica Belgica*, **32**, 136–141.

4 Verstraete, M. (1985) Clinical application of inhibitors of fibrinolysis. *Drugs*, **29**, 236–261.

5 Rybo, G. and Westerberg, H. (1972) The effect of tranexamic acid in postoperative bleeding after conization. *Acta Obstet. Gynec. Scand.*, **51**, 347–350.

6 Landin, L.E. and Werner, E. (1975) Late bleeding after conization. The effect of tranexamic acid (Cyclokapron). *Opuscula Medica*, **20**, 280–284.

7 Horrow, J.C., Hlavacek, J., Strong, M.D. *et al.* (1990) Prophylactic tranexamic acid decreases bleeding after cardiac operations. *J. Thorac. Cardiovasc. Surg.*, **99**, 70–74.

8 Staël von Holstein, C.C.S., Eriksson, S.B.S. and Källen, R. (1987) Tranexamic acid in gastric and duodenal bleeding. *Scand. J. Gastroenterol.*, **22** (Suppl. 137), 71–74.

9 Forbes, C.D., Barr, R.D., Reid, G. *et al.* (1972) Tranexamic acid in control of haemorrhage after dental extraction in haemophilia and Christmas disease. *Br. Med. J.* **2**, 311–313.

10 Baudo, F., DeCataldo F., Landonio, G. and Muti, G. (1988) Management of oral bleeding in haemophilic patients. *Lancet*, **ii**, 1082.

11 Verstraete, M. Hemostatic agents. In: *Meyler's Side Effects of Drugs* (Ed. Dukes, M.N.G.), 11th edn, pp. 776–780. Elsevier Science Publishers, Amsterdam (1988).

12 Achiron, A., Gornish, M. and Melamed, E. (1990) Cerebral sinus thrombosis as potential hazard of antifibrinolytic treatment in menorrhagia. *Stroke*, **21**, 817–819.

13 Vander Salm, T.J., Ansell, J.E., Okike, O.N. *et al.* (1988) The role of epsilon-aminocaproic acid in reducing bleeding after cardiac operation: a double-blind randomized study. *J. Thorac. Cardiovasc. Surg.*, **95**, 538–540.

14 DelRossi, A.J., Cernaianu, A.C., Botros, S. *et al.* (1989) Prophylactic treatment of postperfusion bleeding using EACA. *Chest*, **96**, 27–30.

15 Bartholomew, J.R., Salgia, R. and Bell, W.R. (1989) Control of bleeding in patients with immune and nonimmune thrombocytopenia with aminocaproic acid. *Arch. Intern. Med.*, **149**, 1959–1961.

16 Ruggiero, M. and Lapetina, E.G. (1986) Protease and cyclo-oxygenase inhibitors synergistically prevent activation of human platelets. *Proc. Natl. Acad. Sci. USA*, **83**, 3456–3459.

17 Royston, D., Bidstrup, B.P., Taylor, K.M. and Sapsford, R.N. (1987) Effect of aprotinin on need for blood transfusion after repeat open-heart surgery. *Lancet*, **ii**, 1289–1291.

18 van Oeveren, W., Jansen, N.J.G., Bidstrup, B.P. *et al.* (1987) Effects of aprotinin on haemostatic mechanisms during cardiopulmonary bypass. *Ann. Thorac. Surg.*, **44**, 640–645.

19 Alajmo, F., Calamai, C., Perna, A.M. *et al.* (1989) High-dose aprotinin: hemostatic effects in open heart operations. *Ann. Thorac. Surg.*, **48**, 536–539.

20 van Oeveren, W., Harder, M.P., Roozendaal, K.L. *et al.* (1990) Aprotinin protects platelets against the initial effect of cardiopulmonary bypass. *J. Thorac. Cardiovasc. Surg.*, **99**, 788–796.

21 Angelini, G.D., Cooper, G.J., Lamarra, M. and Bryan, A.J. (1990) Unorthodox use of aprotinin to control life-threatening bleeding after cardiopulmonary bypass. *Lancet*, **335**, 799–800.

22 Bidstrup, B.P., Royston, D., Taylor, K.M. and Sapsford, R.N. (1988) Effect of

aprotinin on need for blood transfusion in patients with septic endocarditis having open-heart surgery. *Lancet*, **i**, 366–367.

23 Neuhaus, P., Bechstein, W.O., Lefèbre, B. *et al.* (1989) Effect of aprotinin on intraoperative bleeding and fibrinolysis in liver transplantation. *Lancet*, **ii**, 924–925.

24 Mallett, S.V., Cox, D., Burroughs, A.K. and Rolles, K. (1990) Aprotinin and reduction of blood loss and transfusion requirements in orthotopic liver transplantation. *Lancet*, **336**, 886–887.

25 Thompson, J.F., Roath, O.S., Francis, J.L. *et al.* (1990) Aprotinin in peripheral vascular surgery. *Lancet*, **335**, 911.

26 Cash, J.D., Gader, A.M.A. and Da Costa, J. (1974) The release of plasminogen activator and Factor VIII by LVP, AVP, DDAVP, AT-III and OT in man. *Br. J. Haematol.*, **27**, 363–364.

27 Mannucci, P.M., Aberg, M., Nilsson, I.M. and Robertson, B. (1975) Mechanism of plasminogen activator and Factor VIII increase after vasoactive drugs. *Br. J. Haematol.*, **30**, 81–93.

28 Mannucci, P.M., Pareti, F.I., Holmberg, L. *et al.* (1976) Studies on the prolonged bleeding time in von Willebrand's disease. *J. Lab. Clin. Med.*, **88**, 662–671.

29 Mannucci, P.M., Ruggeri, Z.M., Pareti, F.I. and Capitanio, A. (1977) DDAVP: A new pharmacological approach to the management of hemophilia and von Willebrand disease. *Lancet*, **i**, 869–872.

30 Castaman, G., Rodeghiero, F., Di Bona, E. and Ruggeri, Z.M. (1989) Clinical effectiveness of desmopressin in a case of acquired von Willebrand's syndrome associated with benign monoclonal gammopathy. *Blut*, **58**, 211–213.

31 Kohler, M., Hellstern, P., Reiter, B. *et al.* (1984) The subcutaneous administration of the vasopressin analogue 1-desamino-8-D-arginine vasopressin in patients with von Willebrand's disease and hemophilia. *Klin. Wochenschr.*, **62**, 543–548.

32 Nilsson, I.M., Vilhardt, H., Holmberg, L. and Astedt, B. (1982) Association between Factor VIII related antigen and plasminogen activator. *Acta Med. Scand.*, **211**, 105–112.

33 Cameron, C.B. and Kobrinsky, N. (1990) Perioperative management of patients with von Willebrand's disease. *Can. J. Anaesth.*, **37**, 341–347.

34 Pfueller, S.L., Howard, M.A., White, J.G. *et al.* (1987) Shortening of bleeding time by 1-deamino-8-arginine vasopressin (DDAVP) in the absence of platelet von Willebrand factor in gray platelet syndrome. *Thromb. Haemost.*, **58**, 1060–1063.

35 Nieuwenhuis, H.K. and Sixma, J.J. (1988) 1-Desamino-8-D-arginine vasopressin (desmopressin) shortens the bleeding time in storage pool deficiency. *Ann. Intern. Med.*, **108**, 65–67

36 Gotti, E., Mecca, G., Valentino, C. *et al.* (1984) Renal biopsy in patients with acute renal failure and prolonged bleeding time. *Lancet*, **ii**, 978–979.

37 Burroughs, A.K., Matthews, K., Qadiri, M. *et al.* (1985) Desmopressin and bleeding time in patients with cirrhosis. *Br. Med. J.*, **291**, 1377–1381.

38 Schulman, S., Johnsson, H., Egberg, N. and Blomback, M. (1987) DDAVP-induced correction of prolonged bleeding time in patients with congenital platelet function defects. *Thromb. Res.*, **45**, 165–174.

39 Kim, H.C., Salva, K., Fallot, P.L. *et al.* (1988) Patients with prolonged bleeding

time of undefined etiology, and their response to desmopressin. *Thromb. Haemost.*, **59**, 221–224.

40 Kobrinsky, N.L., Letts, R.P., Patel, L.R. *et al.* (1987) DDAVP shortens the bleeding time and decreases blood loss in hemostatically normal subjects undergoing spinal fusion surgery. *Ann. Intern. Med.*, **107**, 446–450.

41 Salzman, E.W., Weinstein, M.J., Weintraub, R.M. *et al.* (1986) Treatment with desmopressin acetate to reduce blood loss after cardiac surgery. *New Engl. J. Med.* **314**, 1402–1406.

42 Weinstein, M., Ware, J.A., Troll, J. and Salzman, E. (1988) Changes in von Willebrand factor during cardiac surgery: effect of desmopressin acetate. *Blood*, **71**, 1648–1655.

43 Rocha, E., Llorens, R., Paramo, J.A. (1988) Does desmopressin acetate reduce blood loss after surgery in patients on cardiopulmonary bypass? *Circulation*, **77**, 1319–1323.

44 Hackmann, T., Gascoyne, R.D., Naiman, S.C. *et al.* (1989) A trial of desmopressin (1-desamino-8-D-arginine vasopressin) to reduce blood loss in uncomplicated cardiac surgery. *New Engl. J. Med.*, **321**, 1437–1443.

45 Andersson, T.L.G., Solem, J.O., Tengborn, L. and Vinge, E. (1990) Effects of desmopressin acetate on platelet aggregation, von Willebrand factor, and blood loss after cardiac surgery with extracorporeal circulation. *Circulation*, **81**, 872–878.

46 Hedderich, G.S., Petsikas, D.J., Cooper, B.A. *et al.* (1990) Desmopressin acetate in uncomplicated coronary artery bypass surgery: a prospective randomized clinical trial. *Can. J. Surg.*, **33**, 33–36.

47 Seear, M.D., Wadsworth, L.D., Rogers, P.C. *et al.* (1989) The effect of desmopressin acetate (DDAVP) on postoperative blood loss after cardiac operations in children. *J. Thorac. Cardiovasc. Surg.*, **98**, 217–219.

48 Tyers, G.F.O. (1990) Desmopressin: Do we now know its role? *Can. J. Surg.*, **33**, 5–6.

49 Hutton, R.A., Wickhan, E.A., Reed, J.V. and Tuddenham, E.G.D. (1986) Studies on the action of ethamsylate (Dicynene) on haemostasis. *Thromb. Haemost.*, **56**, 6–8.

50 Louis, J. and Paulus, J.M. (1967) Essai d'un nouvel haemostatique: la Dicynone. *Rev. Med. Liège*, **22**, 649–651.

51 Rennie, J.M., Doyle, J. and Cooke, R.W.I. (1986) Ethamsylate reduces immunoreactive prostacyclin metabolite in low birthweight infants with respiratory distress syndrome. *Early Human Dev.*, **14**, 239–244.

52 Harrison, R.F. and Campbell, S. (1976) A double-blind trial of ethamsylate in the treatment of primary and intra-uterine device menorrhagia. *Lancet*, **ii**, 283–285.

53 Morgan, M.E.I., Benson, J.W.T. and Cooke, R.W.I. (1981) Ethamsylate reduces the incidence of periventricular haemorrhage in very low birthweight babies. *Lancet*, **ii**, 830–831.

54 Daneshmend, T.K., Stein, A.G., Bhaskar, N.K. and Hawkey, C.J. (1989) Failure of ethamsylate to reduce aspirin-induced gastric mucosal bleeding in humans. *Br. J. Clin. Pharmacol.*, **28**, 109–112.

55 Verstraete, M. Haemostatic drugs. In: *Haemostasis and Thrombosis* (Eds Bloom,

A.L. & Thomas, D.P.), 2nd edn, pp. 607–617. Churchill Livingstone, Edinburgh (1987).

56 Koch, H.J., Escher, G.C. and Lewis, J.S. (1952) Hormonal management of hereditary hemorrhagic telangiectasia. *JAMA*, **149**, 1376–1380.

57 Van Cutsem, E., Rugeerts, P. and Vantrappen, G. (1990) Treatment of bleeding gastrointestinal vascular malformations with oestrogen–progesterone. *Lancet*, **335**, 953–955.

58 Van Cutsem, E., Rutgeerts, P., Geboes, K. (1988) Estrogen–progesterone treatment of Osler–Weber–Rendu disease. *J. Clin. Gastroenterol.*, **10**, 676–679.

59 Livio, M., Mannucci, P.M., Vigano, G. *et al.* (1986) Conjugated estrogens for the management of bleeding associated with renal failure. *New Engl. J. Med.*, **315**, 731–735.

60 Bronner, M.H., Pate, M.B., Cunningham, J.T. and Marsh, W.H. (1986) Estrogen–progesterone therapy for bleeding gastrointestinal telangiectasias in chronic renal failure. *Ann. Intern. Med.*, **105**, 371–374.

61 Fish, K.J., Sarnquis, F.H., van Steennis, C. *et al.* (1986) A prospective, randomized study of the effects of prostacyclin on platelets and blood loss during coronary bypass operations. *J. Thorac. Cardiovasc. Surg.*, **91**, 436–442.

Chapter 16
Blood and blood products

WILLIAM G. MURPHY AND JOHN D. CASH

This chapter describes the blood products and bioengineered proteins used in the management of bleeding in surgical patients. Management strategies of bleeding are discussed elsewhere (see Chapters 4 and 17); the intention here is to provide practical information on the use of blood products selected on the basis of such management strategies. Table 16.1 lists the products discussed.

Platelets

Indications

Platelet transfusion is indicated for the prevention and cessation of bleeding in patients with thrombocytopenia or platelet function defects.

Form

Platelets for transfusions are supplied as a suspension of platelets in a fluid medium, usually plasma. Each dose issued for an adult patient will contain approximately 30×10^{10} platelets, and may be derived from a pool of the platelets separated from four to eight individual donor units of blood (random donor pooled), or from one or two donors from whom the platelets have been separated by apheresis (random donor apheresis). For patients who are known to be refractory to platelet transfusions (usually patients who have had recurrent transfusions for chemotherapy-induced marrow aplasia) apheresis platelets will be provided that are either homologous leucocytic antibody (HLA)-matched or crossmatch-compatible.

Platelets for transfusion should be irradiated when they are to be given to patients with profound immune deficiency, or to patients who are first-degree relatives of the donor. It may also be appropriate to provide cytomegalovirus (CMV)-negative platelets to certain recipients such as CMV-negative patients who are awaiting bone-marrow transplant.

Table 16.1 Blood products

Platelets
Random donor pooled
Single donor apheresis
HLA-matched
Crossmatched
Soluble coagulation factor preparations
Plasma
Fresh frozen
Cryoglobulin supernatant
Stored
Cryoprecipitate
Factor concentrates
Factor VIII : C
'Activated' preparations—FEIBA, Autoplex and Factor VIIa
Factors II, IX, X
Factor VII
Factor IX
von Willebrand factor
Antithrombin-III
Fibrin sealant
Intravenous immunoglobulin G
Red-cell preparations
Red-cell concentrate
Whole blood
Fresh whole blood

FEIBA, factor 8 inhibitor bypass activity.

Platelets for transfusion should be ABO and Rh-D compatible.

In surgical patients, platelet transfusions will be required for:

1 Patients with thrombocytopenia or platelet-function disorders undergoing elective or emergency procedures.

2 Patients with abnormal bleeding due to platelet dysfunction and/or thrombocytopenia developing during the course of the disease process, particularly patients developing dilutional thrombocytopenia, disseminated intravascular coagulation, or with persisting microvascular bleeding after cardiopulmonary bypass.

Dose

In theory, the dose of platelets to be transfused is calculated according to the required increment (platelets $\times 10^9$/l) and the surface area or blood volume of the recipient. In reality, particularly in acute situations, platelet doses are determined empirically. A dose of approximately 30×10^{10} platelets is given as a pool of five to six donor units. It would be expected that such a transfusion would raise the platelet count in the clinically stable adult with a blood volume of approximately 5 litres by 40×10^9/l. In general a platelet count of 50×10^9/l is required for relatively minor procedures, while a count of 100×10^9/l is necessary either for surgery in critical areas (eye/brain) or in the presence of microvascular haemorrhage following large-volume transfusion. Spontaneous haemorrhage is uncommon in stable patients when the platelet count is $>10-20 \times 10^9$/l.

In the presence of a platelet function disorder with a normal or high platelet count, the haemostatic effect of platelets given for prophylactic use can be assessed by using the bleeding time. However, the lack of sensitivity and specificity of this test in the management of individual patients limits its usefulness [1].

The necessity for repeated doses of platelet transfusion in these patients can be determined by the clinical response. If unexpected bleeding arises or persists:

1 An inadequate transfusion of platelets has been given. The platelet count should be checked and repeat platelet transfusion given if indicated.

2 The original assessment of a requirement for platelet transfusion was wrong or incomplete. Reassess, check the coagulation screen and consult the Haematology Service.

Ordering and delivery

The time for the blood bank to prepare platelets for issue depends on the following:

1 If the patient's ABO and Rh-D blood groups are known, 15 min. If the blood groups are not known an additional 30 min from receipt of sample at the blood bank.

2 If irradiated products are required—very variable. At the minimum an extra 5 min will be required.

3 If HLA or crossmatched platelets are required, at least 1 day's notice will be necessary.

For elective surgery, platelets should be ordered as far in advance as possible. Failure to do so may compromise patient care due to the logistic realities involved in platelet production.

Storage in ward and theatre

Platelets are optimally stored at 22°C. They must not be refrigerated, but on receipt at the ward or operating theatre may be kept at room temperature for several hours. A pool of units will have a shelf-life of <4 h after issue unless a sterile docking procedure has been used in the preparation. The time of expiry should be stated on the bag label.

Infusion

Platelets should be transfused through a blood (or platelet) giving set; they should not be infused through a giving set that has previously been used for a blood transfusion. A leucocyte-depleting filter may be needed, particularly where surgery is being performed on patients on long-term transfusion support. Platelets may be transfused via mechanical infusion devices: the advice of the manufacturer should be sought.

The duration of the infusion is not critical, but platelets should be transfused over about 30 min. The patient should be observed for fever or other unexpected symptoms or signs during the tranfusion and at 30 min and 1 h afterwards.

Acute complications (see Table 16.4)

Platelet transfusion in surgical patients may be complicated by the following acute reactions:

1 Fever.

2 Urticarial rash.

3 Severe anaphylactic reaction with hypotension, laryngeal and/or bronchial spasm.

4 Respiratory distress due to pulmonary oedema or adult respiratory distress syndrome (transfusion-related acute lung injury).

Fever

Where clinical circumstances permit, stop the transfusion and use paracetamol as an antipyretic. Repeated febrile transfusion reactions are an indication for use of leucocyte-depleted platelets. In critical circumstances, an assessment of the risk of stopping the platelet transfusion must be made. The likelihood is that the fever is due to anti-HLA antibodies in the recipient reacting with white blood cells in the donor platelets, and the possibility that it is a harbinger of a severe allergic, other immune, or septic event is extremely remote.

Urticarial rash

Urticarial reactions to transfusion are usually attributed to preformed antibodies in the recipient to plasma constituents in the donor. The transfusion should be interrupted, and an antihistamine administered before it is restarted.

Severe allergic reactions

The transfusion must be stopped and the patient resuscitated with adrenaline, intravenous antihistamines and hydrocortisone. Adrenaline should be given in a dose of 0.5–1 mg either subcutaneously or intramuscularly, and repeated every 10 min according to blood pressure and pulse. Antihistamines should be given by a slow intravenous injection following adrenaline injection, and should be continued for 24–48 h. Steroids are of secondary value only because of their delayed onset of action, but should be given to prevent further deterioration. Repeat transfusion should not be attempted unless either the exact cause has been determined or washed platelets have been provided.

Respiratory distress syndrome

Infusion of approximately 300 ml of colloid solution over about half an hour can precipitate pulmonary oedema in susceptible individuals. Much more rarely an acute immune reaction can occur in the lungs of the recipient, inducing a condition of diffuse alveolar oedema with cough, dyspnoea and fever, along with palpitations, tachycardia and neutropenia. The reaction is usually precipitated by antileucocyte antibodies in the donor plasma. The condition will usually resolve within 4 days, but mechanical ventilation may be necessary [2].

Plasma preparations

Indications

Plasma therapy may be used in reversal of the warfarin effect, and in the treatment of vitamin K deficiency, acute disseminated intravascular coagulation, thrombotic thrombocytopenic purpura, inherited deficiencies of inhibitors of coagulation and of C1 esterase inhibitor. In addition, plasma is indicated in the presence of bleeding and disturbed coagulation in patients who have received massive transfusion, or with liver disease or following cardiopulmonary bypass surgery.

It should be noted that plasma is only occasionally the only or most appropriate therapeutic agent for bleeding surgical patients.

Cryosupernatant or stored plasma can be substituted for fresh frozen plasma (FFP), where the indication is reversal of the warfarin effect, vitamin K deficiency, thrombotic thrombocytopenic purpura or inherited deficiencies of inhibitors of coagulation and of C1 esterase inhibitor.

Form

Fresh frozen plasma

Plasma is separated from the donor blood or collected by apheresis and frozen within 6 h of withdrawal. All clotting factors are present in approximately physiological concentrations. FFP units are labelled with ABO and Rh-D blood groups. ABO-compatible FFP should be given. In particular, group O FFP should not be given to recipients of blood with groups other than O.

Rh-D-negative patients should receive negative plasma where possible. If the administration of Rh-D-positive plasma to Rh-D-negative females with childbearing potential is inevitable, anti-D immunoglobulin should be given at a dose of 50 iu per unit of FFP transfused.

Cryosupernatant plasma

Plasma is stored after removal of cryoprecipitate for clinical use or fractionation. Such plasma preparations contain about half the physiological concentration of Factor VIII : c, von Willebrand factor and fibrinogen, but other clotting factors are present in physiological amounts.

Stored plasma

This plasma preparation has been separated from whole blood more than 6 h after withdrawal of the donor unit. It is deficient in the labile clotting Factors VIII : c and V.

Dose

Plasma is usually provided in units of approximately 300 ml. The amount used will depend upon the indication and the severity of the underlying disorder. Almost all therapeutic indications in adults will need at least 2–4 units of plasma. The response should be monitored with clinical observation and with measurement of the prothrombin time, partial thromboplastin time, or with specific factor assays where necessary.

Plasma need not be irradiated, or checked for CMV seropositivity [3].

Ordering and delivery

Plasma will be ready for issue from the blood bank in about 30 min after receipt of the request, provided that the patient's ABO and Rh-D group is known. Otherwise, an additional 30 min should be allowed after receipt of the patient's blood sample to allow appropriate determination of these blood groups.

Storage in ward and theatre

Once thawed plasma should be transfused as quickly as practicable, and at least within 4 h of issue from the blood bank. On receipt at the ward or operating theatre, FFP may be refrigerated in a designated blood fridge, or kept briefly at room temperature.

Infusion

Plasma is transfused through a giving set with an in-line 170 μm filter. The patient should be observed for fever or other unexpected symptoms or signs during the transfusion and for 1 h afterwards.

Acute complications (see Table 16.4)

Acute reactions to plasma infusion are similar to those discussed for platelet transfusions above. However, febrile transfusion reactions are less common, because of the absence of cells in plasma.

Cryoprecipitate

Indications

These are:

1 Cryoprecipitate is indicated as a source of fibrinogen in patients with hypofibrinogenaemia or dysfibrinogenaemia that is contributing, or likely to contribute, to bleeding.

2 Cryoprecipitate has been demonstrated to be efficacious in the correction of abnormal platelet function in some uraemic patients.

Form

Cryoprecipitate is prepared by a process of freezing and controlled thawing of plasma separated from whole blood. During the thawing procedure Factor VIII : c, von Willebrand factor, fibrinogen, fibronectin and plasminogen precipitate out, so that about half of the starting amounts of these proteins in the donor plasma unit can be recovered in the final volume of about 30 ml. Each unit of cryoprecipitate contains about 0.15–0.3 g fibrinogen.

Cryoprecipitate that is ABO-compatible with the recipient should normally be given.

Dose

A pool of 10 iu of cryoprecipitate will raise the plasma fibrinogen in an adult with a blood volume of 5 litres by approximately 1 g/l.

Where cryoprecipitate is transfused for correction of dysfibrinogenaemia or hypofibrinogenaemia, a therapeutic effect and correction of clotting times will be observed immediately. In contrast, correction of the bleeding defect in uraemia by cryoprecipitate may take up to 8 h following completion of infusion. In these patients therapeutic effect may be monitored with the bleeding time.

Ordering and delivery

A pool of cryoprecipitate can be prepared within *c.* 15 min provided the patient's ABO and Rh-D blood groups are known.

Storage in ward and theatre

Cryoprecipitate should be transfused immediately on receipt. If essential it may be stored very briefly in a designated blood fridge, or at room temperature. Transfusion should be complete within 4 h of pooling.

Infusion

Cryoprecipitate can be transfused through a giving set without an in-line filter. The patients should be observed for fever or other unexpected symptoms or signs during the transfusion and at 30 min and 1 h afterwards.

Complications (see Table 16.4)

Reactions to cryoprecipitate are essentially identical to those that may arise with plasma infusion.

Coagulation factor concentrates

Indications

Coagulation factor concentrates are indicated in the management of patients with congenital or acquired clotting factor deficiencies. Their use should be monitored in close association with the Haematology Service.

'Activated' preparations are indicated in the treatment of some patients with haemophilia A and antibodies to Factor VIII : C.

Form

Clotting factor concentrates are pharmaceutical preparations usually provided in powdered form for reconstitution in an appropriate diluent, which should be supplied with the concentrate. Appropriate directions for reconstitution, storage and administration will be given in an accompanying product leaflet.

Dose

The dose required will depend on the desired level of clotting factor to be achieved, the preparation in use, and the plasma volume of the patient. Dose and dosage intervals should be determined in consultation with the Haematology Service.

Complications

Modern heat-sterilized products have a very low risk of disease transmission. B19 parvovirus infection, which causes transient red-cell aplasia, may be resistant to current sterilization techniques. Factor II, IX and X concentrates and activated coagulation factor preparations have been associated with thrombogenicity [4], particularly in patients with liver disease or disseminated intravascular coagulation.

Fibrin sealant

Indications

Fibrin sealant has been used as a topical haemostatic agent in a wide range of surgical procedures. It has been reported as being effective in cardiovascular and general vascular surgery, in paediatric cardiovascular surgery, as well as in thoracic surgery, plastic, oral, ear–nose–throat, neurosurgical, trauma, hepatic and orthopaedic surgery. It has also been reported as being haemostatically effective during surgery in patients with acquired coagulation disorders [5].

Form

Fibrin sealant is a pharmaceutical product, and details of preparation, dosage and administration are provided with each kit. The sealant has two main components, a fibrinogen solution and a thrombin solution, which are mixed together at the point of application using a dual syringe device or a spray. The fibrinogen and thrombin solutions are prepared from heat-sterilized powder formulations at the time of use. The fibrinogen is derived from human plasma, and the thrombin is derived either from human or bovine plasma. Aprotinin, Factor XIII and plasminogen are also present in the sealant.

The sealant is applied directly onto the site of action.

Complications (see Table 16.4)

The main theoretical risks are viral disease transmission, which has not been reported, and thrombogenicity, which does not appear to have resulted in significant clinical disease. Use of excess fibrin sealant may impair nerve regeneration and bone repair [6].

Intravenous immunoglobulin G

Indications

Intravenous immunoglobulin G (IVIgG) may be administered for the prophylaxis or treatment of bleeding in surgical patients with immune thrombocytopenias. Where the patient is actively bleeding, platelet transfusion may be given together with the IVIgG.

Form

IVIgG is a pharmaceutical preparation provided as a dried powder for reconstitution in the buffer supplied along with it. Pharmaceutical precautions and directions on reconstitution, storage and administration will be provided in an accompanying product leaflet.

Dose

The usual dose in the management of patients with immune thrombocytopenia is 1–2 g/kg. This infusion takes several hours to administer, and should be supervised by the medical staff of the Haematology Service.

Red-cell preparations

Indications

Red-cell preparations (red-cell concentrate, whole blood, fresh whole blood) are administered to surgical patients to replace oxygen-carrying capacity. In addition, they have limited haemostatic function: *in vitro* platelet function is optimal when the haematocrit is >20; whole blood will provide plasma as well as red cells. Whole blood that has been stored for up to 48 h contains effective haemostatic capacity in terms of functional platelets and adequate plasma levels of clotting factors. Beyond this length of storage time, platelet function is negligible, and in addition the plasma concentration of the labile clotting Factors VIII : C and v are diminished. Very fresh whole blood is extremely difficult to provide other than by autologous transfusion. A recent prospective study in paediatric patients undergoing cardiopulmonary bypass procedures has indicated that the haemostatic ability of fresh whole blood was not superior to whole blood that has been stored for 48 h in this study population [7].

Patients with pre-existing anaemia undergoing elective surgical procedures may require blood transfusion, which should only be considered when haematinics will not correct the anaemia. In a stable patient without pre-existing cardiopulmonary insufficiency, a preoperative haemoglobin level of 70 g/l is not associated with increased morbidity from intraoperative haemorrhage, and in general no requirement exists to transfuse anaemic patients preoperatively to a higher haemoglobin level.

Where preoperative blood transfusion is required, or where blood transfusion is otherwise required in non-bleeding patients, red-cell concentrates should be used.

Form

The forms are as follows (all volumes are approximate):

1 *Whole blood*: volume 500 ml, haematocrit 35–45%.

2 *Red-cell concentrate*: volume 300 ml, haematocrit 65–75%. Most of the donor plasma has been removed from red-cell concentrate after centrifugation, leaving 80 ml of plasma on the red cells.

3 *Red-cell concentrated supplemented*: volume 320 ml, haematocrit 55–65%. Almost all of the donor plasma has been removed, and 100 ml of nutrient solution added back to the red cells.

Dose

In bleeding patients the red-cell requirement is determined by estimates of blood loss. The use of uncrossmatched Group O blood is associated with a low risk of serious transfusion reaction: the use of this product should not be delayed in critical circumstances [8]. However, the patient's initial requirement is maintenance or restoration of perfusion pressure, for which colloid or crystalloid solutions are employed.

The transfusion of one unit of red-cell concentrate to a non-bleeding adult patient should raise the haemoglobin level by 10–15 g/l.

Table 16.2 Time required for the issue of red-cell preparations

Issue of	Time
Group O blood for emergency	Immediate issue. A sample is not needed before issue, but should be drawn before transfusion
ABO group specific blood for emergency transfusion*	5–10 min preparation time. Patient sample needed
Full compatibility testing	Takes about 45 min to 1 h. It will take longer if there are anti-red blood cell alloantibodies present in the patient's serum
Urgent group and screen conversion**	Blood can be issued urgently with a very high degree of safety in 5–10 min. No further patient sample is needed
Standard group and screen conversion**	About 45 min

* The use of ABO-specific blood for emergency transfusion is practised in some areas. The need for correct labelling of the patient sample and meticulous pretransfusion checking must be recognized.

** Group and screen: a patient's blood sample is sent to the blood bank when a requirement for blood is unpredictable, for example patients scheduled for an elective operation that does not usually involved significant blood loss. The patient's ABO and Rh-D groups are determined and the serum is tested for antibodies to red cells. If no antibodies are found blood can be issued with a high degree of safety within 5–10 min of receiving a subsequent request. About 1 in 5000 units of blood prepared by this method will be incompatible and will have a shortened survival in the patient's circulation after transfusion. Significant morbidity from this event is not likely.

Ordering and delivery

Samples for crossmatching must be completely labelled and this labelling must be done at the time the sample is drawn. Failure to do this, particularly in critical situations, can lead to the wrong blood sample being assigned to the intended recipient. Times for the blood bank to prepare red-cell preparations for issue are given in Table 16.2.

Storage in ward or theatre

Red-cell preparations are stored at 4°C in designated blood fridges or specially designed blood boxes. They should not be kept outside such storage for more than 30 min before transfusion. Blood for transfusion must never be placed in a waterbath or on a radiator to warm. Such practice can cause *ex vivo* haemolysis, which has caused death on subsequent transfusion.

Infusion

1 Check that the blood unit to be transfused is intended for the patient about to receive it. Failure to do this is the commonest single cause of ABO incompatibility. The blood unit will be labelled with the recipient's name or other identifier unless uncrossmatched O blood is being used. It is imperative to match the unit label identifier with the patient's identity band.
2 Blood must be transfused through a standard giving set with a 170 μm filter.
3 Rapid blood transfusions of >2 units should be warmed in a designated blood-warming device.
4 In general, blood may be transfused through mechanical infusion devices. However, some peristaltic devices may cause haemolysis of red-cell concentrates, and the manufacturer's specifications must be checked.
5 Transfusion of 1 unit of blood should be complete within 4 h.
6 Saline solution (0.9%), but no other solution or drug, can be mixed with blood in the infusion line. Blood units may be transfused sequentially through the same giving set, which should be changed after 12 h.

The patient should be observed throughout the duration of the blood transfusion for signs of fever, hypotension or rash and, if conscious, for symptoms of distress or dyspnoea, and pain at the infusion site or in the chest or back.

Acute complications (see Table 16.4)

The acute reactions to red cells are similar to those for platelets and plasma with the important additions of acute lysis of infused red cells and the acute metabolic consequences of rapid large-volume blood transfusion.

Acute haemolytic transfusion reactions

These are usually due to ABO mismatch, but may also result from acute haemolysis caused by preformed antibody in the recipient to minor

Table 16.3 Diagnosis and management of suspected haemolytic transfusion reactions

Clinical features

Pain at the infusion site and along the line of the vein, chest pain, back pain
Fever, rigors
Generalized flushing
Hypotension
Haemoglobinuria and haemoglobinaemia
Spontaneous oozing around vascular access sites, injection sites and wounds
Oliguria

Immediate therapy

- Stop the blood transfusion and replace the giving set. Maintain intravenous access with sodium chloride (0.9%). Attempt to induce a diuresis with a fluid challenge of 100–200 ml of intravenous saline and frusemide (150 mg); 100 ml of 20% mannitol should be given intravenously if the initial attempt to induce diuresis is unsuccessful
- Maintain a urine flow at >100 ml/h
- The complications of established renal failure and disseminated intravascular coagulation must be anticipated and treated accordingly

Investigations of cause

1 Ensure that the blood unit has been issued for the patient who is receiving it
2 Send blood for re-crossmatching and serological investigation (5 ml EDTA (ethylenediaminetetra-acetic acid), and 10 ml clotted). Blood samples must be sent immediately for coagulation screen and electrolyte levels. Clinical chemistry and coagulation investigations should be repeated frequently as clinical circumstances dictate
In addition a blood sample should be sent for blood culture

Further transfusion requirements

Further transfusion requirements should be discussed immediately with the blood-bank physician

blood group antigens in the donor. They are almost always caused by human error either at the bedside or in the laboratory. The overall mortality is about 3%, but is higher if >200 ml of blood have been transfused.

The management of a suspected haemolytic transfusion reaction is presented in Table 16.3. Adverse effects of transfusions are given in Table 16.4.

The acute metabolic effects of large-volume blood transfusions include acidosis, citrate toxicity, hypokalaemia and hypothermia.

Table 16.4 Adverse effects of transfusion of blood and blood products

Acute	Delayed
Allergic	Delayed haemolytic
Haemolytic	Infection
Metabolic	*Bacterial*
Respiratory distress (pulmonary oedema or rarely adult respiratory distress syndrome)	Brucellosis
Non-haemolytic febrile reactions	Syphilis
Septic shock from transfusion of bacterially infected units: very rare	*Helminthic*
	Filiariasis
	Protozoal
	Babesiosis
	Chagas' disease
	Kala-azar
	Malaria
	Sleeping sickness
	Toxoplasmosis
	Rickettsial
	Relapsing fever
	Rocky Mountain spotted fever
	Viral
	B19 (may be transmitted by some heat-treated factor concentrates)
	Cytomegalovirus
	Epstein–Barr virus
	HIV-1 & 2
	HTLV-1 & 2
	Hepatitis
	Parvovirus
	Yellow fever
	Sensitization/alloimmunization
	Haemolytic disease of the newborn
	Immune suppression, associated with an apparent increased susceptibility to postoperative infection and with an increased risk of tumour recurrence
	Post-transfusion purpura
	Platelet refractoriness

References

1 Lind, S.E. (1991) The bleeding time does not predict surgical bleeding. *Blood*, **77**(12), 2547–2552.

2 Andrews, A.T., Zmijewski, C.M., Bowman, H.S. and Reihart, J.K. (1976) Transfusion reaction with pulmonary infiltration associated with HLA-specific leukocyte antibodies. *Am. J. Clin. Pathol.*, **66**(3), 483–487.

3 Bowden, R. and Sayers, M. (1990) The risk of transmitting cytomegalovirus infection by fresh frozen plasma. *Transfusion*, **30**(8), 762–763.

4 Kohler, M., Heiden, M., Harbauer, G. *et al.* (1990) Comparison of different prothrombin complex concentrates—*in vitro* and *in vivo* studies. *Thrombosis Res.*, **60**(1), 63–70.

5 Kram, H.B., Nathan, R.C., Stafford, F.J. *et al.* (1989) Fibrin glue achieves hemostasis in patients with coagulation disorders. *Arch. Surg.*, **124**, 385–387.

6 Gibble, J.W. and Ness, P.M. (1990) Fibrin glue: the perfect operative sealant? *Transfusion*, **30**(8), 741–747.

7 Manno, C.S, Hedberg, K.W., Kim, H.C. *et al.* (1991) Comparison of the hemostatic effects of fresh whole blood, stored whole blood, and components after open heart surgery in children. *Blood*, **77**(5), 930–936.

8 Schwab, C.W., Shayne, J.P. and Turner, J. (1986) Immediate trauma resuscitation with type O uncrossmatched blood: a two-year prospective experience. *J. Trauma*, **26**(10), 897–902.

Chapter 17
Surgical management

DAVID W. EASTER AND ALFRED CUSCHIERI

Control of bleeding is one of the most important aspects of surgical practice. Life-threatening haemorrhage necessitating immediate intervention to prevent exsanguination is a common emergency, usually arising on a background of trauma or as a complication of gastrointestinal disease. Meticulous haemostasis is an essential component of modern surgical practice and may pose problems in patients with defective coagulation if adequate haematological and clotting-factor support is not provided. Finally, postoperative bleeding is still a complication of major excisional and transplant surgery which at best delays recovery and often results in serious compromise of organ function.

In addressing these issues effectively, the surgeon must have the necessary knowledge concerning the common pathophysiological mechanisms involved in bleeding states and be familiar with modern techniques which can be employed for the arrest of haemorrhage. This chapter describes, from a surgeon's perspective, the issues surrounding the various management options and the techniques involved, surgical or otherwise, in dealing with the bleeding patient. What needs to be stressed at the outset is the key role of the surgeon in the management of these patients irrespective of presentation, underlying condition or initial treatment. Equally important is the realization that the interests of the patient with a bleeding disorder are best met by a multidisciplinary approach involving the relevant specialties. In the absence of a systemic disorder, control of bleeding can nowadays be achieved by angiographic, endoscopic or direct surgical intervention. Means of controlling bleeding are listed in Table 17.1.

Gastrointestinal bleeding

The stomach and duodenum remain the most common sources of gastrointestinal haemorrhage, including bleeding per rectum. Although the latter usually consists of melaena, when brisk, upper gastrointestinal

Table 17.1 Control of gastrointestinal bleeding

Pharmacological	Non-thermal	Thermal
Glypressin	Balloon tamponade	Monopolar cautery
Somatostatin	Sclerosing agents	Bipolar cautery
Beta-blockers	Adrenaline	Heater probe
Tranexamic acid	Polidocanol	Photocoagulation
	Ethanol	Nd : YAG
	Hypertonic saline	Argon
	Tissue adhesives	Microwave
	Angioembolization	
	Surgical intervention	

haemorrhage can present with red blood per rectum. For this reason, a rational approach to this clinical situation is to perform upper gastrointestinal endoscopy as the first investigation. If unrevealing, this is followed by proctosigmoidoscopy with extension to colonoscopy if the proctosigmoid region is normal. Complete colonoscopy should be performed only after mechanical cleansing of the colon, and with support equipment and personnel available to ensure the successful completion of a meticulous and thorough examination.

Fibreoptic endoscopy establishes the bleeding site in the majority of patients with enteric bleeding. Recourse to visceral angiography (coeliac, superior mesenteric, inferior mesenteric) is made in those rare instances of active gastrointestinal bleeding where endoscopy proves noncontributary. In this setting, visceral angiography can be both diagnostic and therapeutic. Isotope-labelled red blood cell scans play a secondary role limited to the patient with slow or intermittent bleeding. Even when positive, these scans can be difficult to interpret and may mislead the clinician.

Once the source is identified, several management options are available for the control of gastrointestinal bleeding. In addition to surgical intervention, these include pharmacological manipulations, endoscopic control by the local injection of sclerosants or vasoactive agents, application of heat energy and angioembolization (Table 17.1).

Endoscopic control of haemorrhage

During the past 10 years, therapeutic endoscopy has been advocated and used for the control of many types of bleeding lesions: ulcers, varices,

Mallory–Weiss tears, vascular lesions (hereditary or acquired), Dieulafoy lesion and diffuse gastric antral vascular ectasia ('watermelon stomach'). Endoscopic control of bleeding can be achieved by the local injection of sclerosants or vasoactive substances (singly and in combination), and by the local application of thermal energy.

Endoscopic injection of sclerosants and vasoactive substances

A variety of sclerosant agents are used for sclerotherapy such as hypertonic saline, alcohol, sodium morrhuate, and ethamolin. Sclerotherapy by intra- or paravariceal injection of sclerosants is now the first-line treatment in the arrest of bleeding oesophageal varices [1,2] and has been increasingly used during the past 5 years in the control of bleeding ulcers, where its reported efficacy is at least as good as that obtained by the endoscopic thermal methods [3,4]. The most commonly used vasoactive substances for endoscopic injection therapy are adrenaline and polidocanol. Impressive results have also been reported with these vasoactive substances, often injected locally in combination [5].

These direct endoscopic measures must be distinguished from the systemic use of specific agents such as the controlled intravenous infusion of vasopressin (or preferably its analogue, glypressin, which has fewer myocardial effects) and, more recently, the long-acting somatostatin analogues Octreotide (Sandostatin). The latter has been shown in clinical trials to be particularly effective in the control of bleeding oesophageal varices [6]. Beta-blockade with propranolol or nadolol lowers the portal venous pressure and for this reason is used in some centres as a prophylaxis against variceal haemorrhage in patients with portal hypertension. A meta-analysis of the published data on the use of tranexamic acid in upper gastrointestinal bleeding has shown that this fibrinolytic inhibitor can result in a 20% reduction of re-bleeding, a 30% reduction in the need for surgical intervention and a 40% lowering of mortality [7].

Mechanical methods

The best known and well validated is the trilumen tube first introduced by Sengstaken and popularized by Blakemore. Various modern versions are available but the best are made of silicon. These are easier to introduce than the latex varieties and have tougher balloons which are less liable to rupture. With the right precautions, balloon tamponade is still a very effective method of arrest of bleeding varices and may be used following sclerotherapy either routinely or selectively when bleeding continues after injection of sclerosants. Deflation is mandatory after 12 h because of the risk of erosion of the oesophageal walls. Surgical intervention is indicated in the event of renewed or continued bleeding subsequent to deflation. More recently, the concept of balloon compression has been extended to the endoscopic treatment of bleeding duodenal ulcer. A balloon is placed endoscopically distal to the pylorus and thereafter inflated [8]. Although early reports have been favourable, the experience is small and limited to one centre.

Another recently introduced mechanical endoscopic technique is 'band ligation' for oesophageal varices [9]. The small cylindrical device fits on the end of the endoscope. After the varix is sucked inside the cylinder, a trip wire is tugged to dislodge a circular rubber band over the base of the varix. The reported efficacy of endoscopic banding is equivalent to that obtained by sclerotherapy.

Endoscopic thermal methods

The endoscopic thermal haemostatic techniques include the heater probe, monopolar electrocautery, bipolar electrocautery, laser photocoagulation, and more recently the application of microwave energy.

The use of the *endoscopic heater probe* for the control of gastrointestinal bleeding is simple, safe, effective, and one of the least expensive methods. Although electric energy is used to heat the probe, there is no contact of electric current with the tissues. The direct transfer of thermal energy (*c*. 250°C) requires *c*. 3–8 s periods of contact with the bleeding source to achieve the necessary degree of tissue coagulation. In one comparative study, the heater probe technique was found to be as effective and more convenient and safe than Nd : YAG-laser photocoagulation [10].

Electrocautery can be delivered endoscopically using either *monopolar* or *bipolar* ('Bicap') electrodes.

In *monopolar high-frequency electrosurgery*, the current escapes from the electrode tip, dissipates into the receptive tissue, and exits through the grounding pad (neutral electrode). This should have an even surface and is applied to the patient's upper thigh, covering a large area of clean hairless skin. Special efforts are made to ensure that the patient's skin does not come in contact with metal components of the operating tables, chucks and restraining devices or damp clothing. The connecting cables to the neutral and active electrodes must be in perfect condition with respect to their insulation and connector plugs. The potential hazards of electrocoagulation include the unwanted discharge and absorption of low-frequency currents (shocks), high-frequency current burns (to patient and staff) and sparking to unwanted areas. Electrical current leakage can also cause malfunction of pacemakers and monitors. The monopolar high-frequency unit must not be operated in the vicinity of an ECG electrode (minimum distance of 15 cm). The further use of high-frequency monopolar electrosurgery in laparoscopy is discussed below (p. 371).

In *bipolar electrocautery*, heating of the tissue is confined to the area between the two ends of the probe and there is no current flow through the patient. If a combined machine is used, it must have a separate bipolar circuit. Bipolar generators do not require a neutral patient electrode but the combined machines do, and the same safeguards described above with regard to safe application of the neutral electrode must be strictly adhered to. When using bipolar electrocoagulation, only the minimum power necessary is used and every precaution must be taken to avoid contact between the active electrode and metal instruments. The tips of the electrode must be kept clean as encrusted coagulated tissue impairs the coagulation efficiency.

Although the efficacy in achieving haemostatic control is similar, the bipolar system is considerably safer because instead of passing through the patient, the electric current flows the short distance between the tips of the microelectrodes, thereby limiting the chance of deep-tissue damage. Both techniques, which like the heater probe allow application of direct pressure to the bleeding lesion (unavailable with laser devices), are relatively inexpensive and easy to learn.

Photocoagulation using laser energy (argon or neodymium : yttrium aluminium garnet—Nd : YAG) delivered endoscopically as a free beam via an optical fibre is practised in a number of centres. Success at arresting haemorrhage is nearly as good as with electrocautery devices but randomized trials have shown no specific benefit to laser therapy in patients with bleeding peptic ulcers [11,12]. Perforation of tissues is a serious concern, occurring in *c.* 1.0% of cases [13]. Other disadvantages of laser photocoagulation include its expense (in 1992, about £50 000), non-portable bulk, optical hazard, need for a technician to operate the laser machine and the cost of maintenance and repair. More recently, microwave energy has been used endoscopically for tissue coagulation

[14]. Although early results are promising, the reported experience is too limited to enable firm conclusions on its relative efficacy and cost benefit over the established endoscopic methods outlined above.

The efficacy in terms of adequate control of difficult bleeding sites, potential for tissue erosion/perforation, expense and special equipment requirements of the four most commonly used endoscopic thermal methods of tissue cautery (heater probe, bipolar electrocautery, monopolar electrocautery and laser) can be compared in light of the reported series and clinical trials. The heater probe is probably the most efficacious at controlling major vessel bleeding. Bipolar electrocautery is also very good at this, but both laser and monopolar electrocautery fall well short of the ideal. The heater probe and bipolar cautery are also safer (less risk of perforation) than either monopolar electrocautery or laser photocoagulation. The latter is clearly the most expensive method and requires the greatest technical support.

Although benefits in terms of diminished hospital stay, lower surgical intervention rate and reduced transfusion requirements have been reported in clinical trials with endoscopic sclerotherapy or direct electrocoagulation, no study has shown evidence of reduced mortality [15,16]. This simply reflects the very large number of patients (several thousands) which would have to be randomized to detect a mortality difference [17]. In practice this level of recruitment is impossible and mortality is thus an unrealistic endpoint in clinical trials designed to test the efficacy of endoscopic haemostatic techniques in patients with gastrointestinal bleeding.

The 'surgical threshold' in a patient with gastrointestinal bleeding is an important but somewhat arbitrary milestone. However, generally agreed criteria which are used to determine when a bleeding patient becomes a 'surgical candidate' include haemodynamic instability, a visible vessel (bleeding or not) in the base of an ulcer, and the transfusion of >6 units of red cells. Recurrent episodes of bleeding despite rigorous attempts at endoscopic control or medical therapy is also an indication for surgical intervention.

Diagnostic and therapeutic angiography

Selective angiography is useful both in the diagnosis of occult bleeding (usually from the gastrointestinal tract and less commonly from the liver) and in the treatment of difficult bleeding problems where surgical control is difficult and accompanied by high mortality. In this respect, superselective angioembolization with special coaxial catheters has been a significant therapeutic advance, and may avoid the need for surgical intervention or facilitate subsequent surgical control or excision. The advantage of successful angioembolization in this setting includes control of bleeding with preservation of organ function in many patients [18,19].

Difficult bleeding can arise in three ways: acute disease such as necrotizing pancreatitis, trauma and tumours. In the trauma setting, angioembolization is used to control life-threatening bleeding from the pelvis [20], retroperitoneum [21], liver [22]—where it can be used in association with packing in major injuries prior to transport for definitive treatment in major trauma centres—faciomaxillary injuries [23] and bleeding from the posterior nasopharynx [24].

Angiography with selective embolization of the arterial inflow may be employed before surgical removal of certain organs. This applies particularly prior to excision of the pathologically enlarged spleen, especially when the splenic vein is occluded [25]. Preoperative embolization is also used in patients with neoplastic disorders of the pelvis [26], liver [27], breast [28], lung [29], and head and neck [30] and kidneys. Apart from minimizing blood loss or control of a bleeding tumour, angioembolism reduces the dissemination of cancer cells into the blood stream during the surgical dissection and removal of these tumours.

Routine assessment of patients undergoing elective surgery

A preoperative screen is undertaken in all patients. In practice this consists of a history concerning any bleeding tendency and a physical examination, which dictate whether specific haematological and blood-clotting tests are needed in the individual patient. The history-taking should determine the presence of easy bruising, prolonged bleeding with minor trauma, bleeding complications after minor procedures (including dental trauma), or concurrent medical disorders such as liver disease, neoplasia, malabsorption, familial bleeding disorders and drug therapy. These are covered in the relevant chapters of this book. Physical examination of patients in the preoperative setting should specifically search for jaundice, joint disease, ecchymoses, petechiae, mucosal bleeding or friability, and signs of liver disease. In this respect all patients with jaundice, hepatomegaly and splenomegaly must be suspected of harbouring significant problems with the haemostatic mechanisms or their reserves.

Laboratory studies are indicated only in the context of the above screening. A negative history and physical examination require no special blood investigations. Should suspicion arise after history and physical examination, or if major surgery is planned with the potential for substantial blood loss, laboratory screening should at least include a platelet count, prothrombin time and partial thromboplastin time. More extensive investigation will be based upon the risks, suspicion of coagulopathy, and results of routine biochemical screens, but may include fibrin clot stability, thrombin time, bleeding time, clotting-factor levels, platelet function studies and α_2-antiplasmin levels [31].

Intraoperative methods of haemostasis

The dictum 'bad surgery is bloody bad' has a number of important connotations. A bloodless operative field facilitates surgical dissection and ensures a smooth recovery period without compromise of organ function in the postoperative period. The avoidance of perioperative blood transfusion is in this respect an important objective of modern surgical treatment and apart from abolishing the risk of transmission of viral disease, may be important in enhancing the cure rate and disease-free survival after extirpative surgery for cancer [32,33].

Control of blood vessels

Although practice does vary, vessels up to 1.0 mm can be electro- or photocoagulated. Larger vessels (1.0–3.0 mm) must be clipped or tied. Beyond 3.0 mm clipping becomes unsafe and these vessels are best ligated. The tension on a ligature is expressed by the formula

$$T = 3/2\,pr\delta$$

where p is the pressure within the vessel, r the radius of the vessel and δ the radius at the ligature site. This formula, however, underestimates the actual tension on a vascular ligature. The observed ligature tension on a 4.5 mm artery perfused at 140 mmHg on a test rig approximates to 10 g and for a 9.0 mm artery, 55 g [34]. These are lower than generally expected and indicate that knot integrity and durability of the ligature material are more important than the tensile strength of the material in ensuring continued haemostasis after ligature of blood vessels.

In general, vessels are best ligated in continuity before being divided. Cut vessels close to the parenchyma of an organ or accidentally avulsed branches of large vessels are best controlled by suture ligation. Large vessels, particularly those arising close to or directly from the aorta (splenic, left gastric, inferior mesenteric) are usually secured by transfixation. Although generally considered reliable, this technique is unsafe in patients with grossly atherosclerotic vessels as the needle bite may considerably weaken the vessel wall at the point of ligature. In these patients, double ligation of the vessel is safer. Vessels larger than 1.0 cm should be clamped and the proximal end sutured using 4/0 arterial atraumatic material.

Clips should not be applied to vessels greater than 3.0 mm. The principles governing their safe application are well established. Perhaps the most important are adequate clip size such that the approximated clip ends project beyond the vessel wall, disposition at right angles to the axis of the vessel and double proximal clipping for increased safety. The advantages of clips include ease and rapidity of application, especially in relatively inaccessible areas. Previous generation clips manufactured from stainless steel or tantalum caused considerable problems with computed tomography scanning and magnetic resonance imaging. These problems have been overcome to a large extent with the introduction of clips manufactured from titanium or polydioxanone ('Absolok', Ethicon). The advantage of the latter is their biodegradability, although they are rather bulky and more difficult to apply than the titanium variety.

Surface bleeding

Direct pressure on bleeding vessels or organs by dry packs allows time for either complete or partial natural haemostasis. In the latter event, the final control by whatever means is considered appropriate is facilitated, as with the diminished haemorrhage the bleeding point(s) can be identified. Topical haemostatic measures are used for large areas of raw surface bleeding where suture methods are either inappropriate or inadequate. The various agents employed include the application of thrombin concentrates [35], fibrin glue [36,37], amylose succinate [38], calcium alginate [39], oxidized cellulose, absorbable gelatin, microfibrillar collagen, and acrylates [40]. Tissue or fibrin glue is now commercially available from several companies. It consists of two solutions: (i) fibrinogen plus antiprotease (usually aprotinin) and (ii) activated thrombin delivered through a double syringe system with a terminal common channel where the solutions mix and the clotting process starts. Both quick- and slow-setting varieties are available (depending on concentrations of the constituents). As the resultant fibrin polymer incorporates the antiprotease, it is more stable than endogenous fibrin and thus effectively controls bleeding from large raw surfaces, including the cut hepatic parenchyma. Recent experimental studies have, however, indicated that tissue glue impairs wound healing and promotes fibrosis [41]. Histological studies have shown that the stable fibrin resists invasion by vascular granulation tissue, an essential component of the healing process [42].

When surface bleeding occurs over a large raw surface area or from cut tissue parenchyma, the most efficient haemostasis is obtained by the use of the argon gas beamer with the high-frequency generator set in the spray coagulation mode. An alternative method employs infrared coagulation. Though effective, this instrument is bulky to manipulate and the process slow.

Electrosurgery

The underlying principle of electrosurgery involves the passage of an electrical current through the tissue by means of a potential difference (voltage). The resultant flow of electrons excites the tissue molecules, notably water, creating heat energy which causes water evaporation and tissue coagulation. High-frequency currents (>100 000 c.p.s.) are used to minimize the risk of electric shocks. The characteristics of the applied current can be varied from continuous sinewave to modulated, to favour cutting or coagulation, respectively.

High-frequency electrocutting

High-frequency (monopolar) electrocutting is dependent on the production of electric arcs concentrating the entire current onto a single point, where the tissue is immediately vaporized. The operating peak voltage to produce this effect has to be in the 200–500 V range. If the voltage drops to <200 V, tissue cutting cannot be achieved since the electric arcs are not generated. On the other hand, if the voltage rises to >500 V, the electric arcs produced are so intense that the tissue is carbonized and the electrode may be damaged. Within the safe operating range, the depth of the coagulation of the cut edges increases with increasing voltage and intensity of the electric arcs. In practice, the depth of coagulation during electrocutting is determined by the setting of the high-frequency output power and the degree of modulation of the current (blend or mix). It is also influenced by three other factors: (i) thickness of the cutting electrode, (ii) rate and depth of cutting, and (iii) the impedance of the high-frequency generator. With a conventional high-frequency unit having an impedance of 250 Ω, fluctuations in the current on the output voltage and intensity of the electric arcs are produced by variations in the depth and rate of cutting. This may lead to carbonization of the tissue along the cut edges, particularly at the beginning and end of the cut. This problem can be obviated by the use of high-frequency surgical units which incorporate microprocessor-controlled automatic control circuits with sensor electronics (Erbe ACC-450, Tübingen, Germany). This ensures that the intensity of the electric arcs is kept constant irrespective of the cutting rate and depth.

Electrocoagulation

This is produced by a modulated current. When a high-frequency modulated alternating electric current is applied specifically for endogenous heating of living tissue, the temperature rise is proportional to the specific electric resistance of the tissue, the duration of current flow and the square of the root-mean-square of the electrical current density. Largely because of the irregular current density distribution in the tissue, the temperature rises at different rates in various zones in the tissue. As the current density is largest in the zone of contact between the tissue and the electrode, the maximum temperature is reached there, with the temperature decreasing proportionately with the distance from the contact area. On this phenomenon depends the safe feasibility of monopolar electrocoagulation, since the further away the tissue from the contact area, the less likely the damage. Once the temperature of the tissue near the contact surface has reached boiling point, a layer of vapour forms between the tissue and the electrode which impedes further current flow. Thereafter the sequence of changes depends on the peak voltage. If this is <200 V, the coagulation process slows down until the tissue next to the electrode has dried out, when further current flow ceases. If the current is not switched off, the coagulum becomes adherent to the electrode. When this happens, removal of the electrode will dislodge the coagulum and precipitate renewed bleeding. If the peak voltage exceeds 200 V once the tissue next to the contact area has dried out, electric arcs are produced which carbonize and puncture the coagulum, thereby causing the coagulation process to continue unabated until the generator is switched off or the dried up coagulum is so thick that it resists further puncture by the electric arcs.

There are three coagulation modes which can be used: soft, forced and spray. There is no doubt that *soft coagulation* is the safest. As the peak voltage is <200 V, no electric arcs are generated between the coagulating electrode and the tissue during the entire process, with elimination of tissue carbonization. As the reproducibility of the soft coagulation depth increases inversely with the impedance of the high-frequency generator, a unit with automatic voltage control is ideal. Activation of the unit should cease during soft coagulation when vapour formation commences, as beyond this stage the coagulum will desiccate and become adherent to the probe. There are now generator units with an automatic de-activation of the high-frequency current once the end of the coagulation process has been reached. These are ideal for laparoscopic soft coagulation because they eliminate the above problem and the risk of detachment of the coagulum on withdrawal of the probe. In *forced electrocoagulation*, high peak voltages are used (>500 V) to generate electric arcs between the electrode and the tissue in order to obtain deep coagulation. *Spray coagulation* is a non-contact mode where long electric arcs are intentionally generated by strongly modulated high-frequency voltages (a few kilovolts) to surface coagulate raw bleeding areas or achieve haemostasis from inaccessible vessels.

Argon-beam electrocoagulation

This is a recent modification of electrocautery. It utilizes a plasma of argon gas to deliver the electrical current and can be directed in a focused beam to the desired target. The argon-gas beamer works with certain specific generators which are capable of providing a spray coagulating current. The electric arcs from this current produce a conductive channel of ionized argon gas in the centre of the gas cone, resulting in non-contact precise coagulation with minimal charring and depth of tissue necrosis underneath the coagulum. Other advantages of the system method include the displacement of blood and debris by the gas spray, thereby allowing for more direct application of current to the bleeding area and cooling around the coagulating zone by the outer layers of the gas, thereby minimizing lateral thermal damage.

In open surgery, there is an optimal setting of the gas flow in relation to the generator setting used. Thus a flow rate of 4.0 l/min is needed when the power is set at 20–60 W, whereas 8.0 litres of flow are required when the setting is higher, at 60–100 W. When operating on vascular organs such as the liver, spleen and kidneys the argon gas-flow rate must not exceed 10.0 l/min because of the risk of gas embolism. Recent trials have shown benefit from the use of argon gas spray coagulation in terms of blood loss and/or reduced operating time in treating lesions of the kidney [43], head and neck [44], CNS [45], liver and pelvic surgery [46].

Laser photocoagulation

There is great enthusiasm as well as considerable controversy surrounding the use of laser energy for tissue dissection and coagulation. The Nd : YAG laser is the most commonly used source of photocoagulation energy, but many wavelength variations are available that give different characteristics to the photon energy. The wavelengths for Nd : YAG, argon, and CO_2 are 1.06, 0.5 and 10.6 μm, respectively. These wavelengths confer differential properties to the laser energy, and can be selected for such. The Nd : YAG laser is absorbed preferentially by tissue and proteinaceous molecules, coagulates and cuts tissue well, and vaporizes tissue easily by comparison. The argon laser is absorbed more specifically by haemoglobin and melanin molecules, coagulates moderately well, and cuts and vaporizes tissue poorly. The CO_2 laser is absorbed mainly by water, cuts much better than it coagulates, and has a moderate vaporization effect. Thermal necrosis (and perforation potential) is greatest with the non-contact Nd : YAG, followed closely by the argon laser. The CO_2 laser and the Nd : YAG in the contact mode are the least destructive, with thermal necrosis in the 0.5–1.0 mm range [47].

Miscellaneous adjunctive methods for control of surgical bleeding

Numerous methods and devices have been utilized by surgeons in patients with difficult or serious bleeding problems. Such mechanical methods include pressure packing, usually for severe injuries to solid organs and uncontrollable pelvic bleeding [48–51], pneumatic anti-shock garments prior to surgical control of bleeding, usually in trauma victims [52,53], ligation of feeding arteries [54], constricting mesh wraps of biodegradable material such as polyglycollate [55,56], temporary shunts [57], muscle flaps [58], skin and fascia grafts [59], pigskin [60], and even thumbtacks [61].

Surgical control of massive haemorrhage

For many bleeding problems, direct compression is the best first measure to control blood loss. This may require thoracotomy, laparotomy or surgical exploration of the bleeding region (scalp, extremity wounds, etc.). Bleeding from a torn or injured vessel is readily found on adequate surgical exploration, and the vessel is ligated or repaired as necessary.

There are patients who reach the emergency room in extremis with profound hypotension, grossly distended tense abdomen, blotchy lower limbs (due to compression of the iliac veins) and who remain hypotensive (blood pressure <80 mmHg) despite rapid volume replacement. The cause is either a major vascular (vena cava, aorta, iliac artery) or organ injury (liver, spleen) and less commonly fracture of the pelvis. Laparotomy in these patients is usually fatal as the sudden decompression leads to the final fatal exsanguination. Some 30% of these patients can be saved by a prompt crossclamping of the descending thoracic aorta performed quickly through a left anterolateral thoracotomy at the Vth intercostal space. This controls the bleeding and permits effective transfusion to replace the severe volume deficit.

Fortunately these instances are rare but severe bleeding from major liver injuries is relatively common [62–64]. Severe hepatic injuries still carry a high mortality, usually from exsanguination. In this respect, bleeding from injuries extending to involve the retrohepatic vena cava and hepatic veins is particularly difficult to control.

Compression of the hepatoduodenal ligament by the fingers or preferably by a vascular clamp (Pringle's manoeuvre) to temporarily occlude the hepatic artery and portal vein will considerably reduce bleeding from the injured hepatic parenchyma until control is achieved by suture ligation of obvious bleeding vessels or mass suture of the hepatic parenchyma. However, bleeding from the vena cava and/or the hepatic veins is not controlled in this way. Although techniques for the insertion of a variety of tube atriocaval shunts have been described, they are seldom successful and difficult to perform and the best practical advice to a general surgeon faced with this difficult situation is to pack the liver and supracolic compartment and close the wound. This usually controls the bleeding and allows resuscitation and transfer to a specialized hepatobiliary unit. In practice, this affords the best chance of survival for these trauma victims [48,50].

The surgical management of splenic injuries is currently under review. The emphasis in recent years has been on splenic preservation [65–67] because of the postulated risk of postsplenectomy sepsis by encapsulated organisms, particularly *Streptococcus pneumoniae*. Some of these patients, particularly children, are managed conservatively in the first instance, surgery being undertaken only if there is evidence of continued or renewed bleeding [68]. Splenic preservation for type I–III injuries should be attempted only if the condition of the patient is stable and there is no contamination of the peritoneal cavity. The techniques of splenic repair include simple blanket suture taking deep bites of the splenic parenchyma, splenorrhaphy using the greater omentum, partial splenectomy and insertion/compression of the damaged spleen into an absorbable ('Vicryl') mesh bag. When splenectomy is inevitable, as in type IV injuries, autotransplantation of splenic slices in omental pouches is advocated in an attempt at preserving the splenic immune function.

There are no controlled clinical trials comparing splenic preservation versus splenectomy. Thus the controversy remains unsettled. However, two reports [69,70] rightly point to caution before widespread adoption of a conservative (non-surgical) management and indiscriminate attempts at splenic preservation. Since 1978, there have been only three deaths from postsplenectomy sepsis identified in the English-language literature, all in children. Thus the often quoted prevalence of this complication of splenectomy, 1–2%, probably represents a 20-fold overestimation. Patients who are managed conservatively usually require substantially more blood transfusion than those treated initially by surgery. Thus the enhanced risk of hepatitis (6.9% for 1 unit, 10.3% for 2–3 units and 12% for 6–15 units) probably outweighs the potential benefit of prevention of postsplenectomy sepsis, particularly as the long-term mortality from chronic hepatitis is 5–10%.

Bleeding from a hollow viscus can be managed with either resection or enterotomy and oversewing of bleeding areas. Accurate localization is imperative prior to laparotomy if one is to be expedient and confident of a successful outcome. If necessary, intraoperative endoscopy can be directed through the intestines by the surgeon at laparotomy to localize bleeding site(s).

Bleeding from extremity wounds may require the temporary interruption of blood supply to distant tissue, but this is usually tolerated without serious sequelae for up to 6 h in the normothermic non-acidotic patient. Alternatively, temporary shunt catheters can be placed to return blood flow to an injured extremity during vascular reconstruction, tissue debridement and stabilization of fractures. The principles of adequate exposure, inflow and outflow control apply to repair of any vessel, including the ruptured aorta.

Haemostasis during minimal access surgery

Haemostatic measures during laparoscopic surgery are the same as those used during open surgery, but with some important modifications. Tissue exposure, retraction and identification of structures can be problematic. However, with experience, laparoscopic methods can actually improve upon the visualization of structures. Perhaps the most important principle in laparoscopic surgery is the avoidance of bleeding in the first place, by coagulating, clipping or ligating in continuity suspect vascular structures prior to their division. A cut arteriole can retract within surrounding fibro-fatty tissue and prove difficult to identify. The second important principle is to acquire the skill to operate laparoscopically with two hands, such that an atraumatic insulated grasper is always at the operative site, available for immediate grasping or compression of the bleeding point. The value of direct compression of bleeding areas should not be forgotten. Topical haemostatic agents can be delivered through the cannulae on the end of grasping forceps and applied with compression to the troublesome areas. Surgical clips can control bleeding, but can also inflict damage when applied without precise visual control. The principles governing their safe use must be rigidly followed. We now prefer to ligate vessels >3.0 mm in continuity using the modified Roeder slip knot using polydioxanone before division. This provides even greater security than the Roeder knot tied with catgut [71].

Most commonly, however, haemostasis is achieved by the use of thermal energy: high-frequency electrosurgery or laser photocoagulation, described above. Although there are proponents for both systems, there are only scant data with which to compare laparoscopic electrocautery with laser dissection. Early experiences during laparoscopic cholecystectomy seem to favour conventional electrocautery because of its better control of bleeding sites, quicker dissection, and cost advantage [72]. Electrocoagulation is inexpensive and familiar to most surgeons. Electrocautery with monopolar electrodes requires the conduction of electrical current through normal tissues. This can cause undesirable thermal damage. The electrical current can also arc and damage tissue if voltage is applied while the instrument is unknowingly close to vulnerable structures or out of laparoscopic view. These problems are not unfamiliar to most practising surgeons, however, and should be avoided with proper precautions and the use of the appropriate equipment.

There are a number of rules governing the laparoscopic use of high-frequency monopolar electrosurgery which are insufficiently appreciated. In the first instance, soft coagulation (instead of forced) is recommended in minimal access surgery whenever monopolar electrodes are brought into direct contact with tissue. As electric arcs are not generated, sparking injuries are totally avoided. An additional advantage to the use of soft coagulation is preservation of the sharpness of instruments, particularly dissecting scissors.

In using monopolar electrocautery it is important to appreciate that if high-frequency current flows through long segments of tissue with the same cross-section, the entire length of the structure may be electrocoagulated. Furthermore, high-frequency current applied with the monopolar technique flows preferentially through narrow segments. Thus the coagulation starts at the point of constriction of the tissue and not at the point of contact with the electrode.

Another overlooked factor is the use of excessive amounts of isotonic saline which pools in the various recesses and can conduct the return current to adjacent structures. For this reason the electrocoagulating current should be activated in the presence of a dry field. Furthermore, Ringer's lactate is preferable to isotonic saline as it is less conductive. The use of the microprocessor-controlled high-frequency generator with sensor electronics (Erbe ACC-450) provides a measure of safety which is not provided with the usual equipment. If unavailable, the minimum power setting should be employed with any current and this should not be activated until the tissue is grasped and lifted, to ensure that adjacent organs are not in contact with the active electrode. The non-insulated part of the active electrode must not touch any metal—telescope or cannula. Electrocoagulation should be applied to the thinnest point of the structure or adhesion to prevent secondary coagulation from the high current density. If the required coagulation is not achieved, a quick check of the following is made: neutral electrode is in position, all connections are correct, metallic parts of the instruments and electrodes are clean, there is no shorting due to inadvertent contact between active electrode and metal (optics and cannula). This check should be performed before increasing the power output of the generator.

There are now bipolar hooks, loops and forceps which provide the greatest safety margin. The output for these bipolar endoscopic applications should be in the range of 40–80 W.

The argon gas beamer can also be used laparoscopically with the appropriate probe which delivers gas at the rate of 2.0 l/min. The high-frequency generator must be in the spray mode. Its advantages include diminished charring and reduced depth of thermal necrosis. With the present equipment, the gas flow during activation of the beamer leads to hyperinflation of the abdomen, with a substantial rise in intra-abdominal pressure, and periodic deflation is essential for safety. This problem can be overcome by the insertion of a 22-gauge needle through the abdominal wall during its use.

The three lasers commonly used in laparoscopic surgery are argon, Nd : YAG, KTP and holmium : YAG. Most laparoscopic laser dissections are carried out using the contact mode (bare fibre) in preference to the free-beam mode because of the enhanced safety and the tactile feedback. The one major disadvantage of lasers during laparoscopic dissection is the risk of inadvertent damage from the 'past pointing' or 'shoot past' phenomenon, where the laser energy penetrates through the intended target and damages deeper structures. Unintentional damage may also be inflicted by imperfect beam collimation and shake in the non-contact mode. Laser dissection and photocoagulation are also slower than electrosurgical. Other disadvantages include the relative inexperience of most surgeons with this technology and the requirement for additional technical support. It is claimed by some that smoke generation is less than with electrocautery, although there is little evidence for this assertion.

References

1 Lieberman, D.A. (1988) In the eye of the needle: a reappraisal of endoscopic sclerotherapy. *J. Clin. Gastroenterol.*, **10**, 249–252.

2 The Copenhagen Esophageal Varices Sclerotherapy Project (1984) Sclerotherapy after first variceal hemorrhage in cirrhosis: a randomized multicenter trial. *New Engl. J. Med.*, **311**, 1594–1600.

3 Sugawa, C., Fugita, Y., Ikeda, T. and Walt, A.J. (1986) Endoscopic hemostasis of bleeding of the upper gastrointestinal tract by local injection of 98 per cent dehydrated ethanol. *Surg. Gynec. Obstet.*, **162**, 159–163.

4 Hirao, M., Kobayashi, T., Masuda, K. *et al.* (1985) Endoscopic local injection of hypertonic saline–epinephrine solution to arrest haemorrhage from the upper gastrointestinal tract. *Gastrointest. Endosc.*, **31**, 313–317.

5 Soehendra, N., Grimm, H., and Stenzel, M. (1985) Injection of nonvariceal bleeding lesions of the upper gastrointestinal tract. *Endoscopy*, **17**, 129–132.

6 Jenkins, S.A., Baxter, J.N., Corbett, W. *et al.* (1985) A prospective randomized

controlled clinical trial comparing somatostatin and vasopressin in controlling acute variceal haemorrhage. *Br. Med. J.*, **290**, 275–278.

7 Henry, D.A. and O'Connell, D.L. (1989) Effects of fibrinolytic inhibitors on mortality from upper gastrointestinal haemorrhage. *Br. Med. J.*, **298**, 1142–1146.

8 Taylor, T.V. (1988) Isolated duodenal tamponade for treatment of bleeding duodenal ulcer. *Lancet*, **i**, 911–912.

9 Stiegmann, G.V., Goff, J.S., Sun, J.H. *et al.* (1989) Endoscopic variceal ligation: an alternative to sclerotherapy. *Gastrointest. Endosc.*, **35**, 431–434.

10 Johnston, J. (1985) Endoscopic thermal treatment of upper gastrointestinal bleeding — overview and guidelines. *Endosc. Rev.*, **2**, 12–26.

11 Krejs, G.J., Little, K.H. and Westergaard, H. (1985) Laser photocoagulation for the treatment of acute ulcer bleeding: a randomized controlled clinical trial. *Gastroenterology*, **88**, 1457 (Abstract).

12 Johnston, J.H., Sones, J.O. and Long, B.W. (1985) Comparison of heater probe and YAG laser in endoscopic treatment of major bleeding from peptic ulcers. *Gastrointest. Endosc.*, **31**, 175–180.

13 Fleischer, D.E., Roth, B.E. and Larson, D.E. (1983) Therapeutic endoscopy for control of upper gastrointestinal bleeding. *Gastrointest. Endosc.*, **29**, 245–247.

14 Tabuse, K., Katsumi, M., Nagai, Y. *et al.* (1985) Microwave tissue coagulation applied clinically in endoscopic surgery. *Endoscopy*, **17**, 139–144.

15 Fullarton, G.M., Birnee, G.G., MacDonald, A. and Murray, W.R. (1989) Controlled trial of heater probe treatment in bleeding peptic ulcers. *Br. J. Surg.*, **76**, 541–544.

16 Laine, L. (1987) Multipolar electrocoagulation in the treatment of active upper gastrointestinal tract hemorrhage: a prospective controlled trial. *New Engl. J. Med.*, **316**, 1613–1617.

17 Fromm, D. (1987) Endoscopic coagulation for gastrointestinal bleeding. *New Engl. J. Med.*, **316**, 1652–1654.

18 Orzel, J.A., Coldwell, D.M. and Eskridge, J.M. (1988) Superselective embolization for renal hemorrhage with a new coaxial catheter and guidewire. *Cardiovasc. Intervent. Rad.*, **11**, 343–345.

19 Olliff, S., Thomas, S., Karani, J. and Walters, H. (1990) Superselective embolization using a coaxial catheter technique. *Br. J. Radiol.*, **63**, 197–201.

20 Appleton, D.S., Sibley, G.N. and Doyle, P.T. (1988) Internal iliac artery embolisation for the control of severe bladder and prostate haemorrhage. *Br. J. Urol.*, **61**, 45–47.

21 O'Hanlan, K.A., Trambert, J., Godriguez-Rodriguez, L. *et al.* (1989) Arterial embolization in the management of abdominal and retroperitoneal hemorrhage. *Gynecol. Oncol.*, **34**, 131–135.

22 Fandrich, B.L., Gnanadev, D.A., Jaecks, R. and Boyle, W. (1989) Selective hepatic artery embolization as an adjunct to liver packing in severe hepatic trauma: case report. *J. Trauma*, **29**, 1716–1718.

23 Sakamoto, T., Yagi, K., Hiraide, A. *et al.* (1988) Transcatheter embolization in the treatment of massive bleeding due to maxillofacial injury. *J. Trauma*, **28**, 840–843.

24 Hicks, J.N. and Vitek, G. (1989) Transarterial embolization to control posterior epistaxis. *Laryngoscope*, **99**, 1027–1029.

25 Adams, D.B., Mauterer, D.J., Vujic, I.J. and Anderson, M.C. (1990) Preoperative control of splenic artery inflow in patients with splenic venous occlusion. *South. Med. J.*, **83**, 1021–1024.

26 Pisco, J.M., Martins, J.M. and Correia, M.G. (1989) Internal iliac artery: embolization to control hemorrhage from pelvic neoplasms. *Radiology*, **172**, 337–339.

27 Clouse, M.E. (1989) Hepatic artery embolization for bleeding and tumors. *Surg. Clin. N. Am.*, **69**, 419–432.

28 Rankin, E.M., Rubens, R.D. and Reidy, J.F. (1988) Transcatheter embolisation to control severe bleeding in fungating breast cancer. *Eur. J. Surg. Oncol.*, **14**, 27–32.

29 Rabkin, J.E., Astafjev, V.I., Gothman, L.N. and Grigorjev, Y.G. (1987) Transcatheter embolization in the management of pulmonary hemorrhage. *Radiology*, **163**, 361–365.

30 Bhansali, S., Wilner, H. and Jacobs, J.R. (1986) Arterial embolization for control of bleeding in advanced head and neck carcinoma. *J. Laryng. Otol.*, **100**, 1289–1293.

31 Rappaport, S.I. (1983) Preoperative hemostatic evaluation: Which tests, if any? *Blood*, **61**, 229–231.

32 Burrows, L. and Tartter, P.I. (1982) Effect of blood transfusion on colonic malignancy recurrence rate. *Lancet*, **ii**, 662–665.

33 Parrott, N.R., Lennard, T.W.J., Taylor, R.M.R. *et al.* (1986) Effect of perioperative blood transfusion on recurrence of colorectal cancer. *Br. J. Surg.*, **73**, 970–973.

34 Cuschieri, A. and Berci, G. *Laparoscopic Biliary Surgery*. Blackwell, London (1990).

35 Roberts, W.S., Cavanagh, D., Roberts, V.C. *et al.* (1989) Wound hematoma: prophylaxis with topical thrombin. *South. Med. J.*, **82**, 607–609.

36 Hauser, C.J. (1989) Hemostasis of solid viscus trauma by intraparenchymal injection of fibrin glue. *Arch. Surg.*, **124**, 291–293.

37 Baker, J.W., Spotnitz, W.D., Matthew, T.L., *et al.* (1989) Mediastinal fibrin glue: Hemostatic effect and tissue response in calves. *Ann. Thorac. Surg.*, **47**, 450–454.

38 Largis, J.K. and Katz, A.R. (1987) Experimental evaluation of amylose succinate absorbable hemostat in a canine model. *J. Biomed. Mater. Res.*, (A3 Suppl.) **21**, 299–318.

39 Sirimanna, K.S. (1989) Calcium alginate fibre (Kaltostat 2) for nasal packing after trimming of turbinates—a pilot study. *J. Laryng. Otol.*, **103**, 1067–1068.

40 Larson, P.O. (1988) Topical hemostatic agents for dermatologic surgery. *J. Derm. Surg. Oncol.*, **14**, 623–632.

41 van der Ham, A.C., Kort, W.J., Weijma, I.M. *et al.* (1991) Effect of fibrin sealant on the healing colonic anastomosis in the rat. *Br. J. Surg.*, **78**, 49–53.

42 Byrne, D.J., Hardy, J., Wood, R.A.B. *et al.* (1991) The effect of fibrin glue on the mechanical properties of healing wounds. *Br. J. Surg.*, **78**, 841–843.

43 Hernandez, A.D., Smith, J.A. Jr, Jeppson, K.G. and Terreros, D.A. (1990) A controlled study of the argon beam coagulator for partial nephrectomy. *J. Urol.*, **143**, 1062–1065.

44 Ward, P.H., Castro, D.J. and Ward, S. (1989) A significant new contribution to radical head and neck surgery. The argon beam coagulator as an effective means of limiting blood loss. *Arch. Otolaryng. Head Neck Surg.*, **115**, 921–923.

45 Kim, L.Y. Jr, Roxey, T.E. and Day, A.L. (1987) The argon 'contact' laser scalpel: Technical considerations. *Neurosurgery*, **21**, 858–860.

46 Brand, E. and Pearlman, N. (1990) Electrosurgical debulking of ovarian cancer: A new technique using the argon beam coagulator. *Gynecol. Oncol.*, **39**, 115–118.

47 Dixon, J. (1988) Current laser applications in general surgery. *Ann. Surg.*, **207**, 355–371.

48 Hollands, M.J. and Little, J.M. (1989) Perihepatic packing: Its role in the manage-

ment of liver trauma. *Austral. NZ J. Surg.*, **59**, 21–24.

49 Zama, N., Fazio, V.W., Jagelman, D.G. *et al.* (1988) Efficacy of pelvic packing in maintaining hemostasis after rectal excision for cancer. *Dis. Colon Rectum*, **31**, 923–928.

50 Feliciano, D.V., Mattox, K.L., Burch, J.M. *et al.* (1986) Packing for control of hepatic hemorrhage. *J. Trauma*, **26**, 738–743.

51 Saifi, J., Fortune, J.B., Graca, L. and Shah, D.M. (1990) Benefits of intra-abdominal pack placement for the management of nonmechanical hemorrhage. *Arch. Surg.*, **125**, 119–122.

52 Brunette, D.D., Fifield, G. and Ruiz, E. (1987) Use of pneumatic antishock trousers in the management of pediatric pelvic hemorrhage. *Ped. Emerg. Care*, **3**, 86–90.

53 Evers, B.M., Cryer, H.M. and Miller, F.B. (1989) Pelvic fracture hemorrhage. Priorities in management. *Arch. Surg.*, **124**, 422–424.

54 Thavarasah, A.S., Sivalingam, N. and Almohdzar, S.A. (1989) Internal iliac and ovarian artery ligation in the control of pelvic haemorrhage. *Austral. NZ J. Obstet. Gynaecol.*, **29**, 22–25.

55 Lau, J.L., Fowler, J.E. Jr, Stobnick, M. *et al.* (1986) Polyglycollic acid mesh in experimental renal trauma. *J. Urol.*, **136**, 715–718.

56 Brismar, B. and Akerlund, J.E. (1989) Polyglycollic acid (Dexon) mesh for packing to control intra-abdominal bleeding. Case report. *Acta Chir. Scand.*, **155**, 421–422.

57 Pachter, H.L., Spencer, F.C., Hofstetter, S.R. *et al.* (1986) The management of juxtahepatic venous injuries without an atriocaval shunt: preliminary clinical observations. *Surgery*, **99**, 569–575.

58 Arnold, P.G. and Pairolero, P.C. (1988) Intrathoracic muscle flaps in the surgical management of life-threatening hemorrhage from the heart and great vessels. *Plastic Reconstr. Surg.*, **81**, 831–837.

59 Eitan, A., Munichor, M. and Barzilai, A. (1989) Autogenous skin and fascia grafts as topical hemostatic agents in splenic injuries. *Eur. Surg. Res.*, **21**, 60–64.

60 Peper, W.A., Allor, O.R., Peterson, E.L. and Magilligan, D.J. Jr (1986) Pigskin as a topical hemostat in arterial, liver, and splenic injuries. *Surgery*, **99**, 557–563.

61 Khan, F.A., Fang, D.T. and Nivatvongs, S. (1987) Management of presacral bleeding during rectal resection. *Surg. Gynecol. Obstet.*, **165**, 274–276.

62 Cox, E.F., Flancbaum, L., Dauterive, A.H. and Paulson, R.L. (1988) Blunt trauma to the liver. Analysis of management and mortality in 323 consecutive patients. *Ann. Surg.*, **207**, 126–134.

63 Feliciano, D.V., Jordan, G.L., Itondo, C.G. *et al.* (1986) Management of 1000 consecutive cases of hepatic trauma (1979–1984). *Ann. Surg.*, **204**, 438–445.

64 Carmona, R.H., Lim, R.C. Jr and Clark, G.C. (1982) Morbidity and mortality in hepatic trauma. *Am. J. Surg.*, **144**, 88–94.

65 Kidd, W.T., Lui, R.C.K., Khoo, R. and Nixon, J. (1987) The management of blunt splenic trauma. *J. Trauma*, **27**, 977–979.

66 Millikan, J.S., Moore, E.E., Moore, G.E. and Stevens, E. (1982) Alternatives to splenectomy in adults after trauma. Repair, partial resection, and reimplantation of splenic tissue. *Am. J. Surg.*, **144**, 711–716.

67 Barrett, J., Sheaff, C., Abuabara, S. and Jonasson, O. (1983) Splenic preservation in adults after blunt and penetrating trauma. *Am. J. Surg.*, **145**, 313–317.

68 Tom, W.W., Howells, G.A., Bree, R.L. *et al.* (1985) A nonoperative approach to the adult ruptured spleen sustained from blunt trauma. *Am. Surg.*, **51**, 367–371.

69 Ragsdale, T.H. and Hamit, F. (1984) Splenectomy versus splenic salvage for spleens ruptured by blunt trauma. *Am. Surg.*, **50**, 645–648.

70 Luna, G. (1987) Nonoperative observation therapy for splenic injuries: A safe therapeutic option? *Am. J. Surg.*, **153**, 462–468.

71 Nathanson, L.K., Easter, D.W. and Cuschieri, A. (1991) Ligation of the structures of the cystic pedicle during laparoscopic cholecystectomy. *Am. J. Surg.*, **161**, 350–354.

72 Hunter, J.G. (1991) Laser or electrocautery for laparoscopic cholecystectomy. *Am. J. Surg.*, **161**, 345–349.

Index

Page numbers in *italics* indicate an illustration or table appearing on a different page from its text.